Manual of Lipid Disorders

Reducing the Risk for Coronary Heart Disease

SECOND EDITION

Manual of Lipid Disorders

Reducing the Risk for Coronary Heart Disease

SECOND EDITION

Antonio M. Gotto, Jr., MD, DPhil

Dean and Provost of Medical Affairs
Weill Medical College of Cornell University
New York, New York

Henry J. Pownall, PhD

Professor of Medicine
Chief, Section of Atherosclerosis and Lipoprotein Research
Baylor College of Medicine
Houston, Texas

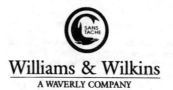

Williams & Wilkins

A WAVERLY COMPANY

BALTIMORE • PHILADELPHIA • LONDON • PARIS • BANGKOK
BUENOS AIRES • HONG KONG • MUNICH • SYDNEY • TOKYO • WROCLAW

Editor: David Charles Retford
Managing Editor: Jennifer Kullgren
Project Editor: Joan Scullin

Copyright © 1999 Williams & Wilkins

351 West Camden Street
Baltimore, Maryland 21201-2436 USA

Rose Tree Corporate Center
1400 North Providence Road
Building II, Suite 5025
Media, Pennsylvania 19063-2043 USA

Printed in the United States of America

First Edition, 1992

Library of Congress Cataloging-in-Publication Data
Gotto, Antonio M.
    Manual of lipid disorders : reducing the risk for coronary heart
disease / Antonio M. Gotto, Jr., Henry J. Pownall. -- 2nd ed.
        p. cm.
    Includes bibliographical references and index.
    ISBN 0-683-30676-6
    1. Lipids--Metabolism--Disorders--Handbooks, manuals, etc.
I. Pownall, Henry J. II. Title.
    [DNLM: 1. Metabolic Diseases--diagnosis. 2. Metabolic Diseases-
-therapy. 3. Lipids--metabolism. 4. Atherosclerosis. 5. Coronary
Disease--prevention & control. WD 200G686m 1999]
RC632.L5668 1999
616.3'997--dc21
DNLM/DLC
for Library of Congress   98-41675
                                                                    CIP

To purchase additional copies of this book, call our Customer Service Department at **(800) 638-0672** or fax orders to **(800) 447-8438.** For other book services, including chapter reprints and large quantity sales, ask for the Special Sales Department.

Canadian customers should call **(800) 665-1148,** or fax **(800) 665-0103.** For all other calls originating outside the United States, please call **(410) 528-4223** or fax us at **(410) 528-8550.**

Visit Williams & Wilkins on the Internet: http://www.wwilkins.com or contact our customer service department at **custserv@wwilkins.com.** Williams & Wilkins customer service representatives are available from 8:30 am to 6:00 pm EST, Monday through Friday, for telephone access.

98 99 00 01 02
1 2 3 4 5 6 7 8 9 10

Contents

Preface

Six years have passed quickly since we prepared the first edition of this manual. In those years we have been privileged to witness tremendous advances in the understanding of atherothrombosis, plasma lipid metabolism and its relation to other metabolic factors, and how to reduce risk for CHD. There has been a sea change in our understanding of how atherosclerotic disease leads to acute clinical events. The unexpected finding that most events arise from angiographically mild or moderate lesions that are unstable and prone to rupture—lesions typified by a large lipid core, a thin cap, and high macrophage density—has led to the concept of using lesion stabilization to reduce risk for disability and death. There has never been a more exciting time in cardiovascular preventive medicine.

The question of whether cholesterol lowering is beneficial has been very clearly resolved now that the HMG-CoA reductase inhibitors (statins) have made it possible to reduce LDL cholesterol very substantially. Gold standard large, randomized, controlled clinical trials of the statins have demonstrated that cholesterol lowering significantly reduces not only CHD morbidity and mortality but also all-cause mortality rates. They clearly support benefit in patients both with and without high cholesterol. Coronary benefit in these trials extended to women, diabetic patients, and elderly patients in addition to men, nondiabetic patients, and younger patients. The results clarify that cholesterol lowering can benefit a wide spectrum of patients and justify expanded use of cholesterol-lowering therapy in clinical practice.

U.S. practice recommendations have also evolved in the past several years, the following among them:

• In June 1993, updated clinical guidelines for cholesterol control and CHD risk reduction were published by the second Adult Treatment Panel of the National Cholesterol Education Program.
• In July 1995, an American Heart Association consensus panel provided a guide to comprehensive risk reduction in patients with known atherosclerotic disease.
• In April 1996, a smoking cessation guide for primary care physicians was published by a panel convened by the Agency for Health Care Policy and Research of the Public Health Service, working with the Centers for Disease Control and Prevention.

- In July 1996, the Surgeon General's first report on physical activity and health was a national call to action for a more active lifestyle among Americans.
- In November 1996 and March 1997, American Heart Association and American College of Cardiology task forces recommended that lipid-lowering drug therapy not be delayed in patients with CHD when LDL cholesterol exceeds 130 mg/dL.
- In July 1997, the American Diabetes Association developed new criteria for diagnosing diabetes, including a lower fasting plasma glucose cut-point.
- In November 1997, revised Joint National Committee guidelines (JNC VI) for the assessment and management of high blood pressure were published.
- In January 1998, the American Diabetes Association added specific recommendations for lipid management in diabetic patients to its clinical practice guidelines.
- In June 1998, the American Heart Association added obesity to the list of major risk factors for CHD, and the first U.S. federal guidelines on the identification, evaluation, and treatment of overweight and obesity in adults were issued by the National Institutes of Health.

All the recommendations were major steps forward and emphasized the need for attention to multiple risk factors. Yet despite these cogent guidelines, compelling clinical data, and the availability of effective interventions, CHD remains the leading killer of both men and women in the United States, as well as in most developed nations. Many patients are still not receiving cost-effective, risk-reducing treatments. Among American adults, 65% of those eligible for lipid-lowering diet or drug therapy are receiving no therapy of any kind. High blood pressure is untreated in 46% and uncontrolled in 73%, and 28% of men and 23% of women still smoke. About 25% of American adults report no leisure-time physical activity, and 55% are overweight or obese. Only about 40% of patients eligible for beta-blocker therapy after acute MI receive such therapy.

This edition of the *Manual of Lipid Disorders* has been designed to help physicians address such shortfalls. While its focus remains the control of dyslipidemia, it also highlights the aforementioned practice recommendations and perspectives regarding smoking, hypertension, obesity, physical inactivity, and the lipid risk of diabetes mellitus. We hope that the reader will find it a thought-provoking yet practical tool for understanding clinical recommendations in the field of CHD risk reduction. The manual begins with Henry Pownall's overview of lipid metabolism (Section I), followed by Tony Gotto's sections on the pathophysiology of atherosclerosis, observational and interventional epidemiologic findings relating dyslipidemia to CHD, clinical recommendations, and CHD risk reduction options (Sec-

tions II–IV). Tony Gotto closes the manual by highlighting the very important area of CHD risk prevention in subpopulations, including women, the
elderly, children and adolescents, U.S. ethnic minorities, patients with diabetes mellitus, and patients with both dyslipidemia and hypertension (Section V). We hope that with such a resource close at hand, physicians will not
miss opportunities to intervene against cardiovascular risk factors and that
this work may contribute to the better care of patients.

We are pleased that the second edition's publication coincides with
the golden anniversaries of the National Heart, Lung, and Blood Institute
and the American Heart Association. Both organizations have had profound influences on the research and treatment advances described
herein.

Acknowledgments

The authors thank Suzanne Simpson, BA, Instructor, for research and writing assistance; Peter H. Jones, MD, Associate Professor, Christie M. Ballantyne, MD, Associate Professor, Joel D. Morrisett, PhD, Professor, Lynne W. Scott, MA, RD/LD, Assistant Professor, John A. Farmer, MD, Associate Professor, and Bassem el-Masri, MD, Assistant Professor, for their helpful commentary; and Jeanne Philbin, BFA, for editorial and graphics assistance. All are colleagues in the Section of Atherosclerosis and Lipoprotein Research, Department of Medicine, Baylor College of Medicine.

Abbreviations

ACAT	acyl:cholesterol acyltransferase
ACE	angiotensin-converting enzyme
ADA	American Diabetes Association
AHA	American Heart Association
apo	apolipoprotein
BMI	body mass index
CABG	coronary artery bypass grafting
CDC	U.S. Centers for Disease Control and Prevention
CETP	cholesteryl ester transfer protein
CHD	coronary heart disease
CI	confidence interval
CK	creatine kinase
CNS	central nervous system
CVD	cardiovascular disease
DBP	diastolic blood pressure
ECG	electrocardiogram/electrocardiography
ERT	estrogen replacement therapy
FCH	familial combined hyperlipidemia
FDA	U.S. Food and Drug Administration
FFA	free (nonesterified) fatty acids
FH	familial hypercholesterolemia
HDL-C	high-density lipoprotein cholesterol
HMG-CoA	3-hydroxy-3-methylglutaryl coenzyme A
ICAM	intercellular adhesion molecule
IDL	intermediate-density lipoprotein
IFN	interferon
IL	interleukin
JNC	Joint National Committee
LCAT	lecithin:cholesterol acyltransferase
LDL-C	low-density lipoprotein cholesterol
Lp[a]	lipoprotein [a]
LPL	lipoprotein lipase
LVH	left ventricular hypertrophy
MI	myocardial infarction
NCEP	U.S. National Cholesterol Education Program
NHANES	U.S. National Health and Nutrition Examination Survey
NHBPEP	U.S. National High Blood Pressure Education Program

NHLBI	U.S. National Heart, Lung, and Blood Institute
NIDDK	U.S. National Institute of Diabetes and Digestive and Kidney Diseases
NIH	U.S. National Institutes of Health
oxLDL	oxidized LDL
PAI-1	plasminogen activator inhibitor 1
PDGF	platelet-derived growth factor
PLTP	plasma lipid transfer protein
PTCA	percutaneous transluminal coronary angioplasty
PVD	peripheral vascular disease
QCA	quantitative coronary angiography
SBP	systolic blood pressure
SMC	smooth muscle cell
TC	total cholesterol
TG	triglyceride
TGF	transforming growth factor
TGRL	triglyceride-rich lipoprotein
TIA	transient ischemic attack
TNF	tumor necrosis factor
VCAM	vascular cell adhesion molecule
VLDL	very low density lipoprotein

Manual of Lipid Disorders

Reducing the Risk for Coronary Heart Disease

SECOND EDITION

Fundamentals of Lipid Metabolism

Models are to be used, not believed.

—E. Thiel, *Advances in Econometrics* (1959)

Sometimes in politics and economics, the process is as important as the product. The same may be said of our models of lipoproteins and their metabolism. All models of lipoprotein structure have their basis in data derived by indirect methods, and over time the models have been refined to accommodate new information. In parallel, models of how lipoproteins are assembled, transported, and catabolized have evolved as new pathways and their attendant proteins have been discovered.

References for Section I (Chapters 1–4) begin on page 52.

Chapter 1

Plasma Lipoproteins: Structure, Nomenclature, and Occurrence

LIPIDS

Physiologically, lipids are simple or complex, the latter derived from the former by covalent association. In human plasma lipoprotein metabolism, the most important simple lipids are fatty acids, sphingosine, and cholesterol (Figure 1.1), whereas cholesteryl esters, triacylglycerol (TG), phosphatidylcholine (lecithin), phosphatidylethanolamine (cephalin), and sphingomyelin are the most important complex lipids (Figure 1.2). Phospholipids, such as monoacylglycerol, diacylglycerol, lysophosphatidylcholine, and ceramide, which are also complex, are metabolic intermediates in the formation or degradation of other complex lipids. As second messengers, these intermediates, which are present in plasma in fairly low abundance, regulate a broad spectrum of cellular activities.

Lipids can be classified as polar or nonpolar; this characteristic is an important determinant of where they are found within a lipoprotein (Segrest and Albers 1986a, 1986b; Small 1986). The major nonpolar lipids are TG and cholesteryl ester, which are miscible and soluble in hydrocarbon solvents. Nonpolar lipids form the core of plasma lipoproteins, and the relative abundance of TG and cholesteryl ester in lipoproteins can affect their physical properties and metabolism (McKeone et al. 1993). TG forms the center of lipid-rich inclusions in adipocytes; cholesteryl ester is the major component of inclusions in macrophage foam cells in arterial lesions. In contrast, polar lipids are not readily soluble in hydrocarbon solvents or in nonpolar lipids but dissolve in polar organic solvents such as ethanol; they can be dispersed in water, where they form micelles or emulsions. Polar lipids are located on lipoprotein and intracellular lipid inclusion surfaces, where they form a barrier between the neutral lipid core and the surrounding aqueous phase. In each instance, the hydrocarbon part of

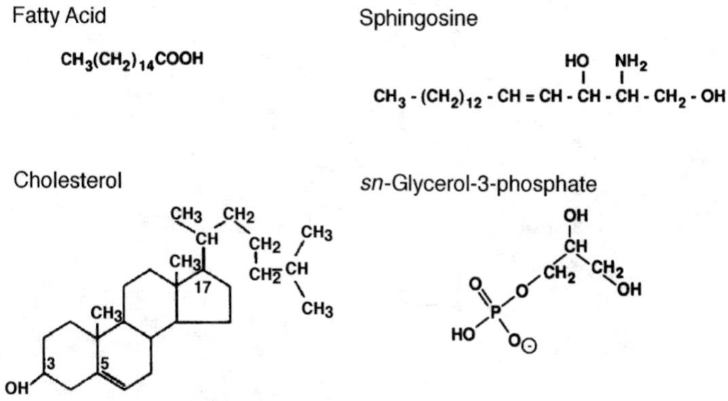
Fatty Acid
CH3(CH2)14COOH
Sphingosine
HO NH2
CH3 - (CH2)12 - CH = CH - CH - CH - CH2 - OH
Cholesterol
CH3 CH2
CH
CH2
CH3
CH3
CH2 CH
17
CH3
CH3
3
5
OH
sn-Glycerol-3-phosphate
OH
CH
CH2
CH2
OH
O
O
P
HO
O

Figure 1.1. Simple lipids.

a polar lipid is in contact with the neutral lipid, whereas the polar head group is in contact with water.

Most of the monoacylated lipids, including fatty acids and lysophosphatidylcholine, are sparingly soluble in water. Their solubility decreases as the length of the attached acyl chain increases. Monoacylated lipids form micelles (Figure 1.3) composed of about 100 lipid molecules. The single hydroxyl moieties of cholesterol and diacylglycerol make them only slightly polar, and their solubility properties are between those of polar and nonpolar lipids. For this reason, cholesterol and diacylglycerol can dissolve in both the nonpolar lipids and the polar lipids that compose the surface film surrounding nonpolar lipids in microemulsions (see Figure 1.3). In the absence of nonpolar lipids, phospholipids sometimes form liposomes or single-bilayer vesicles that have a contained volume of water. All these lipid structures, which are sometimes used as model lipoproteins, share some physical and biochemical properties with native human plasma lipoproteins.

Some important differences in complex lipids are determined by fatty acid composition. There are three major fatty acid classes: saturated, monounsaturated, and polyunsaturated (Figure 1.4). Fatty acids follow several metabolic pathways, which are determined in part by their structure. The differences are important determinants of the effects of fatty acyl components of dietary fat on plasma cholesterol and TG concentrations in the fasting or postprandial state. Although most dietary fatty acids are delivered to cells to satisfy energy and growth requirements, some (most important, the highly unsaturated fatty acids arachidonate and eicosapentaenoate) are precursors to or modulators of bioregulators such as prostaglandins, thromboxanes, and leukotrienes.

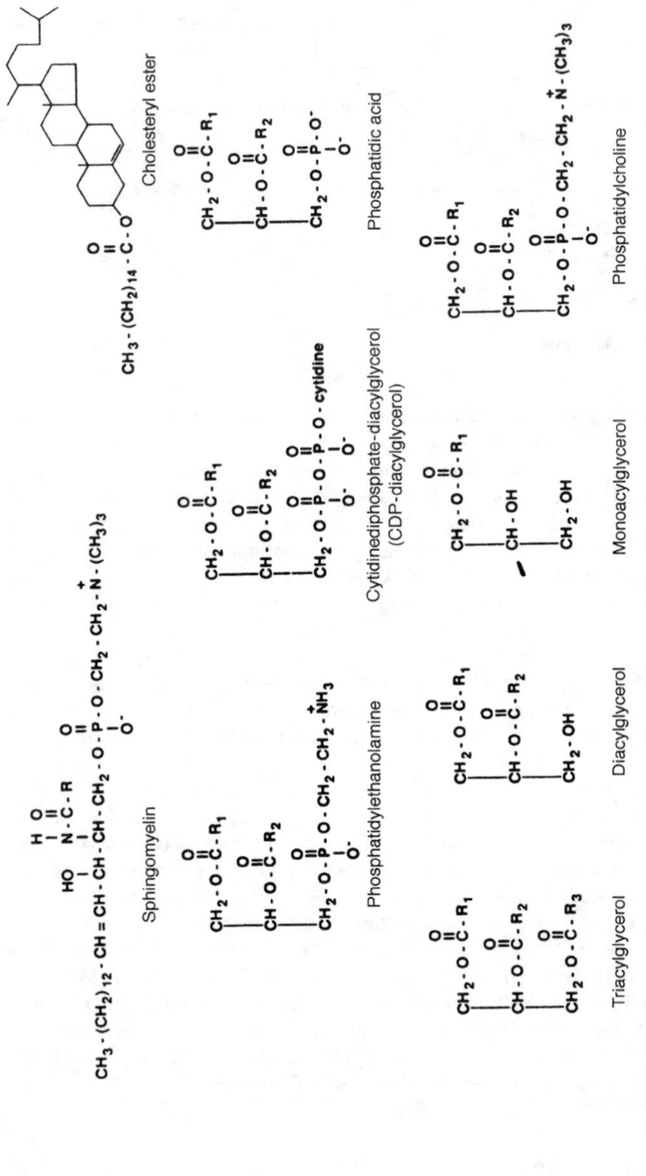

Figure 1.2. Complex lipids.

Single-bilayer vesicle

Micelle

Bilayer disc

Microemulsion

Multilamellar lipsosome

CE + TG

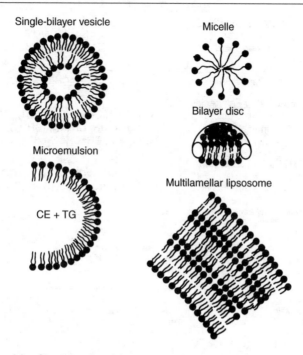

Figure 1.3. Structures of model systems used to emulate plasma lipoproteins. CE, cholesteryl ester.

LIPOPROTEINS

As the name implies, plasma lipoproteins are complexes of lipids and proteins (apolipoproteins; see later). With the exception of free cholesterol, the lipoprotein lipids are always complex; they include cholesteryl esters, TGs, and phospholipids. Lipoproteins are operationally classified according to their densities and electrophoretic mobilities (Table 1.1). In order of decreasing density, they are HDL, LDL, IDL, VLDL, and the chylomicron, a TGRL that appears in the plasma after an oral fat load. The lipoproteins are quasi-distinct structures that are distributed over a characteristic range of densities rather than a single density, which would typify a pure stoichiometric compound. Moreover, HDL is bimodal and appears in two distinct subclasses, HDL_2 and HDL_3 (subclassified as HDL_{2a}, HDL_{2b}, HDL_{3a}, HDL_{3b}, and HDL_{3c}). Another entity, pre-β-HDL, which is composed mainly of apo A-I, cholesterol, and phospholipid, shares HDL's density but migrates with pre-beta rather than alpha mobility. Pre-β-HDL is present in plasma only in very low concentrations but is believed to be an important mediator in the transfer of cholesterol from cells (Castro and Fielding

__Saturated Fatty Acids__
Palmitic acid $CH_3(CH_2)_{14}COOH$
Stearic acid $CH_3(CH_2)_{16}COOH$

__Monounsaturated Fatty Acids__
Oleic acid $CH_3(CH_2)_7CH{=}CH(CH_2)_7COOH$

__Polyunsaturated Fatty Acids (n-6)__
Linoleic acid $CH_3(CH_2)_4(CH{=}CHCH_2)_2(CH_2)_6COOH$
Linolenic acid $CH_3CH_2(CH{=}CHCH_2)_3(CH_2)_6COOH$
Arachidonic acid $CH_3(CH_2)_4(CH{=}CHCH_2)_4(CH_2)_2COOH$

__Polyunsaturated Fatty Acids (n-3)__
Eicosapentaenoic acid $CH_3CH_2(CH{=}CHCH_2)_5(CH_2)_2COOH$
Docosahexaenoic acid $CH_3CH_2(CH{=}CHCH_2)_6CH_2COOH$

Figure 1.4. Major fatty acid classes.

Table 1.1. CLASSIFICATION AND PROPERTIES OF PLASMA LIPOPROTEINS

Lipoprotein class	Major lipid component(s)	Apolipoprotein(s)	Density (g/mL)	Diameter (Å)	Electrophoretic mobility
Chylomicron	TG	A-I, A-II, A-IV, Cs, B-48, E	<0.95	800–5,000	Origin
Chylomicron remnant	CE, TG	B-48, E	<1.006	>500	Origin
VLDL	TG	B-100, Cs, E	<1.006	300–800	Pre-beta
IDL	CE	B-100, Cs, E	1.006–1.019	250–350	Broad beta
LDL[a]	CE	B-100	1.019–1.063	180–280	Beta
HDL					
HDL$_2$	CE, PL	A-I, A-II[b]	1.063–1.125	90–120	Alpha
HDL$_3$	PL	A-I, A-II[b]	1.125–1.210	50–90	Alpha

CE, cholesteryl ester; PL, phospholipid.
[a]A usually minor but variable fraction of LDL is complexed to apo[a] and constitutes a lipoprotein subclass termed Lp[a].
[b]Minor apolipoproteins of HDL are C-I, C-II, C-III, A-IV, and D.

Table 1.2. FATTY ACID COMPOSITION OF PLASMA LIPIDS FROM HUMANS ON A DIET HIGH IN SATURATED FATTY ACIDS

		Fatty acid								
Lipid	Lipo-protein	14:0	16:0	16:1	18:0	18:1	18:2	18:3	20:4	Other
CE	VLDL	2.7	18.	2.5	1.6	17.	51.	0.70	4.8	2.1
	LDL	0.48	11.	1.6	0.89	18.	58.	0.02	8.6	2.0
	HDL_3	0.45	12.	1.7	1.1	16.	58.	0.15	9.0	1.9
TG	VLDL	2.2	27.	5.1	2.4	35.	26.	0.95	1.0	0.80
	LDL	2.5	23.	4.2	4.3	39.	25.	0.62	2.5	0.10
	HDL_3	1.6	24.	3.0	4.4	38.	26.	1.3	2.0	0.30
PL	VLDL	0.79	30.	1.7	15.	11.	22.	0.00	12.	8.3
	LDL	0.55	32.	0.24	19.	8.8	20.	0.00	10.	9.4
	HDL_3	1.5	27.	0.61	15.	8.0	21.	0.03	14.	12.

CE, cholesteryl esters; PL, phospholipids.
Note: Fatty acids are represented as n:m, where acyl chains have n carbons and m double bonds. Values are reported to two significant figures.
Source: Data from Pownall et al. 1995.

1988; Fielding and Fielding 1995a). Its plasma concentration has not yet been linked to risk for CHD.

The plasma lipoproteins can be altered in structure and composition by various types of hyperlipidemia. Density can shift according to changes in composition, and electrophoretic mobility can be altered by changes in the charges on the proteins. β-VLDL, which is found in familial type III hyperlipidemia and is enriched in cholesteryl ester and apo E, represents such an alteration (Weisgraber et al. 1990). LDL can be modified by the covalent attachment of apo[a], yielding Lp[a]. Apo[a] is a highly polymorphic protein whose molecular weight can vary greatly according to the number of kringle units in its primary structure (Koschinsky et al. 1990).

Lipid fatty acid compositions for VLDL, LDL, and HDL_3 are shown in Table 1.2. In all lipoproteins, the major fatty acids are linoleate, oleate, and palmitate in cholesteryl esters; palmitate, stearate, oleate, and linoleate in phospholipids; and oleate, palmitate, and linoleate in TGs. Typically, saturated fatty acids are located at the *sn*-1 position, whereas the *sn*-2 position contains almost all monounsaturated and polyunsaturated fatty acids. Each complex lipid is quite similar in composition among VLDL, LDL, and HDL. Where differences exist in fatty acid composition, LDL and HDL are more similar to each other than to VLDL. This can be attributed to the activity of CETP, which exchanges TG and cholesteryl ester between lipoproteins (Tall 1995). The lifetimes of LDL and HDL (>3 days) are sufficiently long for equilibration to occur. In contrast, VLDL TG is rapidly removed by lipolysis, before equilibration. The fatty

Table 1.3. MAJOR LIPIDS IN FASTED HUMAN PLASMA

Lipid	Concentration	
	mmol/L	mg/dL
TC	5.2	200
Free cholesterol	1.4	54
Cholesteryl ester	3.8	250
Total phospholipid	3.1	230
TG	1.6	140
FFAs	0.4	11

Note: The SI data are from Mayes 1993. Molecular weights of 387 for cholesterol, 650 for cholesteryl ester, 750 for phospholipid, 886 for TG, and 273 for fatty acid were used for conversion to conventional units.

acid compositions shown in Table 1.2 are representative of those found in a person on a diet high in saturated fatty acids. Compositions vary as dietary intake changes. More unusual fatty acids, such as the omega-3 fatty acids found in cold-water fish, occur in each of the lipid and lipoprotein classes in amounts related to dietary intake (Pownall et al. 1995). Omega-3 fatty acids are precursors to important bioregulatory molecules such as leukotrienes.

Human plasma concentrations of lipids vary greatly according to nutritional status and genetically determined interindividual differences. In the plasma of subjects who have fasted, the predominant lipids are cholesteryl esters, followed by phospholipids and TGs (Table 1.3). Following dietary intake of fat, the TG concentration initially increases dramatically, then declines after about 4 hours. Elevated plasma TG is associated with certain clinical disorders, discussed in later chapters. Much of the interest to date in plasma lipids has been related to the predictivity of plasma cholesterol concentration for CHD. Plasma cholesterol concentration is determined by complex metabolic relations among many other lipids in the plasma compartment and the regulation of cellular cholesterol synthesis by plasma factors that include both lipids and proteins. There is a growing focus on the role of TG as a cardiovascular risk factor, including its role in the structure and metabolism of all lipoprotein subclasses in insulin resistance syndrome.

PROTEINS

Apolipoproteins (apoproteins) are a specialized group of proteins that associate with lipids and mediate several biochemical steps associated with plasma lipid metabolism. The apolipoproteins are designated by letters and Roman numerals, for example, apo A-I and apo C-II. The designa-

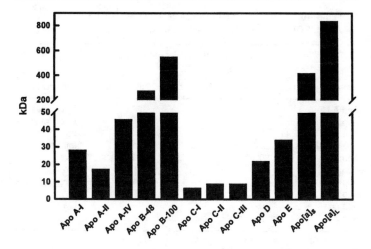

Figure 1.5. Molecular masses of the apolipoproteins that are most abundant in human plasma. Apo[a] encompasses a range of masses; masses are shown for only the smallest (S) and largest (L) isoforms.

tions arose from two sources. First, it was once thought that apolipoproteins composed families, so those forming a family were given the same letter prefix. The scheme has remained even though its basis is no longer widely accepted. The numbers refer simply to the order in which the fractions that contain them emerge from a chromatographic column in their isolations.

The apolipoproteins encompass a wide range of molecular masses, from less than 6 kDa for apo C-I to more than 500 kDa for some B apolipoproteins and apo[a] (Figure 1.5). The relative abundance, distribution, and site of synthesis for the apolipoproteins are shown in Table 1.4. Most of the apolipoproteins are soluble and spontaneously associate with lipid surfaces in vitro and in vivo. Others are insoluble and are markers of the fates of the secreted particles that contain them. An early view was that apolipoproteins were simply vehicles for solubilization and transport of lipids in the plasma compartment. More recent evidence indicates that many of them contain determinants that regulate several activities essential to normal lipid metabolism. Some apolipoproteins stimulate enzymes that degrade plasma lipids. Others contain the ligands that mediate the binding of lipoproteins to cell surface receptors; binding is succeeded by the internalization of all or part of a lipoprotein and the regulation of intracellular lipid synthesis.

Other lipid-binding proteins in the plasma compartment play important roles as well in lipid metabolism. Foremost is serum albumin, which

Table 1.4. ABUNDANCE, DISTRIBUTION, AND SOURCES OF APOLIPOPROTEINS IN HUMAN PLASMA

Apolipo-protein	Plasma concentration (mg/dL)	Percentage for each apolipoprotein				Tissue source(s)
		HDL	LDL	IDL	VLDL	
Apo A-I	130	64				Liver, intestine
Apo A-II	40	20				Liver, intestine
Apo A-IV	—					Liver, intestine
Apo B-48	—					Intestine
Apo B-100	80		95	63	36	Liver
Apo C-I	6	6		1	3	Liver
Apo C-II	3	1		4	7	Liver
Apo C-III	12	4		15	40	Liver
Apo D	10	3	—	—	—	Liver
Apo E	5	2	<5	14	13	Liver

Source: Smith et al. 1983; used with permission.

binds to FFAs and many other hydrophobic substances, including certain drugs. However, in certain pathologic states in which plasma FFA may be elevated (e.g., insulin resistance syndrome) or plasma albumin concentrations are very low (e.g., nephrotic syndrome), the excess fatty acids can be diverted to lipoprotein surfaces, where they modify lipoprotein structure and catabolism (Cistola and Small 1991). Several transfer proteins that mobilize specific lipids between phospholipid surfaces in the plasma compartment also occur (see "Suggested Reading" in Chapter 3).

Suggested Reading

Fielding CJ, Fielding PE. Molecular physiology of reverse cholesterol transport (review). J Lipid Res 1995;36:211–228.

Koschinsky ML, Beisiegel U, Henne-Bruns D, et al. Apolipoprotein (a) size heterogeneity is related to variable number of repeat sequences in its mRNA. Biochemistry 1990;29:640–644.

McKeone BJ, Patsch JR, Pownall HJ. Plasma triglycerides determine low density lipoprotein composition, physical properties, and cell-specific binding in cultured cells. J Clin Invest 1993;91:1926–1933.

Chapter 2

Intracellular Lipid Synthesis and Lipoprotein Assembly

Although protein folding is considered a complex process, it is simple compared with the assembly of multiple proteins and lipids into the quasi-discrete structures of lipoproteins. The major secreted lipoproteins are VLDL, which is assembled in the liver, and the chylomicron, which is formed in the intestine. Both lipoproteins undergo substantial remodeling in the plasma compartment; thus, remnants or mature forms of the circulating particles are found under fasting conditions.

LIPID SYNTHESIS

One common component of the assembly of lipoproteins is the synthesis of their lipids. A description of the biosynthesis and regulation of lipids could fill many volumes. Here, the focus is on two aspects: the parts of the pathway altered in hyperlipidemia, and those parts thought to be important in the regulation of plasma lipid concentrations by drugs and diet. The biosynthesis of lipids involves four major pathways, which are the focus of this chapter. Each of the four pathways, similar in most tissue sites, leads to one of four compounds: fatty acids, glycerol lipids, cholesterol and its esters, and sphingolipids.

Lipogenesis is the synthesis of fatty acids from glucose (Figure 2.1). It is highly regulated through the interaction of insulin, glucagon, and somatostatin and through the concentration of the initial substrate and of the product of this pathway. The pathway leads to the synthesis of palmitic acid, which, through a series of elongation and desaturation reactions, forms long-chain unsaturated fatty acids. The hypertriglyceridemia that frequently accompanies diabetes mellitus is, in part, due to the oversynthesis of fatty acids in the liver. Fatty acids are incorporated into TGs and secreted as VLDL particles, which are further remodeled through hydrolysis in the plasma compartment to FFAs. They in turn are incorporated into adipose tissue.

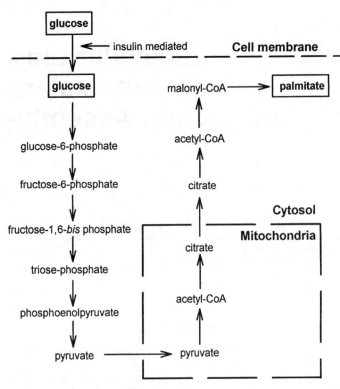

Figure 2.1. Schema of lipogenesis.

Most glycerol lipids, the second of the four products, are derived from glycerol-*sn*-3-phosphate and the coenzyme A (CoA) derivatives of a variety of fatty acids (Figure 2.2). Two successive acylations of glycerol-*sn*-3-phosphate produce phosphatidic acid, which is converted first to a specific phosphatase and then to diacylglycerol. Diacylglycerol may enter one of three pathways. When fatty acid concentrations are low, a large fraction of the diacylglycerol is converted to phosphatidylcholine, the most abundant phospholipid in plasma lipoproteins, or to phosphatidylethanolamine through the transfer of cytidine 5'-diphosphate (CDP)-choline and CDP-ethanolamine, respectively. Phospholipids are necessary for the formation of cell membranes and, thus, are critical to cell survival. As available fatty acid increases, the pathways for phospholipid synthesis become saturated, and an increasing fraction of the TG is diverted to the synthesis of triacyl-

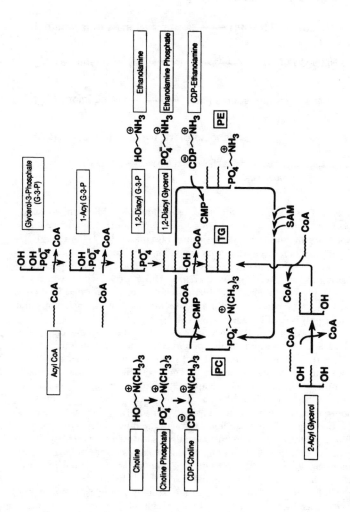

Figure 2.2 Glycerolipid synthesis.

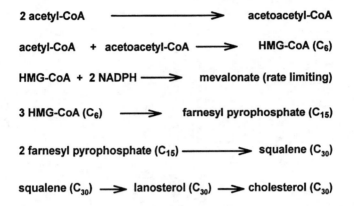

Figure 2.3. Selected steps in cholesterol biosynthesis. The number of carbon atoms is shown in parentheses.

glycerol. This hierarchy is the result of the lower K_m (Michaelis constant) associated with phospholipid synthesis and the much higher maximum velocity for the diacylglycerol acyltransferase that forms TG. Although the relevant mechanisms have not yet been identified, the relative amounts of TG and phospholipid formed by this route appear to be important in determining whether TG is secreted as VLDL or is retained as cytoplasmic lipid droplets. Additional phosphatidylcholine can be formed by methyl transfer from S-adenosyl-methionine to phosphatidylethanolamine, but this pathway is usually considered to be minor.

The specificity of the enzymes involved in the synthesis of glycerol lipids leads to a nonrandom distribution of saturated and unsaturated fatty acids. Fatty acyl groups at the sn-1 and sn-3 positions of glycerol are almost always saturated, whereas the fatty acyl group at the sn-2 position is usually unsaturated. As discussed in Chapter 3, this distribution is important to those lipolytic enzymes in the plasma compartment whose substrates are lipoproteins. An additional route for the formation of TG exists in the intestine. Because the passage of lipids through the intestinal mucosa is largely a function of their solubility, intestinal lipases hydrolyze fatty acids at the sn-1 and sn-3 positions of glycerol lipids; this produces water-soluble FFAs and 2-monoacyl-glycerol. The acylation of 2-monoacylglycerol then produces TG, which forms part of the neutral lipid core of chylomicrons.

Cholesterol, the third of the four pathway products, is one of the most studied biomolecules. Its biosynthesis has been investigated by many of the most famous scientists of this century. Although they are complex, its synthetic pathways have been elucidated in considerable detail. The steps of cholesterol biosynthesis germane to the examination of lipoproteins and lipid disorders are shown in Figure 2.3. Endogenous cholesterol is derived from acetate through a rate-limiting intermediate step—the

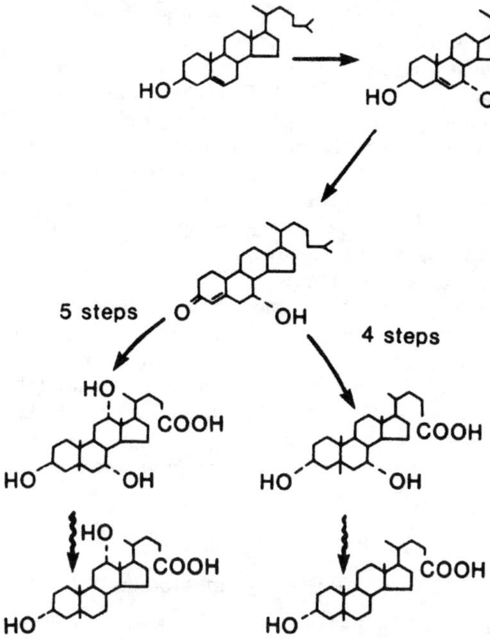

Figure 2.4. Major steps in the formation of bile salts from cholesterol.

conversion of HMG-CoA to mevalonic acid by HMG-CoA reductase. As discussed in Chapter 17, this key step is inhibited by the HMG-CoA reductase inhibitor drugs, or statins, which results in a dramatic reduction in the rate of cholesterol biosynthesis and an increase in LDL receptors. The liver and intestine are the major sources of endogenously derived lipoprotein cholesterol. A variable fraction of cholesterol can be derived from diet, and in normal subjects its occurrence in cells down-regulates cholesterol biosynthesis. Both endogenous cholesterol and dietary cholesterol are involved in several important processes, including biogenesis of cell membranes, production of steroid hormones, and formation of bile acids. The last serve as fat emulsifiers in the digestive tract.

The major steps in the formation of bile salts from cholesterol are shown in Figure 2.4. These steps include those that occur in the liver and those that require catalysis by intestinal enzymes. For example, in the rate-limiting step, the enzyme 7-α-hydroxylase is the catalyst. This pathway is important in the reduction of plasma TC and LDL-C concentrations by bile acid sequestrant drugs. In the absence of sequestrants, there is substantial reabsorption of the bile acids, which can be recycled; in the presence of sequestrants, reabsorption is greatly reduced. Because cholesterol is a bile acid precursor, an additional fraction of cholesterol must be diverted into this pathway for the synthesis of more bile acid. Such diversion lowers the amount of cellular cholesterol and increases the number of LDL receptors (see Chapter 4). Free cholesterol is a substrate for plasma and for intracellular enzymes that form cholesteryl esters (see Chapter 3). ACAT is a membrane-bound enzyme that resides in the rough endoplasmic reticulum. One of its substrates, cholesterol, is membrane bound. The other, acyl CoA, is amphophilic: Part of it resides in the cytoplasm as a free monomeric species or is bound to a fatty acyl–binding protein; the remainder, which is membrane bound, is thought to be part of the acyl CoA pool that is used by ACAT.

Sphingolipids are the fourth and last of the lipid synthesis pathway products. Sphingomyelin, the second most abundant phospholipid component of plasma lipoproteins, is synthesized from palmitoyl CoA, as shown in Figure 2.5. Ninety percent of cellular sphingomyelin resides in the plasma membrane. Even though LDL particles and atherosclerotic lesions are richer in sphingomyelin than are other plasma lipoproteins and healthy arterial tissue, relatively little attention has been paid to this lipid in terms of pathophysiology.

LIPOPROTEIN ASSEMBLY

Very Low Density Lipoproteins

The secretion of VLDL by the liver is the best understood of the lipoprotein secretory pathways (Bamberger and Lane 1988, 1990; Boren et al. 1992). Some questions still remain, and two not entirely reconcilable models have been proposed. These are shown in Figure 2.6. In the first model (Figure 2.6A), the TG-rich principal component of VLDL is assembled in the smooth endoplasmic reticulum. It migrates to junctions with the rough endoplasmic reticulum, where apo B-100 and ACAT-derived cholesteryl esters are incorporated. The enlarged particle continues its migration through the Golgi apparatus, where most of the glycosylation occurs. The particle then enters secretory vesicles within the plasma membrane. After the vesicles release their contents into the space of Disse, the VLDL particles diffuse to the sinusoids and into the bloodstream. There they acquire other proteins and undergo massive remodeling by plasma lipid transfer proteins and lipases.

The alternative model (Figure 2.6B) differs primarily in the site of VLDL assembly and in the mechanism involved. In this model, VLDL begins as a lens of TG between the bilayers that form the membrane of the endoplasmic reticulum. As additional TG synthesis occurs, the lens grows to a sphere of TG that is surrounded by the polar lipids on the inner leaflet of the endoplasmic reticulum. Apo B-100 may be incorporated as a component of the membrane as the TG core continues to grow, or, as Figure 2.6B suggests, the protein may be transferred to the preformed TG particle. At first glance, the process might appear to be

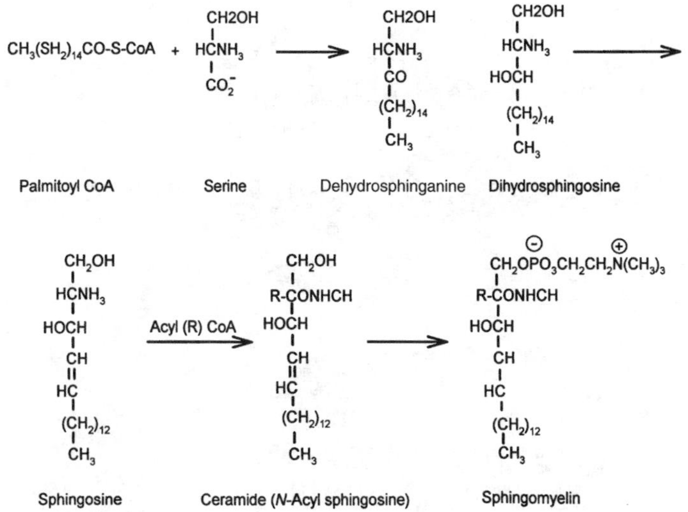

$$CH_3(SH_2)_{14}CO\text{-}S\text{-}CoA \;+\; \underset{\text{Serine}}{\overset{\displaystyle CH_2OH}{\underset{\displaystyle CO_2^-}{\mid HCNH_3 \mid}}} \;\longrightarrow\; \underset{\text{Dehydrosphinganine}}{\overset{\displaystyle CH_2OH}{\mid HCNH_3 \mid CO \mid (CH_2)_{14} \mid CH_3}} \;\; \underset{\text{Dihydrosphingosine}}{\overset{\displaystyle CH_2OH}{\mid HCNH_3 \mid HOCH \mid (CH_2)_{14} \mid CH_3}} \;\longrightarrow$$

Palmitoyl CoA   Serine   Dehydrosphinganine   Dihydrosphingosine

Sphingosine
CH2OH
HCNH3
HOCH
CH
HC
(CH2)12
CH3

→ Acyl (R) CoA →

Ceramide (N-Acyl sphingosine)
CH2OH
R-CONHCH
HOCH
CH
HC
(CH2)12
CH3

→

Sphingomyelin
CH2OPO3CH2CH2N(CH3)3
R-CONHCH
HOCH
CH
HC
(CH2)12
CH3

Figure 2.5. Sphingomyelin biosynthesis.

unlikely because it would require the passage of more than 4,000 amino residues through the aqueous phase separating the membrane and the particle. However, many such processes can be facilitated by the local synthesis of phosphatidylcholine, which appears to be a requirement for the assembly of secretion-competent VLDL (Vance 1985; Vance and Vance 1985, 1986). This phospholipid might provide the additional surface lipid components that allow VLDL to "bud out" into the lumen, or it might simply act as a detergent that allows apo B-100 to transfer from the membrane to a preformed particle.

More recent in vitro evidence supports a stepwise process that is dependent on adequate lipidation of a "prenascent" VLDL. Lipidation is dependent on a supply of fatty acids for TG synthesis and on an activity that transfers newly synthesized TG into a prenascent VLDL. That activity resides in the microsomal TG transfer protein (MTP), which catalyzes the initial lipidation of prenascent VLDL but is not required for the subsequent addition of most of the TG (Gordon et al. 1996). In the absence of adequate lipidation, some apo B-100 degradation occurs in the endoplasmic reticulum (Ingram and Shelness 1996), whereas the remainder occurs in cytosol through the ubiquitin-proteasome pathway, which is regulated by the molecular chaperone heat shock protein 70 (Fisher et al. 1997). The importance of the first step in the lipidation of apo B-100 is emphatically supported by the recent elucidation of the structural defect in abetalipoproteinemia (Du et al. 1996). Mutations in the MTP gene are

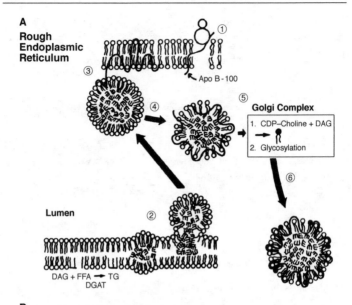

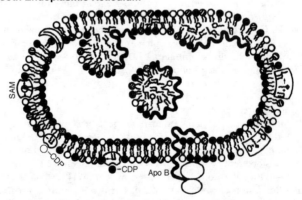

Figure 2.6. Synthesis and assembly of hepatic VLDL components in the endo-plasmic reticulum. (A) Stepwise assembly of preformed TG droplet with apo B-100. (B) Concerted TG synthesis and assembly with apo B-100. DAG, diacylglycerol; DGAT, diacylglycerolacyltransferase; SAM, *S*-adenosylmethionine.

responsible for that autosomal recessive disorder, characterized by the inability of the liver and intestine to secrete apo B. The loss of MTP occurring in patients with abetalipoproteinemia leads to a complete, but specific, block in apo B secretion (Du et al. 1996).

Chylomicrons

Chylomicrons are formed in enterocytes from fatty acids and monoglycerides extracted from the intestinal lumen. Chylomicron assembly has not been as well characterized as that of VLDL in the liver. Certain parallels do exist, including a requirement for fatty acids and MTP (Moberly et al. 1990; Mathur et al. 1997). For example, VLDL particles and chylomicrons contain a TG core surrounded by a surface coat of phospholipids and proteins. In addition, they are substrates for lipolytic processes in plasma that set in motion a series of reactions that form or modify other lipoproteins.

There are three major differences, however. First, because chylomicrons are much larger than VLDL particles, they scatter more light. Thus, during postprandial lipemia, plasma becomes much cloudier, even when TG concentrations are only doubled. Second, the fatty acid composition of chylomicrons is similar to that of the dietary fat load (Pownall 1994). The liver contains lipogenic enzymes that can synthesize new fatty acids. Through elongation and desaturation, a fatty acid profile relatively insensitive to diet is formed. For individuals on a high-carbohydrate diet, increased lipogenesis leads to an elevated plasma VLDL concentration. Third, there is an unusual editing mechanism in the translation of the apo B-100 gene in the intestine (Chen et al. 1987). This editing leads to truncation of the expression, producing a protein that has only 48% of the mass of normal apo B-100, which is found in VLDL and LDL. This apo B-48 is considered a valid marker for lipoproteins of intestinal origin. Although there have been unconfirmed reports that traces of apo B-100 are secreted by the intestine, the liver secretes only apo B-100. Unlike VLDL, retinyl palmitate is found in the chylomicrons of an individual after a dietary fat load containing retinol. Retinyl palmitate transfers very slowly between lipoproteins. It is frequently used as a marker to distinguish between TGRLs of hepatic origin and those of intestinal origin. Because neither apo B-100 nor apo B-48 transfers between lipoproteins, both are valid markers for monitoring the degradation and removal of the particles with which they are associated.

Other chylomicron components synthesized in the intestine include apo A-I, apo A-II, and apo A-IV. These three apolipoproteins transfer freely between chylomicrons, HDL, and the aqueous compartment of plasma. The C apolipoproteins transfer between chylomicrons, HDL, and VLDL.

High-Density Lipoproteins

Origin is not as clear for HDL as for VLDL particles and chylomicrons because there is no reliable nontransferable marker for HDL. On the basis of animal models, clinical correlations, and in vitro tests, two probable sources of HDL have been identified. Perfusion studies suggest that the liver secretes a nascent HDL that is a bilayer disk. The disk is rapidly converted to a mature lipoprotein by plasma enzymes and transfer proteins. Another possible synthetic route by which a substantial fraction of HDL is derived—either instead of or in addition to a route involving plasma enzymes and transfer proteins—involves lipolysis of TGRLs (VLDL and chylomicrons) in the plasma compartment (Patsch et al. 1978). This hypothesis is supported by the observation, discussed in Chapter 3, that HDL-C is increased in individuals who have low plasma TG, presumably because of very efficient lipolysis. This hypothesis continues to gain support from studies that show a strong correlation between lipolysis and HDL-C concentration.

Suggested Reading

Bamberger MJ, Lane MD. Assembly of very low density lipoprotein in the hepatocyte: differential transport of apoproteins through the secretory pathway. J Biol Chem 1988;263:11868–11878.

Fisher EA, Zhou M, Mitchell DM, et al. The degradation of apolipoprotein B-100 is mediated by the ubiquitin-proteasome pathway and involves heat shock protein 70. J Biol Chem 1997;272:20427–20434.

Gordon DA, Jamil H, Gregg RE, et al. Inhibition of the microsomal triglyceride transfer protein blocks the first step of apolipoprotein B lipoprotein assembly but not the addition of bulk core lipids in the second step. J Biol Chem 1996;271:33047–33053.

Moberly JB, Cole TG, Alpers DH, Schonfeld G. Oleic acid stimulation of apolipoprotein B secretion from HepG2 and Caco-2 cells occurs post-transcriptionally. Biochim Biophys Acta 1990;1042:70–80.

Vance JE, Vance DE. Specific pools of phospholipids are used for lipoprotein secretion by cultured rat hepatocytes. J Biol Chem 1986;261:4486–4491.

Remodeling of Lipoproteins in the Plasma Compartment

APOLIPOPROTEIN STRUCTURE

Some of the apolipoprotein genes are closely linked. Those for apo A-I, apo A-IV, and apo C-III are within 22 kbp on chromosome 11. Those for apo C-I, apo C-II, and apo E are all on chromosome 19. The genes for plasminogen and apo[a] are closely linked on chromosome 6. Those for apo A-II, apo B-100, and apo D are on chromosomes 1, 2, and 3, respectively.

The plasma apolipoproteins can be divided into three groups according to shared protein and gene structures. Group 1 comprises the soluble apolipoproteins that reversibly associate with lipid surfaces, namely, apo A-I, A-II, A-IV, C-I, C-II, C-III, and E. The gene structures of these proteins, which belong to the same multigene family, are shown in Figure 3.1. It can be seen that all these proteins are coded by a gene that contains four exons and three introns. With the exception of exon 4, there is high homology among respective exons in all seven genes. Exon 1 codes for part of the 5'-untranslated region of the apolipoprotein. Exon 2 codes for the remainder of the 5'-untranslated region and a portion of the leader sequence that usually characterizes secreted proteins. Exon 3 codes for the remainder of the leader sequence, approximately 40 residues of the primary polypeptide structure, and a pro-sequence in apo A-I, apo A-II, and apo C-II. Exon 4 codes for the region that gives each applicable apolipoprotein its distinct physiologic character.

Additional similarities in the primary structures of the group 1 apolipoproteins are revealed through the application of two very common algorithms: the Chou-Fasman probability algorithm and the helical hydrophobic moment algorithm. The Chou-Fasman probability algorithm predicts that numerous regions in all the group 1 apolipoproteins will have a high probability of being helical (Krebs and Phillips 1983; Pownall et al.

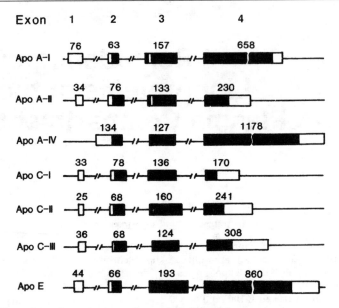

Figure 3.1.   Gene structures of group 1 apolipoproteins.

1983). The helical hydrophobic moment algorithm adds that these helical regions are amphophilic; that is, the amino acid residues on one helical face are polar, whereas those on the opposing helical face are nonpolar. Inspection of the primary structure of the group 1 apolipoproteins reveals that there are, in fact, repeat sequences composed of amphophilic sequences that are 11 or 22 residues in length. Evolution of an apolipoprotein from a small, 11- or 22-residue helical domain into a much larger molecule occurs through gene duplication.

The recognition of putative amphophilic helical regions in the plasma apolipoproteins nearly 20 years ago gave rise to the hypothesis that these regions are responsible for binding apolipoproteins to a lipid surface in lipoproteins. According to this model, as shown in Figure 3.2, the helix associates with a lipoprotein with its axis parallel to the lipoprotein surface. The nonpolar side of the helix penetrates into the lipids beneath the lipoprotein surface; the polar residues remain in contact with the polar head groups of the phospholipids and the surrounding aqueous phase. Thus, by forming a surface film around the neutral lipids, apolipoproteins and phospholipids make the lipids soluble in an aqueous environment. On examination of the location of these helical regions within the gene structure, the distinct roles of exons in apolipoproteins become more evident. For example, as can be seen from the alignment of hydrophobic and

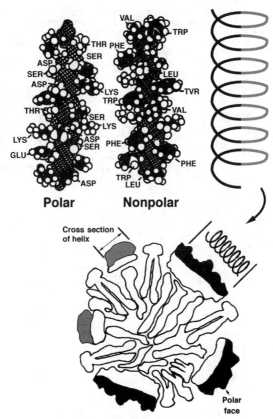

Figure 3.2.   Helical group 1 apolipoproteins are thought to bind at their amphophilic regions to the lipid surfaces of lipoproteins.

polar amino acid residues in Figure 3.3, the portion of the protein encoded by exon 3 contains three amphophilic helices that are important in attaching the apolipoprotein to the lipid surface. Recent evidence supports the amphophilic helical model of the soluble apolipoproteins. X-ray crystallography of the LDL receptor–binding domain of apo E reveals a protein that forms an elongated, four-helix bundle, with the helices stabilized by a tightly packed hydrophobic core that includes leucine zipper-type interactions and by salt bridges on a charged surface (Wilson et al. 1991). The crystal structure of the truncated analogue of human apo A-I, composed of residues 44–243, is almost entirely a continuous, amphipathic,

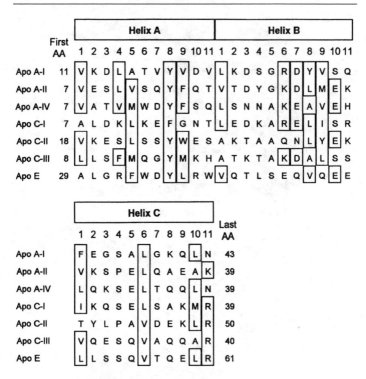

Figure 3.3. Internal repeats in human plasma apolipoproteins (exon 3) showing three amphophilic helices (A–C).

alpha-helix that is interrupted by proline kinks at regularly spaced intervals (Borhani et al. 1997).

Apo B-100 and apo B-48 form the group 2 plasma apolipoproteins. The two apolipoproteins are grouped together because they are very large and are associated with the cholesteryl ester–rich lipoproteins and TGRLs. Although some amphophilic helical regions have been found in these proteins, they are not the dominant structural motifs that they are in the group 1 apolipoproteins. Apo B-100 contains a proline-rich 25-amino-acid residue repeat unit and a hydrophobic 52-amino-acid residue repeat unit (Yang et al. 1986; DeLoof et al. 1987) (Figure 3.4). The physiologic role of these repeats remains to be determined.

Apo B-100 also contains several lipid-binding domains (Figure 3.5). They have been identified in a tryptic digestion, in heparin-binding domains, and in multiple sites of glycosylation. Apo B-100 contains 25 cysteines, some of which are located in a disulfide cluster within the first 500

Consensus 25–Residue Repeat Sequence

Phe- Gln- **Met-** Pro- Ser- **Phe-** His- **Val-** Pro- Glu-
Thr- Asp- **Leu-** Glu- **Val-** Pro- Ser- **Ile-** Thr- **Ile-**
Glu- **Val-** Pro- Ala- **Leu-**

Consensus 52–Residue Repeat Sequence

Leu- Asp- Ser- **Leu-** Lys- Ala- **Leu-** Asp- **Met-** Pro-
Thr- **Phe-** His- **Ile-** Pro- Ser- Ser- Asp- **Phe-** Arg-
Leu- Pro- Ser- **Ile-** Thr- **Ile-** Pro- Glu- Pro- Thr-
Ile- Glu- **Ile-** Pro- Lys- **Leu-** Lys- Asn- Ser- Gln-
Val- Pro- ------ Ala- **Leu-** Ser- **Ile-** Pro- Asp- **Phe-**
Gln- Glu- **Leu-**

Figure 3.4.   Amino acid residue repeats contained in apo B-100.

amino acid residues of the primary structure. One of the cysteines forms a disulfide link with apo[a]; this is the means by which apo[a] is attached to LDL. Apo B-48 is the amino terminal 48% of apo B-100. Although a single gene codes for both proteins, mRNA editing machinery in the intestine substitutes a stop codon for one that codes for an amino acid (Chen et al. 1987). Apo B-48 contains some of the glycosylation and heparin-binding sites as well as the disulfide cluster of apo B-100, but it does not contain the receptor-binding domain of apo B-100 that targets LDL to cell surface receptors.

Group 3 is the remainder of the apolipoproteins for which no unifying structural or functional determinant has been identified. These are apo D and apo[a], neither of which has any obvious connection with lipid metabolism. Apo D belongs to a broad family of proteins that bind to and transport various ligands (Drayna et al. 1987a; Peitsch and Boguski 1990; Pevsner et al. 1988). The family includes retinol-binding protein and alpha$_2$-macroglobulin. Although it was once thought that apolipoproteins in this family played a role in cholesteryl ester transfer, it is now known that this activity is performed by another protein. Apo D contains no internal repeats of amphipathic helices.

Apo[a], which is bound to a minority of LDL particles, belongs to a family of proteins involved in fibrinolysis. Highly polymorphic, it bears little resemblance to any of the other apolipoproteins. One of the fundamental subunits of apo[a] is the kringle (Figure 3.6); this structure is widely distributed among the proteins of the fibrinolysis pathway. A

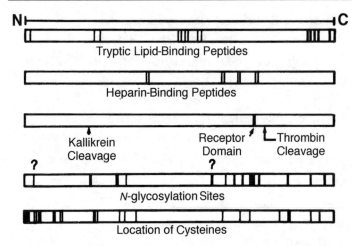

Figure 3.5. Functional regions of apo B-100.

kringle is a protein domain that contains about 80 amino acid residues that are cross-linked by three internal disulfide bonds. Having several cross-links within such a small domain contorts it, yielding the characteristic kringle structure (named for a looped Scandinavian pastry). The molecular weight of apo[a] varies greatly; the various polymorphs largely differ because of differences in the number of kringles (Koschinsky et al. 1990). Apo[a], which contains from 17 to more than 30 kringles, has been likened to Glu-plasminogen, which contains 790 amino acid residues and 5 kringles that precede a serine protease domain. Although the catalytic triad that characterizes serine proteases is present in apo[a], the potential activation site that is cleaved by tissue plasminogen activator is modified and may not be activated.

The general hypothesis of lipoprotein structure, which is applicable to all lipoprotein classes, is the "oil drop" model (Shen et al. 1977) (Figure 3.7). A polar surface containing the apolipoproteins and phospholipids is thought to surround an oily core containing the neutral lipids (TGs and cholesteryl esters). Most of the free cholesterol in a small lipoprotein such as HDL is near the surface; in lipoproteins with a larger core, a greater fraction is partitioned into the core. Protein and lipid compositions of HDL_3, HDL_2, LDL, and VLDL are shown in Figure 3.8; because lipoproteins are only quasi-discrete structures whose compositions reflect genetic and dietary differences, however, the values given there are only nominal. Nevertheless, the compositional range is sufficiently narrow that there are clearly recognizable differences between lipoproteins found in hyperlipidemic and healthy subjects. In most hyper-

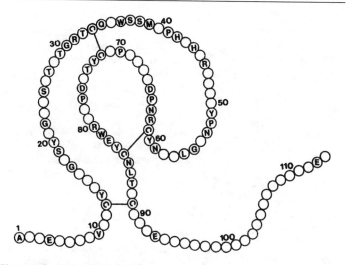

Figure 3.6. Typical extended kringle found in apo [a].

triglyceridemic subjects, there is a higher than normal ratio of protein to neutral lipids in the LDL fraction. In FH, there is an elevation in the cholesteryl ester content of LDL. Moreover, even in normolipidemic subjects, slight enrichment of HDL with TG derived from VLDL is sufficient to alter its density significantly.

The details of the organization of apolipoproteins on the surface of lipoproteins are not known. The fact that the apolipoproteins in HDL are more helical when associated with lipid than when in solution supports the idea that the amphophilic helix is important in binding some of these proteins to lipoproteins. It is probable that the proline residues that frequently appear between helical segments are needed to form some of the turns that allow a single polypeptide chain as long as apo A-I to surround a compact HDL particle.

Although all mature lipoproteins have a uniform surface monolayer of apolipoproteins and phospholipids, there is considerable heterogeneity in apolipoprotein ratio depending on the metabolic state of the subject. Larger VLDL particles contain apo B-100, C apolipoproteins, and apo E. Smaller VLDL particles contain less C apolipoprotein. Virtually all of the protein component of IDL is apo B-100 and apo E. An LDL particle contains one molecule of apo B-100 as its sole protein; addition of apo[a], as noted in Chapter 1, yields Lp[a]. HDL$_2$ and HDL$_3$ also vary in apolipoprotein stoichiometry; the latter is enriched in apo A-I. Postprandially, HDL is slightly less dense, presumably reflecting the transfer of C apolipoproteins from HDL to chylomicrons.

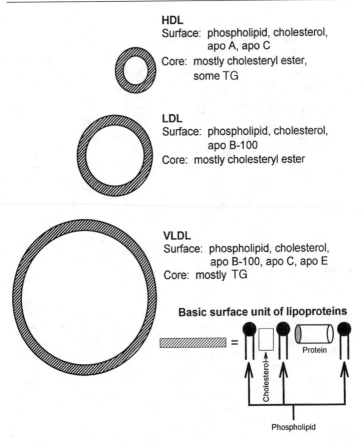

HDL
Surface: phospholipid, cholesterol, apo A, apo C
Core: mostly cholesteryl ester, some TG

LDL
Surface: phospholipid, cholesterol, apo B-100
Core: mostly cholesteryl ester

VLDL
Surface: phospholipid, cholesterol, apo B-100, apo C, apo E
Core: mostly TG

Basic surface unit of lipoproteins

Protein

Cholesterol

Phospholipid

Figure 3.7. "Oil drop" model of lipoproteins. The core contents shown are for unmodified lipoproteins.

SPONTANEOUS LIPID AND PROTEIN TRANSFER

Spontaneous lipid transfer—especially the transfer of cholesterol—is undoubtedly an important physiologic event (Phillips et al. 1987). Transfer of molecules between lipoproteins occurs by spontaneous transfer or protein-mediated transfer. Spontaneous transfer of cholesterol from cells in the vascular wall is probably the initial step in the process known as reverse cholesterol transport. Recent studies implicate the caveolae, which are clathrin-free cell surface organelles active in transmembrane transport, as a site of preferential cholesterol efflux (Fielding and Fielding 1995a, 1995b, 1997).

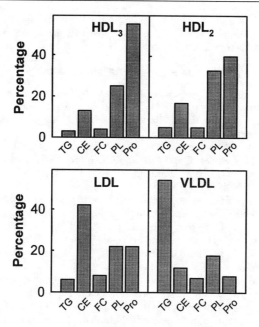

Figure 3.8. Nominal composition for four lipoproteins. CE, cholesteryl ester; FC, free cholesterol; PL, phospholipid; Pro, protein.

Apolipoproteins are transferred between plasma lipoproteins by a spontaneous mechanism. Many lipids that contain a polar moiety, including cholesterol and phospholipids, are sparingly soluble in water. In contrast, cholesteryl esters and TGs are insoluble in water. Both cholesterol and phospholipids transfer between lipoproteins as aqueous monomers that are formed by rate-limiting desorption of the lipid from the lipoprotein surface into the surrounding aqueous phase (Phillips et al. 1987; Pownall et al. 1987). The time required for transfer is inversely proportional to the aqueous solubility of the transferring species. Solubility decreases with increasing length and saturation of its acyl chains. Transfer of a typical phosphatidylcholine such as 1-palmitoyl-2-oleoylphosphatidylcholine between HDL particles is on the order of 15 hours at 37°C. The corresponding time for transfer of free cholesterol, which is more soluble, is about 5 minutes.

Transfer time for a given lipid or protein decreases as a function of increasing diameter of the donor lipoprotein. The transfer half-times for cholesterol from LDL (molecular weight = 2×10^6) and HDL_3 (molecular weight = 10^5) to other lipoproteins are about 45 minutes and 3 minutes, respectively. For the C apolipoproteins, the transfer half-times are less than

1 second. Transfer of apo A-I and apo A-II out of HDL models is more complicated in kinetics and slower. It is likely that the C apolipoproteins spontaneously transfer rapidly between HDL, VLDL, and chylomicrons.

KEY PLASMA PROTEINS OF LIPID TRANSPORT

LPL, a 448-residue glycoprotein, is the major TG-hydrolyzing activity in human plasma. It is synthesized in tissue parenchymal cells and is secreted and transported to the capillary endothelium, where it is bound to heparin sulfate. High concentrations of LPL are found in adipose tissue and striated muscle. The active form of LPL appears to be a dimer that has two bound molecules of apo C-II; apo C-II is required for its maximum activity against TG lipoproteins. Unlike hepatic lipase (HL), LPL is inhibited by 1 M NaCl. LPL hydrolyzes the 1(3)-position of TGs and diglycerides. The resulting monoglyceride is sufficiently water soluble to transfer to tissues, where cellular lipases complete the hydrolysis. In adipose tissue, LPL activity is induced by insulin. HL and LPL belong to a multigene family whose members have identical active-site sequences. HL, a 477-residue glycoprotein, is synthesized in hepatocytes and transported to hepatic endothelial cells, where it is bound by means of heparin sulfate. Its major role appears to be the hydrolysis of TGs and phosphoglycerides of HDL and IDL, which usually lack the activator for LPL, apo C-II.

LCAT, a 416-residue polypeptide synthesized in the liver, is the only known cholesterol-esterifying activity in human plasma, where it is found in a complex with phospholipids, CETP, apo D, and the apo A-I in VHDL. LCAT has two activities, as shown in Figure 3.9. One is the formation of cholesteryl esters from phosphatidylcholine and cholesterol. The other, which occurs in the absence of cholesterol and other potential acyl acceptors, is a phospholipase A_2 activity. The unsaturated acyl chain at sn-2 is usually cleaved in this reaction, although some of the cholesteryl esters and FFAs are also derived from the sn-1 position. The major esters formed by this reaction are a function of the abundance and reactivities of various molecular species of phosphatidylcholine. The reactivity of acyl groups decreases with increasing unsaturation of the fatty acid chains in the acyl donor. Both activities are activated by apolipoproteins. Apo A-I is the most important of the LCAT activators because of its high abundance and its high stimulatory potency.

Both cholesteryl esters and TGs are too hydrophobic to be transferred between lipoproteins by a spontaneous mechanism. In addition, spontaneous phospholipid transfer is too slow to be important in the turnover of the TGRLs, which are relatively short-lived. CETP and PLTP are factors found in the lipoprotein-free fraction of human plasma that transport lipids between lipoproteins. Both transfer proteins exhibit broad specificity with respect to lipid type and fatty acid composition (Morton 1986; Jarnagin et al. 1987; Swenson et al. 1988). Although CETP transfers cholesteryl esters, TGs, and phospholipids, phospholipid transfer appears to be less important than neutral lipid transfer. On the other

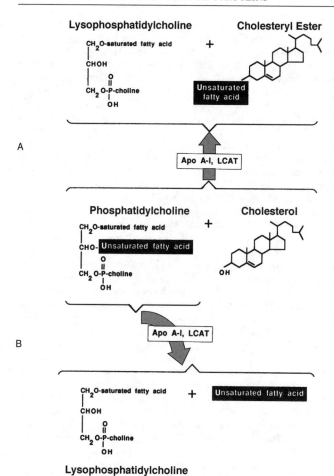

Figure 3.9. LCAT can (A) form cholesteryl esters from phosphatidylcholine and cholesterol or (B) in the absence of acyl acceptors cleave phosphatidylcholine to form lysophosphatidylcholine and an unsaturated acyl chain.

hand, PLTP does not transfer neutral lipids but does transfer a broad spectrum of phospholipids, sphingolipids, and diglyceride (Huuskonen et al. 1996; Rao et al. 1997). In addition, PLTP transfers lipopolysaccharide (Hailman et al. 1996) and alpha-tocopherol (Kostner et al. 1995).

CETP has been characterized in some detail. CETP is a 74-kDa glycoprotein with 476 amino acid residues (Drayna et al. 1987b). Its gene resides on chromosome 16. CETP does not share much structural homology with the apolipoproteins, and the distribution of hydrophobic regions that might bind to neutral lipids is very different from those found in lipolytic enzymes and plasma lipoproteins. The isolation of a CETP-lipid complex in vitro suggests that CETP operates by binding lipid monomers and moving between the surfaces of donor and acceptor lipoproteins. The relative amounts of cholesteryl ester and TG that are transported by CETP are a function of the composition of these two lipids in the surface monolayer of lipoproteins. This supports the idea that there is rapid exchange of neutral lipids between the core and surface region and that most lipolytic and transfer activities occur in the surface region. CETP has the potential to carry cholesteryl esters from HDL into the apo B-100–containing lipoproteins, where they are removed from plasma with the acceptor particle. CETP is also important in the transfer of TG from VLDL to HDL and LDL, and it appears that it mediates this process in the production of TG-rich HDL and LDL in hypertriglyceridemic subjects. The transfer activity of CETP is rather slow (half-time ≥ 4 hours), but still fast by the time scale for HDL and LDL turnover (about 5 days and 3 days, respectively). As a consequence, HDL and LDL are virtually identical in cholesteryl ester fatty acid composition. This observation does not hold for VLDL, the metabolism of which is fast compared with the activity of CETP. CETP deficiency in humans produces a lipoprotein profile that simulates that found in species that lack this activity. The deficiency is associated with the production of HDL particles that are much larger than normal; species that lack CETP are usually resistant to atherosclerosis.

Plasma PLTP is an acidic, 476-amino-acid protein with a protein mass of 54,719 Da and an apparent molecular weight of 78,000. The discrepancy between the protein mass and observed molecular mass is due to glycosylation at one or more of its six N-glycosylation sites and numerous O-glycosylation sites. PLTP belongs to a family of lipid transfer proteins that includes CETP, bactericidal/permeability-increasing protein, and lipopolysaccharide-binding protein (Day et al. 1994; Lagrost et al. 1998). It was originally found as a second phospholipid transfer activity during purification of CETP (Tall et al. 1983; Tollefson et al. 1988). Recent studies suggest that PLTP also plays an important role in lipoprotein turnover and reverse cholesterol transport, and that HDL is the primary target for its transfer and remodeling activity (Jauhiainen et al. 1993; Huuskonen et al. 1996; Rao et al. 1997). PLTP is probably important in cholesterol transport because it facilitates the transfer of phosphatidylcholine. Overexpression of PLTP in mice is associated with a virtual disappearance of plasma HDL and apo A-I (Foger et al. 1997). Hypothetically, PLTP could be a key protein in the net transfer of phospholipids from membranes and other lipoproteins into HDL precursors. Successive rounds of transfer and esterification by LCAT could lead to a growing particle that is a net acceptor of cholesterol and that matures into HDL_2 and HDL_3.

Serum albumin, which is a globular protein composed of nearly 600 amino acid residues cross-linked by 17 disulfide bridges, transports small hydrophobic molecules. Like the apolipoproteins, albumin contains multiple helical loops separated by prolines, which are located at turns in the structure and allow the helical structures to fold into the globular shape of the protein. The major physiologic role of albumin is the transport of FFAs among the major tissue sites that require them for membrane biogenesis, energy production, and the synthesis of bioregulators such as eicosanoids and thromboxanes. FFAs, which have a plasma turnover time of about 3 minutes, bind to albumin with association constants between 10^{-7} and 10^{-9}; binding increases as a function of acyl chain length. The major source of binding energy is hydrophobic; a small component is derived from the head group.

Although albumin is frequently viewed as a transporter of FFAs in plasma, it does not catalyze this process in the same way that CETP transfers neutral lipids. The major difference is that the aqueous solubilities of neutral lipids are so low that virtually none are in the aqueous phase, and a transport protein is required to move them between lipid surfaces. In contrast, most FFAs are water soluble and can move among lipid surfaces and proteins through the aqueous phase. In fact, the diffusion rate of albumin is more than two orders of magnitude greater than is typical for FFAs. Albumin has another important role: It is a buffer that keeps plasma FFAs and lysolipid concentrations low enough to minimize their cytolytic effects on tissues in contact with the plasma compartment.

LIPOPROTEIN CATABOLISM

The remodeling of lipoproteins in the plasma compartment by various plasma enzymes and transfer proteins is an important determinant of their metabolic fate and potential atherogenic or cardioprotective potential. Regarding the modification of lipoproteins by processes that are thought to increase their atherogenicity, the process may be more important than the product.

Many proteins are required for the processing and eventual removal of lipoproteins from plasma. They include enzymes that modify the covalent structure of lipids in the secreted lipoproteins, thereby giving rise to the usual spectrum of lipoproteins found in fasting plasma. Others are the lipid transfer factors CETP and PLTP, which together with the lipolytic enzymes are important to the maturation of a lipoprotein into the form that is eventually transferred through both specific and nonspecific mechanisms from the plasma compartment to cells in contact with plasma. The most important of the specific mechanisms are those mediated by cell surface receptors and receptor ligands within the primary structure of some of the apolipoproteins. As noted above, lipids are also transferred between cell and lipoprotein surfaces by means of a nonspecific spontaneous mechanism, which does not depend on energy or transfer proteins. Specific apolipoproteins are activators for some of the key enzyme activities in plasma. The activities that modify plasma lipoproteins, and the receptor-mediated uptake of lipoproteins are both a function of the structure of the lipoprotein, especially the apolipoprotein component, the fluidity of the lipid surface, and the covalent structure of the individual molecules cleaved by these enzymes.

It is important to re-emphasize that lipoproteins are quasi-discrete structures that do not have a single characteristic density or a distinct stoichiometry of lipids and proteins. This may be due to the nature of the low-energy forces that hold lipoproteins together and to the constant modification of even some of the more homogeneous fractions by lipolysis and spontaneous lipid transfer. Thus, interconversions of lipoprotein subfractions are, by the very nature of the particles involved, a continuum that extends across a spectrum of intermediates that may begin with a nascent lipoprotein, such as VLDL, and end with the mature product (LDL in the case of VLDL). Theoretically, each bond cleavage that is produced by a lipolytic enzyme and every molecule that is added to or removed from a lipoprotein could give rise to another lipoprotein subfraction. In spite of these detailed differences, we adhere to a broader definition that involves measurable changes in composition and structure.

PROCESSING OF VERY LOW DENSITY LIPOPROTEINS

Lipolysis by LPL is the initiating event in the catabolism of the TGRLs (Figure 3.10). In the case of VLDL, apo C-II that is bound to the lipoprotein surface activates LPL, which is located in the capillary endothelium. Lipolysis liberates fatty acids and lysophospholipids, which are transferred to albumin. The hydrolysis of the TGs causes a reduction in the size of the nonpolar core of the particle. Concurrently, there is some hydrolysis of the phosphoglycerolipids in the surface of the particle. The lipolytic activity leads to a reduction in the size of the VLDL particle, and during the loss of lipids and the shrinkage of its dimensions the C apolipoproteins are transferred back to HDL, where most of them were derived immediately after secretion. This results in IDL, which contains almost exclusively one molecule of apo B-100 and variable amounts of apo E. Even after the loss of the C apolipoproteins, lipolytic activity, which may be through the action of HL, hydrolyzes more of the TGs and phosphoglycerolipids, and the remaining complement of apo E is transferred to either HDL or nascent VLDL. This forms LDL. Relative to VLDL, LDL is rich in sphingomyelin, which is not transferred very efficiently to other lipoproteins and for which there is no known hydrolytic activity in plasma.

CHYLOMICRON PROCESSING

The catabolism of chylomicrons is similar in some respects to that of VLDL. Apo C-II stimulates the activity of LPL in the capillary endothelium and releases the lipolytic products to albumin. Chylomicron hydrolysis is much faster than that of VLDL, and its contribution of TGs to other lipoproteins has not been quantified but is probably small. The product of

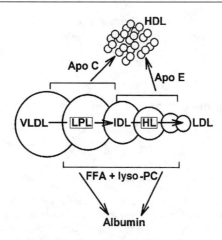

Figure 3.10. Lipolytic cascade for VLDL, showing the transfer of FFAs and lysophosphatidylcholine (lyso-PC) to serum albumin and the transfer of C apolipoproteins from VLDL to HDL and of apo E from IDL to HDL, yielding mature LDL. Lipolysis of VLDL is catalyzed by LPL, and lipolysis of IDL is catalyzed by HL.

chylomicron hydrolysis is the chylomicron remnant, which is removed from plasma by means of a chylomicron remnant receptor in hepatocytes. Nascent chylomicrons contain apolipoproteins B-48, A-I, A-II, A-IV, and E. Almost immediately after chylomicron secretion, apo A-I and apo A-II are transferred to HDL either by spontaneous transfer or as a part of a surface remnant that is released during lipolysis. Concomitantly, apo A-IV is transferred to the aqueous phase and is not strongly associated with any lipoprotein class. The apo B-48 remains with the chylomicron and is a marker for its catabolism because it does not transfer to the aqueous phase or to other lipoproteins. Although the apo E transfers from chylomicron remnants to HDL, a sufficient amount remains with the remnant to mediate its binding to remnant receptors in the liver.

PROCESSING OF HIGH-DENSITY LIPOPROTEINS

Because there are no nonexchangeable markers for HDL remodeling and catabolism, the mechanistic picture of HDL processing is fairly murky, particularly with respect to the initial step. There are putative routes for the first step. One of these is the hepatic secretion of a nascent, discoidal particle. A second is liberation of the surface components of TGRLs during lipolysis. In either instance, an HDL particle that has pre-beta mobility and is rich in phospholipid and apo A-I is processed to mature HDL through the activities of LCAT, HL, and PLTP (Fielding and

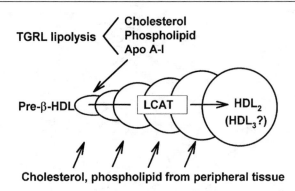

Figure 3.11. Conversion of pre-β-HDL to mature forms of HDL. As TGRLs undergo lipolysis, their surface components, including cholesterol, phospholipid, and apo A-I, are transferred to the expanding HDL particle. In addition, an HDL particle obtains cholesterol and phospholipid from cells in contact with the plasma compartment. The formation of HDL$_3$ by this mechanism is unconfirmed.

Fielding 1995a). This pre-β-HDL is a preferred acceptor of cholesterol from peripheral tissue. As shown in Figure 3.11, phosphatidylcholine and cholesterol are converted by LCAT to lysophosphatidylcholine and cholesteryl esters, thereby increasing the volume of the core. At the same time, some of the surface phospholipid lost through LCAT is replaced by other proteins or by phospholipids delivered by spontaneous transfer or the activity of PLTP. Through additional cycles of cholesterol and phospholipid transfer to HDL and the conversion of these lipids to cholesteryl ester, the remodeled HDL continues to increase in size, ultimately forming HDL$_2$ and HDL$_3$. The relation between HDL$_2$ and HDL$_3$ in normolipidemic subjects is not clear. In vitro studies have shown that PLTP activity converts large particles into small particles (Rao et al. 1997), which are better acceptors of cholesterol. As discussed below, in hypertriglyceridemic subjects, who typically have little or no HDL$_2$, HDL$_2$ is a likely precursor of HDL$_3$. Both HDL$_2$ and HDL$_3$ particles are cleared from the circulation through putative receptors on hepatocytes.

SOURCES OF PLASMA FREE FATTY ACIDS

FFA flux into the plasma compartment is highly variable and is a function of the activities of hormone-sensitive lipase, LCAT, LPL, and HL (Figure 3.12); these enzymes liberate water-soluble products, which are transferred to albumin. Another source of fatty acids is adipose tissue, in which TG lipolysis by hormone-sensitive lipase liberates FFAs, which are then secreted into the plasma compartment. All these enzymes can contribute to the hepatic FFA pool that synthesizes VLDL TG. Through product inhi-

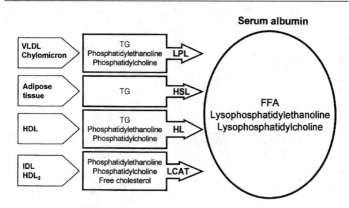

Figure 3.12. LPL, hormone-sensitive lipase (HSL), hepatic lipase (HL), and LCAT liberate water-soluble molecules that are transferred to albumin in the plasma from VLDL, chylomicrons, adipose tissue, HDL, IDL, and HDL$_2$.

bition, plasma FFA concentration can modify the activities of the enzymes that liberate them and of the plasma transfer proteins in particular.

COORDINATION OF LIPOLYSIS WITH LIPID AND PROTEIN TRANSFER

From the time that VLDL is secreted until it is removed from plasma by cellular uptake, there are additional remodeling processes that are mediated by CETP. Although VLDL contains a small amount of cholesteryl ester, during its conversion to LDL it obtains additional cholesterol from HDL. At the same time, some of the TG and a small amount of the VLDL cholesteryl ester are returned to HDL. Some major differences are particularly evident in subjects who are hypertriglyceridemic, and the plasma profile can be further modified when hypertriglyceridemia is combined with insulin resistance syndrome (see also Chapter 8). In hypertriglyceridemia with most of the excess TG in VLDL, CETP mediates the exchange of VLDL TG for cholesteryl ester of LDL and HDL. LDL and HDL become TG enriched: at very high plasma TG concentrations, 65% and 90% of the neutral lipid cores of LDL and HDL are composed of TG.

There are a number of consequences of the elevation of TG content in LDL and HDL. First, the compositional change makes them both substrates for HL, which removes much of the TG core by hydrolysis. With the decrease in the amount of lipid, both particles become smaller; TG-rich HDL$_2$ is converted to HDL$_3$, which remains TG-rich through the concomitant CETP-mediated acquisition of additional TG from VLDL. Replacement of HDL cholesteryl ester with TG reduces the amount of cholesterol

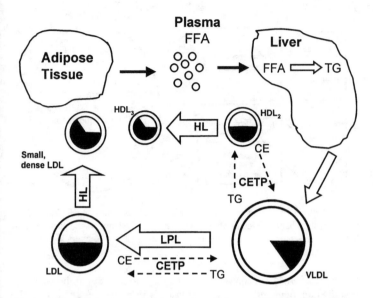

Figure 3.13. Mechanism by which elevation of plasma FFAs derived from hypersecretion or impaired uptake by adipose tissue could lead to derangements in the plasma profile of major lipoprotein classes. The increased plasma FFA concentration leads to enhanced hepatic extraction and to synthesis of VLDL TG. The VLDL particles, increased in size and number, provide a pool of TG that is exchanged for cholesteryl ester (CE) in LDL and HDL_2, a process that is mediated by CETP. TG-rich LDL and HDL_2 are substrates for HL, whose activity removes TG from the core of the particles, giving rise to small, dense LDL and to HDL_3, respectively. In the lipoprotein cores, white indicates CE and black indicates TG.

carried by HDL; this mechanism explains why two risk factors for CHD—elevated plasma TG and low plasma HDL-C—are frequently associated. Moreover, it explains the virtual absence of HDL_2, the larger HDL subclass, in moderate to severe hypertriglyceridemia.

A similar mechanism explains the occurrence of small, dense LDL in hypertriglyceridemic subjects. Exchange of LDL cholesteryl ester for VLDL TG makes LDL a substrate for HL, which converts it to a smaller, denser particle. Small, dense LDL may be associated with enhanced risk for atherosclerosis (see Chapter 8). TG-rich LDL from hypertriglyceridemic subjects contains a structurally altered apo B-100 whose interaction with the LDL receptor is impaired (McKeone et al. 1993).

The initiating factor in the clustering of risk factors that may be referred to as insulin resistance syndrome (see Chapter 8) could be impaired uptake of plasma FFAs by peripheral tissue (Figure 3.13), leading to elevated plasma FFA (Reaven et al. 1988; McGarry 1992). The higher plasma FFA concentration enables a higher hepatic extraction rate, which is associated with the secretion of VLDL increased in size and number. The resulting hypertriglyceridemia leads to changes in LDL and HDL structure and composition, as described above. Another factor that can enhance the CETP exchange of VLDL TG for HDL cholesteryl ester is the stimulation of CETP activity by FFAs. This has been observed both in vitro and in vivo (Barter et al. 1990; Lagrost et al. 1995) and under conditions in which FFA concentration is increased by LPL activity (Tall et al. 1984). In addition, specific activity of plasma CETP in patients with insulin resistance syndrome is elevated (Bagdade et al. 1991). The reduced LPL concentrations seen in insulin resistance syndrome may be due to regulation of LPL synthesis and secretion by plasma FFAs, but this remains to be shown. The high occurrence of insulin resistance syndrome in obese individuals strongly suggests that adipose tissue is the main site of impaired FFA uptake.

Suggested Reading

Borhani DW, Rogers DP, Engler JA, Brouillette CG. Crystal structure of truncated human apolipoprotein A-I suggests a lipid-bound conformation. Proc Natl Acad Sci U S A 1997;94:12291–12296.

Fielding CJ, Fielding PE. Intracellular cholesterol transport. J Lipid Res 1997;38:1503–1521.

McGarry JD. What if Minkowski had been ageusic? An alternative angle on diabetes. Science 1992;258:766–770.

Chapter 4

Lipoprotein Catabolism

Lipoprotein transport out of the plasma compartment is a function of the composition and structure of lipoproteins and of the cell surfaces that are in contact with the plasma compartment and other cell types immediately adjacent to those lining the plasma compartment. Some lipoproteins are removed as intact particles by means of cell surface receptors that recognize a specific ligand within the lipoprotein. Some particles are also internalized by cells through nonspecific mechanisms. Finally, some of the sparingly soluble components of lipoproteins, such as the apolipoproteins, cholesterol, and phospholipids, can transfer from the lipoprotein to cell surfaces by desorption into the surrounding aqueous phase. This is followed by diffusion to the plasma membrane, where they are adsorbed onto the plasma membrane and translocated by various mechanisms into the cell. Studies in this area can be divided into those involving interaction of whole isolated lipoproteins or reassembled lipoproteins with cells in culture; uptake of lipoproteins in organ perfusion experiments; and in vivo turnover of lipoproteins in animal models and in healthy and dyslipidemic human subjects.

MONOMERIC LIPID TRANSPORT

Some components of lipoproteins transfer directly to cells through desorption into the surrounding aqueous phase and subsequent diffusion-controlled association with cell membranes. The mechanism and regulation of this physicochemical process are identical to those described in Chapter 3 for lipid and protein transfer between lipoproteins. The process is reversible and is probably of great importance for molecules such as cholesterol and FFAs. When those lipids are available in excess, intracellular enzymes in the endoplasmic reticulum convert them to cholesteryl ester and TG, which are much less cytotoxic. At low cholesterol and FFA concentrations, cholesteryl esterases and lipases convert the neutral lipid inclusions back to cholesterol and FFAs, both of which are readily transported by spontaneous transfer. Although lipid transfer proteins mobilize cholesteryl ester and TG between lipoproteins, there is little evidence that this is a major pathway between lipoproteins and cells, although the question remains open.

RECEPTOR-MEDIATED UPTAKE OF LIPOPROTEINS

A major route for the removal of lipoproteins from plasma involves receptors located on the surfaces of cells in contact with blood. The receptors are recognized by a specific ligand (a protein or protein fragment) on the lipoprotein surface, and in many instances their expression is regulated by the status of the cell—that is, whether the cell needs more of the lipids that are in a given lipoprotein. Unlike monomeric lipid transfer, receptor-mediated internalization of a lipoprotein transports many lipid molecules into a cell in a single step. In the case of LDL, each particle that enters a cell carries with it more than 1,000 molecules of cholesteryl ester and 500 molecules of free cholesterol. Particle endocytosis is an efficient route for the incorporation of lipids into cells.

Apo E and apo B-100 are the ligands that mediate the removal of plasma IDL and LDL, respectively, by means of hepatic cell surface receptors. Although VLDL contains both apo E and apo B-100, the protein conformations are not completely receptor competent. On lipolytic conversion of VLDL to IDL, the particle becomes smaller, the C apolipoproteins are transferred to HDL, and apo E undergoes changes in its conformation and environment that make it receptor competent. Mutations in the LDL receptor are associated with type II hyperlipidemia. In type III hyperlipidemia, mutations in the ligand-binding region of apo E are associated with impaired uptake of IDL and elevations of plasma IDL (VLDL remnants). A chylomicron remnant with its complement of TG and cholesteryl ester is internalized by means of a receptor ligand in apo E; defects in apo E can lead to plasma elevations of chylomicron remnants. Expression of lipoprotein receptors differs among tissue sites and is determined by the requirements of the cells at each site for different lipids.

Low-Density Lipoprotein Receptor Family

Low-Density Lipoprotein Receptor

The LDL (apo B/E) receptor is the best characterized of all the lipoprotein receptors. Its protein family also includes receptors for VLDL and the chylomicron (Figure 4.1). The work of Michael S. Brown and Joseph L. Goldstein has done much to elucidate the LDL receptor pathway and its role in lipid metabolism and atherogenesis as well as the molecular genetics of FH. In FH homozygotes, competent LDL receptors are absent. Defects can occur in a number of structural subunits in the LDL receptor.

Each LDL contains one molecule of apo B-100 as its only protein. Most dividing cells have receptors that bind to LDL by means of a specific ligand in apo B-100. The binding begins a series of processes schematized in Figure 4.2. LDL binds to receptors located within coated pits on the cell surface. A coated pit closes to form a coated vesicle, which is converted to an endosome that dissociates into an LDL vesicle and an LDL

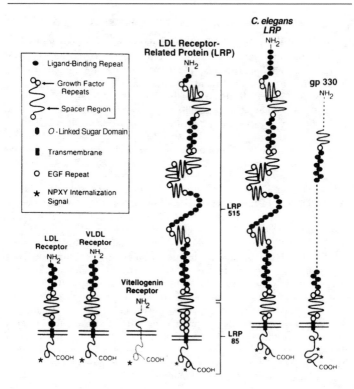

Figure 4.1. The LDL receptor gene family. All members of the family consist of the same basic structural motifs. (From Krieger and Herz 1994; used with permission.)

receptor vesicle. The receptor vesicle recycles to the cell surface, and the remaining endosome is converted into a lysosome. Within the lysosome, acid esterases and proteases hydrolyze the lipids and proteins, respectively, to FFAs, free cholesterol, and amino acids. The free cholesterol, if in excess, is converted into cholesteryl esters. Within the endoplasmic reticulum, free cholesterol down-regulates the production of LDL receptors and the rate-limiting enzyme of cholesterol biosynthesis, HMG-CoA reductase. Down-regulation occurs through the association of cholesterol with proteins that affect the activity of mRNA regulatory binding proteins for both HMG-CoA reductase and the LDL receptor. When there are inadequate supplies of cellular cholesterol, additional receptors are synthesized. After modification in the Golgi compartment, they move to the cell surface.

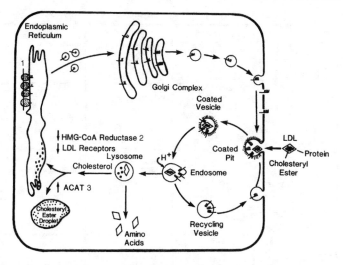

Figure 4.2. The LDL (apo B/E) receptor pathway. (From Brown and Goldstein 1985; used with permission.)

From this model it is easy to understand how LDL receptor activity regulates plasma cholesterol concentration and how the absence of LDL receptors leads to an elevation in plasma cholesterol. In the absence of receptor binding, there is no efficient means of removing LDL from plasma, and the plasma LDL concentration rises. Also, since there is no cholesterol from LDL within the cell to down-regulate cholesterol biosynthesis, the cell continues to produce and secrete cholesterol even though it is not needed. Were it not for nonspecific LDL uptake, plasma TC concentrations would rise even higher than the values of more than 700 mg/dL found in homozygous FH. In normal subjects, about 70% of plasma LDL particles are cleared through the liver by the LDL receptor pathway. The remainder are cleared by nonspecific uptake.

A model for the molecular interaction of the apo B-100 molecule of LDL with the LDL receptor has been proposed on the basis of our knowledge about the structure of the receptor (Figure 4.3) and its ligands. There is a great deal of regional homology between the LDL receptor and proteins of other families. The extracellular part of the LDL receptor is composed of an amino end that contains the ligand-binding domain, which is made up of seven repeats of about 40 amino acids that are arranged head to tail. Near the carboxyl terminus of each repeat, there is a cluster of negatively charged fatty acids that bind to the positively charged amino acids of apo E and apo B, as shown in Figure 4.4. Site-directed mutations of this domain have shown that the receptor determi-

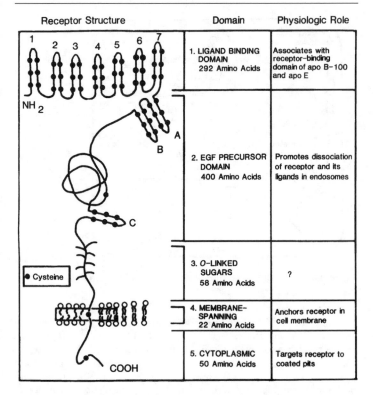

Figure 4.3. Receptor Structure / Domain / Physiologic Role

Receptor Structure	Domain	Physiologic Role
	1. LIGAND BINDING DOMAIN 292 Amino Acids	Associates with receptor-binding domain of apo B-100 and apo E
	2. EGF PRECURSOR DOMAIN 400 Amino Acids	Promotes dissociation of receptor and its ligands in endosomes
	3. O-LINKED SUGARS 58 Amino Acids	?
	4. MEMBRANE-SPANNING 22 Amino Acids	Anchors receptor in cell membrane
	5. CYTOPLASMIC 50 Amino Acids	Targets receptor to coated pits

Figure 4.3. The LDL (apo B/E) receptor protein. (From Yamamoto et al. 1984; used with permission.)

nants for the binding of LDL and β-VLDL are distinct. The second domain is highly homologous to epidermal growth factor (EGF) precursor. It is required for the acid-dependent dissociation of the receptor and ligand within the endosome. It is not required for binding β-VLDL. The role of the third domain, which is small and rich in serine and threonine residues that contain O-linked sugars, is not known. The fourth domain is the 22-residue, membrane-spanning domain that characterizes many integral membrane proteins. The carboxyl terminal domain is intracellular and targets the recycling receptor to the coated pits.

Chylomicron Remnant Receptor

Much of our understanding of chylomicron catabolism is inferred from animal and cell studies. Because different animal and cell models have

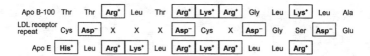

Apo B-100	Thr	Thr	Arg⁺	Leu	Thr	Arg⁺	Lys⁺	Arg⁺	Gly	Leu	Lys⁺	Leu	Ala
LDL receptor repeat	Cys	Asp⁻	X	X	X	Asp⁻	Cys	X	Asp⁻	Gly	Ser	Asp⁻	Glu
Apo E	His⁺	Leu	Arg⁺	Lys⁺	Leu	Arg⁺	Lys⁺	Arg⁺	Leu	Leu	Arg⁺		

Figure 4.4. Putative electrostatic interaction of the positively charged receptor-binding domains of apo B-100 and apo E with the negatively charged consensus repeat within the ligand-binding domain of the LDL receptor.

been used, there is no consensus about the mechanism by which chylomicron remnants are processed. As described in Chapter 2, chylomicrons are TG-rich particles that are secreted by the intestine after a dietary fat load. In the plasma compartment, chylomicron TG is hydrolyzed by LPL. The hydrolysis products, FFAs, are transferred to albumin and subsequently to adipose tissue or skeletal muscle, where they are stored or used. This process leaves a remnant particle that is enriched in cholesterol, cholesteryl esters, phospholipids, apo B-48, and apo E. According to one model (Figure 4.5), reduction in the size of the particles during hydrolysis permits them to pass through the endothelial fenestrae and into the space of Disse, where the remnants are removed directly by receptors (de Faria et al. 1996; Choi and Cooper 1993; Cooper 1997). Some remnants are transiently bound to proteoglycans by means of apo E; others can be sequestered by cell surface HL by means of apo B-48. In each instance they are transferred from their sites of sequestration to the LDL receptor. Remnant uptake stimulated by HL is independent of lipolysis (de Faria et al. 1996; Krapp et al. 1996). Alternatively, the sequestered remnant can acquire additional hepatically derived apo E, which triggers particle recognition by the LDL receptor–related protein (LRP), which is also the receptor for alpha$_2$-macroglobulin (Strickland et al. 1990). Apo E is required for rapid hepatic removal of remnants by means of LRP. Binding of lipoproteins by LRP is inhibited by apo C-I, which presumably competes with apo E.

Very Low Density Lipoprotein Receptor

The VLDL receptor binds lipoproteins that contain apo E and consists of five functional domains that resemble those of the LDL receptor (Jingami and Yamamoto 1995; Krieger and Herz 1994). The VLDL and LDL receptors are almost the same in gene structure and organization. Despite the presence of sterol regulatory element 1–like sequences in the VLDL receptor gene, the transcription of the gene is not down-regulated by sterols. The physiologic role of the VLDL receptor in mammals is unresolved. Animal studies show a high level of expression of its mRNA and protein in nonhepatic tissues, especially endothelial cells. The expression in endothelial cells suggests that the receptor plays a role in the transport of VLDL or another constituent from the plasma compartment to adjacent tissues (Wyne et al. 1996). The VLDL receptor might also be responsible

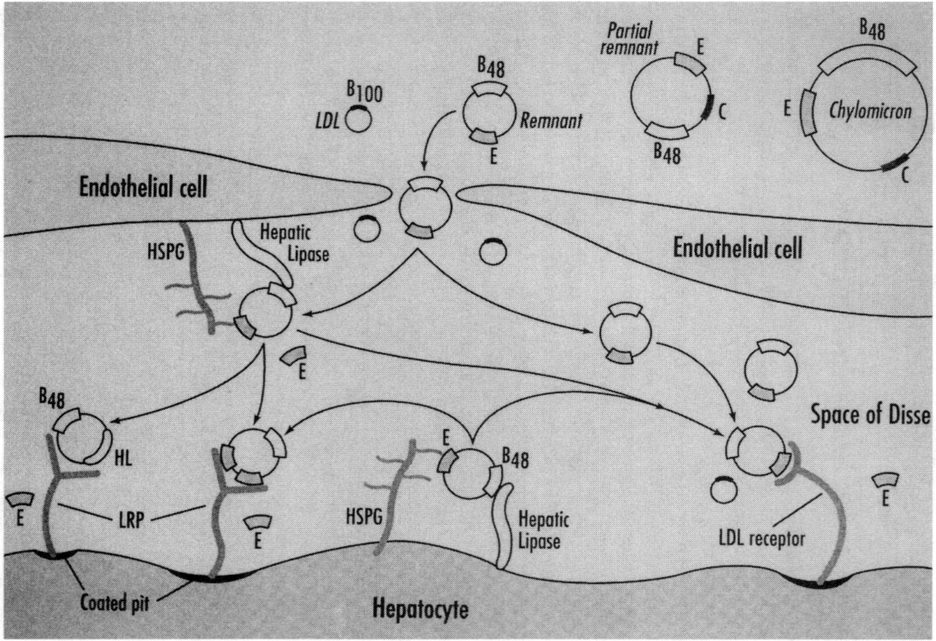

Figure 4.5. The possible pathways that a chylomicron remnant may follow on reaching the liver. If of appropriate size, it enters the space of Disse (here expanded, actually more like a fenestra). The remnant may (1) be taken up directly by the LDL receptor; (2) acquire additional apo E and be taken up directly by the LDL receptor-related protein (LRP); or (3) become sequestered by binding to heparan sulfate proteoglycans (HSPGs) (mediated by apo E) or HL (mediated by apo B). Sequestered particles may then be transferred to the LDL receptor or LRP after further modifications. In the absence of apo E, hepatic lipase might serve as a ligand for LRP. (From Cooper 1997; used with permission.)

for VLDL catabolism in muscle and adipose tissue; VLDL receptor mRNA is highly expressed in tissues that actively metabolize fatty acids as their source of energy. A major ligand for the receptor is VLDL; studies have also shown it to mediate the uptake of Lp[a] (Argraves et al. 1997). The VLDL receptor is expressed in macrophages in human atherosclerotic lesions, and endocytosis of Lp[a] by way of this receptor could lead to cellular accumulation of lipid within macrophages and may represent a molecular basis for the atherogenic effects of Lp[a].

Other Receptors

High-Density Lipoprotein Receptor

Unlike in lipoproteins that contain apo B, all components of HDL are exchangeable through protein-mediated or spontaneous transfer mechanisms. Therefore, the lipids and proteins of HDL can be catabolized independently of one another and of the HDL particle. For example, studies in rats have shown the kidney to be a site of selective uptake of apo A-I, whereas little or no lipid is catabolized in the kidney (Glass et al. 1983; Ponsin et al. 1986; Pownall et al. 1991). Other studies have shown that HDL cholesteryl ester is selectively removed by the adrenal glands and liver (Khoo et al. 1995), and a receptor for this process has been identified: the class B, type I scavenger receptor (SR-BI), which binds HDL (Acton et al. 1996). SR-BI mediates selective uptake of HDL cholesteryl ester by cultured cells, and its expression is coordinately regulated with steroidogenesis in several sites, including the adrenal gland, ovary, and testis. Interestingly, adenovirus-mediated hepatic overexpression of SR-BI in mice results in the virtual disappearance of plasma HDL and increased biliary cholesterol (Kozarsky et al. 1997). SR-BI is the first molecularly well-defined cell surface HDL receptor described. It mediates transfer of lipid from HDL to cells by selective lipid uptake, a mechanism distinct from receptor-mediated endocytosis by means of clathrin-coated pits and vesicles. Free or lipid-bound apo A-I, apo A-II, and apo C-III associated specifically with SR-BI–expressing cells with high affinity and competed for the binding of HDL (Xu et al. 1997). SR-BI is fatty acylated, a property shared with other proteins that concentrate in caveolae. SR-BI colocalized with caveolin 1 (Babitt et al. 1997). In Chinese hamster ovary cells stably transfected with murine SR-BI, overexpression of SR-BI promoted HDL-mediated cellular cholesterol efflux (Ji et al. 1997). In sum, SR-BI colocalizes with caveolae and facilitates both lipid influx and efflux.

Scavenger Receptors

Oxidatively modified LDL (oxLDL) is very different from unmodified LDL in composition, structure, and metabolism. Its content is higher in fatty acid and lysophosphatidylcholine as a result of the action of an LDL-associated phospholipase A_2. OxLDL is characterized as well by reactive aldehydes, reduced cholesterol content with a reduction in the number of reactive amino groups on apo B-100, an increase in oxysterols, and fragmentation of apo B-100. OxLDL or its fragments have been found in animal and human atheromatous lesions (Steinberg 1997). The differences in the structure of oxLDL may contribute to its cytotoxicity toward fibroblasts, SMCs, and endothelial cells, a cytotoxicity that may be relevant to its effects in the arterial wall (see also Chapter 6).

Monocytes/macrophages do not express LDL receptors. Rather, they contain a receptor that binds to and mediates the removal of modified lipoproteins (Krieger and Herz 1994). This receptor, which was originally identified as the acetyl LDL receptor, is now known as macrophage scavenger receptor A because of its broad ligand specificity. Early experiments showed that acetylated LDL is rapidly internalized by macrophages, so that cholesteryl ester–rich inclusions are produced in the cytoplasm (Goldstein et al. 1979). Other studies showed that the uptake of acetylated LDL by macrophages is mediated by a distinct class of scavenger receptors.

All known scavenger receptor ligands are negatively charged, although ligand charge alone does not ensure receptor recognition. Two scavenger receptor isoforms, SRA-I and SRA-II, are generated by the alternative splicing of mRNA encoded by one gene (Emi et al. 1993). Structural analysis based on predictive algorithms and biophysical methods has yielded models of these isoforms (Kodama et al. 1990; Rohrer et al. 1990). SRA-I is a homotrimeric, membrane-bound protein composed of monomers of 451–454 amino acid residues. The proposed structure (Figure 4.6) contains three extracellular C-terminal cysteine-rich domains connected to the transmembrane domain by a long, fibrous stalk. The stalk structure, composed of an alpha-helical coiled-coil and a collagen-like triple helix, has not previously been observed in an integral membrane protein. SRA-II is identical to the type I receptor except that the cysteine-rich domain is replaced by a six-residue C terminus (see Figure 4.6). Despite this truncation, the type II receptor mediates endocytosis of chemically modified LDL with high affinity and specificity, similar to the type I receptor (Rohrer et al. 1990). High-affinity, saturable endocytosis of acetylated LDL and oxLDL was observed in stable Chinese hamster ovary cell transfectants expressing high levels of either the type I or type II bovine scavenger receptor. This was succeeded by the formation of oil red O–staining lipid droplets reminiscent of those in macrophage foam cells (Freeman et al. 1991). This suggests that other macrophage-specific genes are not required for production of the foam cell phenotype. Scavenger receptor overexpression in mice increases hepatic parenchymal cell uptake of acetylated human LDL and produces a twofold increase in the clearance of ^{125}I-acetylated LDL (Wolle et al. 1995). Scavenger receptor expression suppressed the diet-induced rise in lipoproteins containing apo B, suggesting that hepatic overexpression of scavenger receptors may play a cardioprotective role in diet-induced hyperlipidemia.

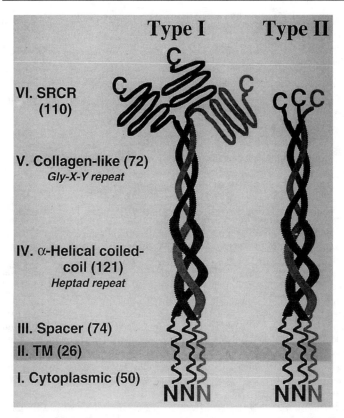

Figure 4.6. Models of the predicted quaternary structures of the type I and type II macrophage scavenger receptors. Here the coiled-coil domains IV and V are overwound to emphasize their triple helical structures. The number of amino acids is shown in parentheses. (From Krieger and Herz 1994; used with permission.)

Physiologically, the putative ligand for the scavenger receptor is oxidized lipoproteins, mainly LDL. Much of the supporting evidence was obtained in vitro, and there has always been some question about the relevance of oxidatively modified lipoproteins in human atherosclerosis. One study in LDL receptor–deficient mice (Palinski et al. 1995) correlated titers of autoantibody against epitopes of oxLDL with the severity of atherosclerosis. Another study in mice, however, showed that the clearance of oxLDL from blood occurs through a mechanism that is independent of SRA (Ling et al. 1997). Additional work on the mechanism by which modified lipoproteins are formed and catabolized in both normal and pathologic states is needed to clarify the role of scavenger receptors and of modified lipoproteins in atherogenesis.

Human monocytes/macrophages also contain a high-affinity, saturable specific binding site for VLDL from hypertriglyceridemic subjects (Gianturco et al. 1988). The site (or sites), which has been identified as two proteins of 200 and 235 kDa, binds to hypertriglyceridemic VLDL, trypsinized VLDL, and chylomicrons from normal subjects through a mechanism that is independent of LPL and apo E (Gianturco et al. 1994). It is not known whether the putative receptor belongs to the LDL receptor family.

REGULATION OF LIPID SYNTHESIS

Receptor-mediated uptake of lipoproteins by cells can increase cellular cholesterol content according to the number of lipoproteins endocytosed and the number of cholesterol molecules per lipoprotein particle. Transfer of cholesterol from cells to lipoproteins by spontaneous transfer will reduce the cellular cholesterol content. Through the release of sterol-sensitive transcription factors, these changes in cellular free cholesterol can indirectly alter several pathways that are connected to lipid and lipoprotein metabolism. Cells contain a group of cholesterol-sensitive transcription factors called sterol regulatory element–binding proteins (SREBPs). SREBPs found so far include several forms, designated SREBP-1a, SREBP-1b, and SREBP-1c, which differ in transcriptional activity and the transcription rate of the LDL receptor gene (Yokoyama et al. 1993). The release of the transcription factor occurs through tandem proteolytic cleavage of two sites in SREBPs. The first of the proteolytic steps, which takes place within the lumen of the endoplasmic reticulum, occurs when cells have been depleted of sterols. Proteolytic cleavage at the first site is abolished when cells are overloaded with sterol by incubation with LDL. Proteolytic cleavage at the second site is not directly regulated by sterols but requires previous cleavage at the first site.

Interestingly, transcription is also affected for a host of other genes of lipid metabolism (Figure 4.7). These include HMG-CoA reductase (Vallett et al. 1996), LDL receptor, HMG-CoA synthase, farnesyl diphosphate synthase (Spear et al. 1994; Ericsson et al. 1996), acetyl CoA carboxylase (Lopez et al. 1996), fatty acid synthase (Bennett et al. 1995; Magana and Osborne 1996), and glycerol-3-phosphate acyltransferase (Ericsson et al. 1997), which is the committing step in glycerol lipid synthesis. The coordinate regulation of so many genes associated with lipid metabolism is of great interest. A thorough understanding of the regulation of these and other genes by sterols will guide the design of improved pharmacologic agents for the management of lipid disorders and atherosclerosis.

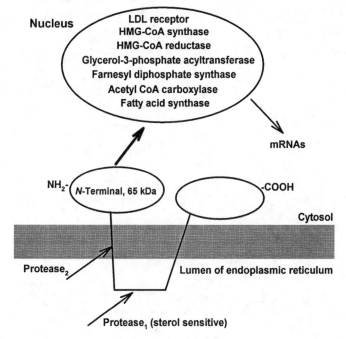

Figure 4.7. Regulation of gene transcription by sterols.

Suggested Reading

Acton S, Rigotti A, Landschulz KT, et al. Identification of scavenger receptor SR-BI as a high density lipoprotein receptor. Science 1996;271:518–520.

Brown MS, Goldstein JL. The SREBP pathway: regulation of cholesterol metabolism by proteolysis of a membrane-bound transcription factor (review). Cell 1997;89:331–340.

Cooper AD. Hepatic chylomicron remnants. J Lipid Res 1997;38:2173–2192.

Krieger M, Herz J. Structures and functions of multiligand lipoprotein receptors: macrophage scavenger receptors and LDL receptor-related protein (LRP). Annu Rev Biochem 1994;63:601–637.

Pownall HJ, Hickson-Bick D, Massey JB. Effects of hydrophobicity on turnover of plasma high density lipoproteins labeled with phosphatidylcholine ethers in the rat. J Lipid Res 1991;32:793–800.

Steinberg D. Oxidative modification of LDL and atherogenesis. Lewis A. Conner Memorial Lecture (review). Circulation 1997;95:1062–1071.

Wolle S, Via DP, Chan L, et al. Hepatic overexpression of bovine scavenger receptor type I in transgenic mice prevents diet-induced hyperbetalipoproteinemia. J Clin Invest 1995;96:260–272.

REFERENCES

Acton S et al. Science 1996;271:518–520.

Argraves KM et al. J Clin Invest 1997;100:2170–2181.

Babitt J et al. J Biol Chem 1997;272:13242–13249.

Bagdade JD et al. Eur J Clin Invest 1991;21:161–167.

Bamberger MJ, Lane MD. J Biol Chem 1988;263:11868–11878.

Bamberger MJ, Lane MD. Proc Natl Acad Sci U S A 1990;87:2390–2394.

Barter PJ et al. Atherosclerosis 1990;84:13–24.

Bennett MK et al. J Biol Chem 1995;270:25578–25583.

Boren J et al. J Biol Chem 1992;267:9858–9867.

Borhani DW et al. Proc Natl Acad Sci U S A 1997;94:12291–12296.

Brown MS, Goldstein JL. Curr Top Cell Regul 1985;26:3–15.

Brown MS, Goldstein JL. Cell 1997;89:331–340.

Castro GR, Fielding CJ. Biochemistry 1988;27:25–29.

Chen SH et al. Science 1987;238:363–366.

Choi SY, Cooper AD. J Biol Chem 1993;268:15804–15811.

Cistola DP et al. J Clin Invest 1991;87:1431–1441.

Cooper AD. J Lipid Res 1997;38:2173–2192.

Day JR et al. J Biol Chem 1994;269:9388–9391.

de Faria E et al. J Lipid Res 1996;37:197–209.

DeLoof H et al. J Lipid Res 1987;28:1455–1465.

Drayna DT et al. DNA 1987a;6:199–204.

Drayna D et al. Nature 1987b;327:632–634.

Du EZ et al. J Lipid Res 1996;37:1309–1315.

Emi M et al. J Biol Chem 1993;268:2120–2125.

Ericsson J et al. J Biol Chem 1996;271:24359–24364.

Ericsson J et al. J Biol Chem 1997;272:7298–7305.

Fielding CJ, Fielding PE. J Lipid Res 1995a;36:211–228.

Fielding PE, Fielding CJ. Biochemistry 1995b;34:14288–14292.

Fielding CJ, Fielding PE. J Lipid Res 1997;38:1503–1521.

Fisher EA et al. J Biol Chem 1997;272:20427–20434.

Foger B et al. J Biol Chem 1997;272:27393–27400.

Freeman M et al. Proc Natl Acad Sci U S A 1991;88:4931–4935.

Gianturco SH et al. J Clin Invest 1988;82:1633–1643.

Gianturco SH et al. J Lipid Res 1994;35:1674–1687.

Glass C et al. Proc Natl Acad Sci U S A 1983;80:5435–5439.

Goldstein JL et al. Proc Natl Acad Sci U S A 1979;76:333–337.

Gordon DA et al. J Biol Chem 1996;271:33047–33053.

Hailman E et al. J Biol Chem 1996;271:12172–12178.

Huuskonen J et al. Biochim Biophys Acta 1996;1303:207–214.

Ingram MF, Shelness GS. J Lipid Res 1996;37:2202–2214.

Jarnagin AS et al. Proc Natl Acad Sci U S A 1987;84:1854–1857.

Jauhiainen M et al. J Biol Chem 1993;268:4032–4036.

Ji Y et al. J Biol Chem 1997;272:20982–20985.

Jingami H, Yamamoto T. Curr Opin Lipidol 1995;6:104–108.

Khoo JC et al. J Lipid Res 1995;36:593–600.

Kodama T et al. Nature 1990;343:531–535.

Koschinsky ML et al. Biochemistry 1990;29:640–644.

Kostner GM et al. Biochem J 1995;305 (pt 2):659–667.

Kozarsky KF et al. Nature 1997;387:414–417.

Krapp A et al. J Lipid Res 1996;37:926–936.

Krebs KE, Phillips MC. Biochim Biophys Acta 1983;754:227–230.

Krieger M, Herz J. Annu Rev Biochem 1994;63:601–637.

Lagrost L et al. Arterioscler Thromb Vasc Biol 1995;15:1388–1396.

Lagrost L et al. Curr Opin Lipidol 1998;9:203–209.

Ling W et al. J Clin Invest 1997;100:244–252.

Lopez JM et al. Proc Natl Acad Sci U S A 1996;93:1049–1053.

Magana MM, Osborne TF. J Biol Chem 1996;271:32689–32694.

Mathur SN et al. J Lipid Res 1997;38:61–67.

Mayes PA. In: Murray RK et al., eds. Harper's biochemistry, ed. 23. Norwalk, CT: Appleton and Lange, 1993.

McGarry JD. Science 1992;258:766–770.

McKeone BJ et al. J Clin Invest 1993;91:1926–1933.

Moberly JB et al. Biochim Biophys Acta 1990;1042:70–80.

Morton RE. J Lipid Res 1986;27:523–529.

Palinski W et al. Arterioscler Thromb Vasc Biol 1995;15:1569–1576.

Patsch JR et al. Proc Natl Acad Sci U S A 1978;75:4519–4523.

Peitsch MC, Boguski MS. New Biol 1990;2:197–206.

Pevsner J et al. Science 1988;241:336–339.

Phillips MC et al. Biochim Biophys Acta 1987;906:223–276.

Ponsin G et al. J Clin Invest 1986;77:559–567.

Pownall HJ. J Lipid Res 1994;35:2105–2113.

Pownall HJ et al. FEBS Lett 1983;159:17–23.

Pownall HJ et al. In: Gotto AM Jr, ed. Plasma lipoproteins. New comprehensive biochemistry, vol. 14. Amsterdam: Elsevier, 1987:95–127.

Pownall HJ et al. J Lipid Res 1991;32:793–800.

Pownall HJ et al. In: Pownall HJ, Spector AS, eds. Omega-3 fatty acids in nutrition, vascular biology and medicine. Dallas: American Heart Association, 1995:64–78.

Rao R et al. Biochemistry 1997;36:3645–3653.

Reaven GM et al. Diabetes 1988;37:1020–1024.

Rohrer L et al. Nature 1990;343:570–572.

Segrest JP, Albers JJ, eds. Plasma lipoproteins. Part A: preparation, structure, and molecular biology. Methods Enzymol 1986a;128.

Segrest JP, Albers JJ, eds. Plasma lipoproteins. Part B: characterization, cell biology, and metabolism. Methods Enzymol 1986b;129.

Shen BW et al. Proc Natl Acad Sci U S A 1977;74:837–841.

Small DM. The physical chemistry of lipids: from alkanes to phospholipids. Handbook of lipid research, vol. 4. New York: Plenum Press, 1986:89–96.

Smith LC et al. In: Pifat G, Herak JN, eds. Supramolecular structure and function. New York: Plenum Press, 1983:205–244.

Spear DH et al. J Biol Chem 1994;269:25212–25218.

Steinberg D. Atherosclerosis 1997;131(suppl):S5–S7.

Strickland DK et al. J Biol Chem 1990;265:17401–17404.

Swenson TL et al. J Biol Chem 1988;263:5150–5157.

Tall AR. Annu Rev Biochem 1995;64:235–257.

Tall AR et al. J Biol Chem 1983;258:2174–2180.

Tall AR et al. J Biol Chem 1984;259:9587–9594.

Tollefson JH et al. J Lipid Res 1988;29:1593–1602.

Vallett SM et al. J Biol Chem 1996;271:12247–12253.

Vance DE. In: Vance DE, Vance JE, eds. Biochemistry of lipids and membranes. Menlo Park, CA: Benjamin/Cummings, 1985:242–270.

Vance JE, Vance DE. Can J Biochem Cell Biol 1985;63:870–881.

Vance JE, Vance DE. J Biol Chem 1986;261:4486–4491.

Weisgraber KH. Ann N Y Acad Sci 1990;598:37–48.

Wilson C et al. Science 1991;252:1817–1822.

Wolle S et al. J Clin Invest 1995;96:260–272.

Wyne KL et al. Arterioscler Thromb Vasc Biol 1996;16:407–415.

Xu S et al. J Lipid Res 1997;38:1289–1298.

Yamamoto T et al. Cell 1984;39:27–38.

Yang CY et al. Nature 1986;323:738–742.

Yokoyama C et al. Cell 1993;75:187–197.

Atherosclerosis

By striking near the root of the disorder in many patients, lipid lowering may overcome the daunting maze of individual cytokines and growth factors, and re-establish a homoeostatic balance within atheromatous lesions.
—Peter Libby (1996)

References for Section II (Chapters 5–10) begin on page 151.

Chapter 5

Atherosclerosis: Overview and Histologic Classification of Lesions

In the past several years, intensified clinicopathologic investigations, the development of improved animal models, and studies at the level of cell and molecular biology have enabled immense advances in our understanding of how atherosclerosis develops and leads to clinical sequelae such as angina pectoris, MI, sudden cardiac death, stroke, and the gangrene of PVD. Not long ago, atherosclerosis was viewed as a steadily progressive process in which fairly inert components relentlessly collected until an artery was (or was not) occluded. Now it is known that most clinical events arise from lesions causing only mild to moderate angiographic stenosis (typically from plaque rupture leading to thrombosis), and that lesion progression can be slowed, stopped, or even regressed. The endothelium, long considered merely a semipermeable membrane, is now viewed as the largest endocrine organ, with endocrine, autocrine, and paracrine effects responsible for several regulatory and antiatherosclerotic functions (Vogel 1997). It is recognized that a variety of cell types actively exchange messages that regulate functions critical to lesion initiation and progression and the development of clinical events (Libby 1996). Indeed, the AHA's dedicated journal on vascular diseases, *Arteriosclerosis,* became *Arteriosclerosis and Thrombosis* in 1991 and then *Arteriosclerosis, Thrombosis, and Vascular Biology* in 1995, illustrating the shift in thinking during this decade.

Nevertheless, we are at only the beginning of a new paradigm of mechanisms of atherosclerosis initiation and progression. Many ideas remain hypothetical, and much evidence is indirect and circumstantial. The disease is extremely complex, and whether clinical manifestations develop depends on a variety of factors. It has been remarked that there may be as many factors as there are scientists working on the question (Kruth 1997). Libby (1996) has written that, on the one hand, the many factors described offer multiple targets for novel interventions, but on the other hand, the multiplicity and redundancy of the signaling pathways suggest a complexity that may stymie a coherent therapeutic approach. He notes that interventions targeting a single growth factor or cytokine may be insufficient to modify the evolution of a lesion. But he also concludes, as highlighted in the epigraph of this section, that lowering lipid concentrations may modify sufficient pathways to strike at the root of the problem. Evidence is overwhelming that elevations in plasma cholesterol and LDL-C contribute to the formation of atherosclerosis. During that development, lipids derived from circulating lipoproteins accumulate in the artery wall, and in most animal models atherosclerosis can be induced by a high-fat or high-cholesterol diet. Although additional interventional strategies will emerge as the basic mechanisms of atherosclerosis are further elucidated, data have already demonstrated the major benefit of cholesterol lowering in the prevention and treatment of CHD.

Although this short manual cannot encompass the full spectrum of proposed mechanisms and must include simplifications, it provides a working model of the development and progression of atherosclerosis through a selection of key concepts.

LEADING HYPOTHESIS

In the prevalent view, atherosclerosis is considered an immune/inflammatory, or healing, response of the intima to injury (Davies 1998; Fuster et al. 1992). The current hypothesis of response to injury, synthesized by Ross, was first formally advanced in 1973 and has been continually updated (Ross and Glomset 1973, 1976; Ross 1993, 1998). It integrates the encrustation hypothesis of Rokitansky (1855) and the lipid insudation hypothesis of Virchow (1856). Rokitansky suggested fibrin deposition and secondary lipid accumulation as a mechanism of atherogenesis, and he included the concept that subclinical thrombi contribute to lesion progression. Virchow viewed lipid deposition as the major mechanism. He proposed that some form of injury to the artery wall associated with an inflammatory response gave rise to what was then considered a degenerative lesion (Ross 1998). Before the Ross elaboration, the response-to-injury idea was extended by many investigators, among them Anitschkov, Duguid, French, and Mustard and Packham (Ross and Glomset 1976).

The current response-to-injury hypothesis assigns a primary role to endothelial injury. Earlier models of traumatic denudation have been replaced by concepts of more subtle forms of damage in which early injury is generally characterized by modulation of endothelial cell function without loss of cells (Buja 1995). As is discussed in Chapter 6, the earliest lesion appears to develop under endothelium that is structurally intact, with the increased adherence of circulating monocytes to the endothelium representing a very early response to hypercholesterolemia.

Entry of the adherent monocytes into the subendothelial space leads to foam cell formation. Other factors that may contribute to lesion initiation or progression include hypertension, cigarette smoking, immunologic mechanisms, and viral injury (Buja 1995). The chronic inflammatory condition may eventually be converted to an acute clinical event by plaque rupture that leads to thrombosis (Fuster et al. 1992). Roles for immunologic mediators are highlighted in Chapter 9.

GENETIC FACTORS

Hegele (1997) has provided a cogent review of considerations in the dissection of the genetic components of atherosclerosis. Genetic factors determine the limits under which the disease develops, whereas environmental factors position the individual's risk within those limits.

Several hundred candidate genes for the study of the genetic component of atherosclerosis have been listed, but whereas in some families or isolated groups the effect of a single gene on susceptibility to atherosclerosis may be great (e.g., familial hypercholesterolemia from mutations in the gene encoding the LDL receptor), given candidate genes have small effects in whole populations. Identification of genetic components can also be confounded by the ability of a gene to manifest itself in more than one way (pleiotropy) and the interaction of genes at different loci (epistasis, which may result in the lack of expression or masking of a hereditary character). Nevertheless, Hegele considers that genetic information might be useful in the clinical recognition of individuals susceptible to atherosclerosis, particularly if as yet undiscovered candidate genes are found to be important disease determinants. Hegele also considers that prediction of onset of clinical manifestations in an individual will not be possible because of the confounding influence of other factors, for example, lifestyle factors, nonlinear interactions between genes and environment, and perhaps even biologic chaos.

Sing et al. (1995) have conceptualized environmental factors as having a time-line impact on the progression of atherosclerosis as either chronic adverse influences (e.g., a diet customarily high in fat) or acute bursts of intense environmental influences (e.g., a particularly bad dietary period). Genetic factors may act in the atherosclerotic process (1) at baseline level of risk (e.g., familial hypercholesterolemia), (2) during lesion progression (e.g., individuals resistant to environmental factors), (3) in the capacity of the artery wall to recover after acute stress, and (4) in the threshold for clinical manifestations (e.g., development of collateral vessels or the ability of tissue to withstand oxygen deprivation).

PATHOLOGY

Although classified as a systemic disorder, atherosclerosis occurs at specific, so-called lesion-prone sites, principally in the elastic arteries (aorta, carotid, and iliac) and some of the large and medium-sized muscular arteries (coronary and popliteal) (Woolf and Davies 1992; Schwartz et al. 1993; DeBakey et al. 1985; Vallabhajosula and Fuster 1997) (Figure 5.1). Most heavily involved are the coronary arteries, the popliteal arteries, the descending thoracic aorta, the internal carotid arteries, and the vessels of the circle of Willis. Among the major coronary vessels, the left anterior descending (LAD) artery has been described as most commonly involved by atherosclerosis at necropsy in patients who had symptomatic CHD (58% of arteries involved in patients aged 41–89 years), followed by the right (33%) and left (25%) circumflex arteries, with the left main coronary artery least frequently involved (16%) (Waller 1989). The disease dominance of the LAD artery persists irrespective of patient age at death, and the artery's sobriquets include "the widowmaker artery" and "the PTCA artery" (Waller et al. 1992b).

Involvement of the intima by atherosclerosis is focal rather than diffuse, producing individual lesions often called plaques. For an individual case the severity of atherosclerosis in one artery does not predict the severity in another, but in population studies the average predilection to advanced lesions in one artery is similar to that in other arteries (Strong 1992). The latter finding is consistent with environmental or lifestyle factors as the key determinant of disease prevalence in a population.

Atherosclerosis has been documented in Egyptian mummies dating from as early as the 15th century BC (Ross 1998). In the so-called Iceman, an approximately 5,300-year-old, completely preserved corpse found in glacial ice in the South Tyrol, computed tomographic studies have demonstrated focal calcification in the neck consistent with carotid calcification (W. A. Murphy, Jr., personal communication, March 1998).

Atherosclerosis is sometimes indiscriminately called "arteriosclerosis," but it may be considered a subset of that disease group, which also includes Mönckeberg's arteriosclerosis (medial calcific sclerosis) and arteriolosclerosis. About 2,000 years ago, Celsius gave "atheroma" the meaning of fatty tumor (the etymology traceable to the Greek *athēra*, "gruel"). "Atheromatosis" appeared in 1815, used by Hodgson. "Arteriosclerosis" was defined by Lobstein, from Strasbourg, in 1833 (via Latin from Greek *sklēros*, "hard"). It was Marchand, from Leipzig, who combined the concepts of a fatty lesion and hardening to propose "atherosclerosis" in 1904 (Cottet and Lenoir 1992).

CHD in this manual refers to atherosclerotic CHD, both symptomatic and asymptomatic. Atherosclerotic disease is by far the most common cause of coronary artery luminal narrowing and related clinical events, but multiple nonatherosclerotic causes of such narrowing also exist (e.g., congenital anomalies, emboli, dissection, spasm, trauma, and arteritis). Approximately 4–7% of all patients with acute MI do not have atherosclerotic CHD as demonstrated by angiography, necropsy, or both (Waller 1998).

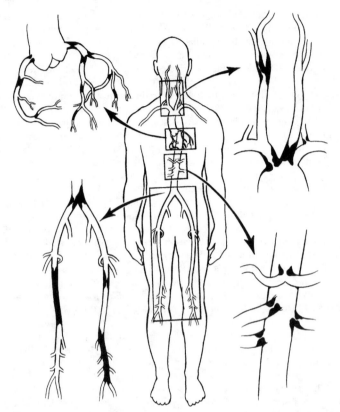

Figure 5.1. Predominant anatomic locations of atherosclerotic occlusive disease: coronary arteries (*top left*), major branches of the aortic arch (*top right*), major visceral branches of the aorta (*bottom right*), and major branches of the terminal aorta (*bottom left*), as developed by DeBakey et al. (1985) by review of the records of 13,827 patients admitted to The Methodist Hospital in Houston from 1948 to 1983. (Reprinted with permission from DeBakey and Gotto, *The New Living Heart,* 1997.)

The Normal Intima

The artery wall comprises three concentric layers: an inner (luminal) layer, the tunica intima, which includes the endothelial surface; a middle layer, the tunica media; and an outer (external) layer, the tunica adventitia (Waller et al. 1992a). Atherosclerosis is a primarily intimal disease.

The intima consists of the vascular endothelium and a thin layer of collagen and elastin fibers that anchor it to the internal elastic lamina

(Waller et al. 1992a); endothelial cells and SMCs are the principal cellular components of human intima (Stary et al. 1992). The internal elastic lamina is generally considered part of the media and may not be well defined in some geometric transition areas of vessels such as bifurcations, branch vessels, and curvatures (Stary et al. 1992).

Amounts of smooth muscle and fibroelastic tissue in the intima are a function of age (Waller et al. 1992b). After birth, the intima, which is not well developed in fetal coronary arteries, progressively thickens, so that it is as thick as the media by late adolescence and thicker than the media after adolescence. It is typically during middle age that the intima may become markedly thickened by atherosclerosis. Often in old age the coronary arteries are tortuous and have an increased luminal diameter, thinned media, and increased calcification.

Watson and Demer (1996) provided evidence to support the hypothesis that arterial calcification in arteriosclerosis is not merely a passive, degenerative process, but also an active, regulated process similar to organized bone formation. They discovered in bovine aortas a subpopulation of artery wall cells, very similar to osteoblasts in many respects, that were capable of producing hydroxyapatite mineral in vitro (Bostrom et al. 1993; Watson et al. 1994). TGF-β and the oxidized sterol 25-hydroxycholesterol, one of the oxidized lipids found in atherosclerotic lesions, were found to be potent enhancers of mineralization by these cells, named calcifying vascular cells. A role for lipids in the mineralization process may help explain why arterial calcification is almost exclusively associated with atherosclerosis. (Calcification in coronary arteries in the elderly does not correlate with severity of atherosclerotic disease, however [Waller et al. 1992b].) The Demer group has also provided results suggesting that specific oxidized lipids may be the common factors in the pathogenesis of vascular calcification and osteoporotic loss of bone mineral, which frequently occur together (Parhami and Demer 1997; Parhami et al. 1997).

The intima is not of uniform thickness. Adaptive increases in thickness occur (Figure 5.2), and are classified as eccentric (relatively abrupt and focal increases associated with vessel branches and orifices) or diffuse (spread-out, often circumferential patterns not clearly related to specific geometric configurations of arteries) (Stary et al. 1992). These adaptive increases, which do not obstruct the lumen, correspond to regions of altered mechanical stress, namely, reduced (Stary et al. 1992) or variable (O'Rourke 1995) wall shear stress, increased wall tensile stress, or both. Thus, the intima may thicken to reduce lumen diameter in an effort to increase flow velocity. Lesions of atherosclerosis form first in some regions with adaptive intimal thickening but are not confined to these regions. Under the influence of atherogenic stimuli, it is at these so-called atherosclerosis-prone locations that lesions form earlier and more rapidly than elsewhere and that symptomatic lesions tend to occur (Stary et al. 1992). Mechanical forces play a role throughout the development of atherosclerosis, including in plaque progression and rupture (Glagov et al. 1995b, 1997; Gibbons and Dzau 1994; Gibson et al. 1993).

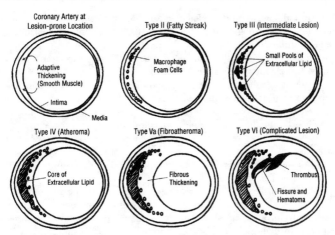

Figure 5.2. Drawings of cross sections of the identical, most proximal part of six LAD coronary arteries. The morphologic features of the intima range from adaptive intimal thickening always present in this lesion-prone location to a type VI lesion with thrombosis in advanced atherosclerotic disease. (Adapted from Ambrose and Weinrauch 1996. Copyright 1996, American Medical Association. The Ambrose and Weinrauch figure was adapted from Stary et al. 1995.)

American Heart Association
Histologic Classification of Lesions

Whereas debate surrounds the exact mechanisms of atherosclerosis, most of the morphologic facts about the disease are well established. Any atherogenesis framework must be related to the natural history, topography, and major established risk factors of the disease (Strong 1992). The AHA has provided a practical classification of human atherosclerotic lesions based on their histologic composition and structure (presented in a series of three papers on the normal arterial intima, the fatty streak and intermediate lesions, and advanced lesions: Stary et al. 1992, 1994, 1995). Lesion types I–III are silent precursors of advanced lesions (types IV–VI) (see Figure 5.2). It is the advanced lesions that give rise to clinical sequelae. An evolutionary sequence is implicit in the AHA categories (Davies 1996a).

In the first three decades of life, lesion composition is predominantly lipidic and relatively predictable, but typically after that time composition becomes unpredictable (Fuster et al. 1992). Formation of atherosclerotic lesions covering the intima in the aorta and coronary arteries accelerates at about ages 25–30 in men and 40–45 in women according to autopsy examinations in western populations (Kagan and Uemura 1976).

Atherosclerosis develops at different rates in populations according to environmental factors, including lifestyle (Strong 1992). Nearly all the major risk factors for CHD (e.g., age, male sex, hypercholesterolemia, hypertension, smoking, and diabetes mellitus) are related to both the prevalence and extent of lesions at autopsy (Solberg and Strong 1983; Reed et al. 1989; Robertson and Strong 1968; Pathobiological Determinants of Atherosclerosis in Youth [PDAY] Research Group 1990, 1993), and average disease extent in a population can change in a relatively short period (Newman et al. 1988). In all geographic populations, the mean number of coronary plaques at autopsy in death from all causes predicts the incidence of ischemic heart disease (Davies 1998). Some risk factors apparently affect one lesion type or arterial segment more than another (Strong 1992). Known risk factors do not account for nearly all the variability in lesions, however, leaving room for other influencing variables (Strong 1992).

Precursor Lesions

Evidence is compelling that lipid accumulation in the intima elicits specific cell reactions and is the fundamental event in the initiation of lesions. As lipid accumulation continues, lesion size and complexity increase. The morphologic features of the precursor lesions and the time in life at which each lesion type tends to be found provide strong presumptive evidence that types I, II, and III are successive steps in the development of atherosclerosis. It may be that each type stabilizes temporarily or permanently and that progression to the next type requires an additional stimulus (Stary et al. 1994).

Type I Lesions. The first microscopically and chemically detectable lipid deposits in the intima and the cell reactions associated with such deposits form type I lesions, which may not be visible to the unaided eye. These lesions appear to be most frequent in infants and children, although they are also found in adults, particularly in lesion-resistant locations of arteries and in individuals without advanced lesions (Stary et al. 1994).

Type II Lesions, Including Fatty Streaks. Type II lesions contain macrophage foam cells as their primary component, stratified in adjacent layers rather than being present as only isolated groups of a few cells. Intimal SMCs now also contain lipid droplets, and T lymphocytes and isolated mast cells have been identified. Most of the lipid in the lesion is intracellular. Fatty streaks, which on gross inspection may be visible as yellow-colored streaks, patches, or spots on the intimal surface, are among type II lesions. Some type II lesions colocate with adaptive intimal thickenings (described earlier) in predictable locations and are deemed progression prone, or type IIa, whereas IIb indicates progression-resistant lesions (Stary et al. 1994).

Type II lesions typically erupt in the coronary arteries around puberty (Stary et al. 1994). It has not been determined what factors elicit the dramatic increase in these lesions at that time, although in adolescents and young adults plasma cholesterol concentrations were found to be higher when there were many rather than few type II lesions (Newman et al. 1987). Not all fatty streaks progress (Strong 1992; Davies and Woolf 1993).

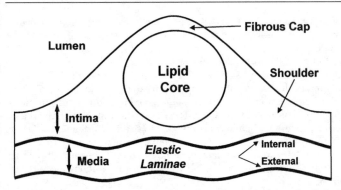

Figure 5.3. Diagrammatic representation of an advanced atherosclerotic lesion without surface disruption, hemorrhage, or thrombosis. (Modified from Libby et al. 1997; used with permission.)

Type III Lesions. Also known as intermediate lesions, transitional lesions, or preatheromas, type III lesions form a morphologic and chemical bridge between type II lesions and atheromas. Microscopically visible extracellular lipid droplets and particles are characteristic, and small pools of lipid form among the layers of SMCs of the generally colocalized adaptive intimal thickening. Type III lesions and the first atheroma-type lesions tend to be found in young adults and at the same vessel locations as type IIa lesions (Stary et al. 1994).

Advanced Lesions

The advanced lesions of atherosclerosis generally contain extracellular lipid deposits of an extent to disrupt and deform the intima, and in very advanced stages the deposits may affect the media and adventitia. Thrombotic mechanisms of progression become predominant in many lesions (Stary et al. 1994). It is the advanced lesions that can give rise to ischemic events. They may or may not narrow the arterial lumen and may or may not be visible by angiography, but lack of arterial narrowing does not preclude clinical significance because complications may develop suddenly (Stary et al. 1995). Major components of an uncomplicated advanced lesion are diagramed in Figure 5.3.

Type IV Lesions. A lipid core characterizes type IV lesions, also known as atheromas. Further lipid deposition and the confluence of the isolated pools of extracellular lipid seen in type III lesions appear to give rise to the dense accumulation of extracellular lipid. Macrophages and SMCs (with and without lipid droplet inclusions), and in some cases lymphocytes and mast cells, are found between the lipid core and the endothelial surface; an increase in fibrous tissue is not a feature. Containing macrophage foam cells, proteoglycans, minimal collagen, and only isolated SMCs, this area may be susceptible to fissure formation (Stary et al. 1995). Type IV lesions, when they first appear in younger people (20s and upward), occur in the same locations as adaptive intimal thickening of the eccentric type (Stary et al. 1995).

Type V Lesions. The formation of prominent new fibrous connective tissue distinguishes type V lesions. In type Va, sometimes called fibroatheroma, the lipid core is also present; in type Vb, the lipid core and other parts of the lesion are calcified; in type Vc, a lipid core is absent and lipid in general is minimal. With type V lesions, arteries are variously narrowed, generally more than with type IV lesions. Type V, like type IV, lesions may develop fissures, hematoma, or thrombus, to become type VI (Stary et al. 1995).

The type Vc lesion, with its uniform structure, is one of two types of plaque that do not fit with the concept of healing after disruption of lipid-rich lesions (Davies 1996a). The other is the so-called gelatinous lesion: a soft, brown, raised intimal lesion composed of fibrinogen-rich edematous fluid. Fibrinogen is found in all types of atherosclerotic plaque; like LDL, it passes freely into the intima. The SMC proliferation in type Vc lesions could arise from stimulation by fibrinogen alone rather than by both LDL and fibrinogen. When the conversion of fibrinogen to fibrin exceeds the removal of fibrin by plasminogen, or when plasminogen activation is deficient, SMC proliferation may ensue (Davies 1996a).

Type VI Lesions. Type VI lesions—or complicated lesions, representing complicated type IV and V lesions—may be subdivided by superimposed features: type VIa, disruption of the surface; type VIb, hematoma or hemorrhage; and type VIc, thrombosis (type VIabc indicates the presence of all three features). The morbidity and mortality of atherosclerosis largely arise from these complications (Stary et al. 1995). Advanced lesions containing thrombi or the remnants of thrombi are frequent from the fourth decade of life on (Stary et al. 1995).

Suggested Reading

Fuster V, Badimon L, Badimon JJ, Chesebro JH. The pathogenesis of coronary artery disease and the acute coronary syndromes. N Engl J Med 1992;326: 242–250.

Hegele RA. Candidate genes, small effects, and the prediction of atherosclerosis (review). Crit Rev Clin Lab Sci 1997;34:343–367.

Ross R. Factors influencing atherogenesis. In: Alexander RW, Schlant RC, Fuster V, eds. Hurst's the heart arteries and veins, 9th ed., vol. 1. New York: McGraw-Hill, 1998:1139–1159.

Stary HC, Blankenhorn DH, Chandler AB, et al. A definition of the intima of human arteries and of its atherosclerosis-prone regions. Circulation 1992; 85:391–405.

Stary HC, Chandler AB, Dinsmore RE, et al. A definition of advanced types of atherosclerotic lesions and a histological classification of atherosclerosis.

A report from the Committee on Vascular Lesions of the Council on Arteriosclerosis, American Heart Association. Circulation 1995;92:1355–1374.

Stary HC, Chandler AB, Glagov S, et al. A definition of initial, fatty streak, and intermediate lesions of atherosclerosis. A report from the Committee on Vascular Lesions of the Council on Arteriosclerosis, American Heart Association. Arterioscler Thromb 1994;14:840–856.

Strong JP. Atherosclerotic lesions: natural history, risk factors, and topography. Arch Pathol Lab Med 1992;116:1268–1275.

Waller BF, Orr CM, Slack JD, et al. Anatomy, histology, and pathology of coronary arteries: a review relevant to new interventional and imaging techniques—part I. Clin Cardiol 1992;15:451–457.

Waller BF, Orr CM, Slack JD, et al. Anatomy, histology, and pathology of coronary arteries: a review relevant to new interventional and imaging techniques—part II. Clin Cardiol 1992;15:535–540.

Chapter 6

Evolution of Lesions

The hallmark of atherosclerosis is the accumulation of cholesterol in the artery wall, and oxidation or other modifications of LDL particles appear to be important events in atherogenesis. A sea change has occurred in our understanding of how atherosclerotic disease leads to acute clinical events. The unexpected finding that most events arise from angiographically mild or moderate lesions that are unstable and prone to rupture (see also Chapter 7) has led to the concept of using lesion stabilization to reduce the risk for disability and death (see Chapter 10).

ENDOTHELIAL INJURY

Endothelial function is critical to maintaining blood flow and vascular integrity, and healthy endothelium tends to favor vasodilation, antithrombosis, fibrinolysis, and monocyte disadhesion (Buja 1995; Vogel 1997). Mechanisms of gene activation in the endothelium's expression of humoral mediators are under active investigation (Buja 1995). Among those mediators are cytokines (which are multipotent intercellular mediators), growth factors, and vasodilatory factors. The best characterized and most powerful of the last category is endothelium-derived relaxing factor (EDRF), which is believed to be nitric oxide (Vanhoutte 1997).

In certain parts of the arterial tree, chronic minimal endothelial injury can result in dysfunctional endothelium characterized by increased uptake of LDL and monocyte recruitment into the vessel wall, which are both pivotal initiating events in atherosclerosis (Fernández-Ortiz and Fuster 1996). Systemic factors that can induce such injury include hypercholesterolemia, especially minimally modified LDL (see later), and active and passive cigarette smoking, which may lead to endothelial dysfunction through an increased production of superoxide radicals by the endothelium, resulting in deactivation of EDRF/nitric oxide (Plotnick et al. 1997; Ohara et al. 1993; Shiode et al. 1996) as well as enhancement of lipoprotein oxidation (Graham et al. 1993). Abnormal vasoconstriction is now increasingly recognized as one of the earliest manifestations of endothelial dysfunction. Also, lysolecithin, which is formed by peroxidation of LDL particles, may play a role in the development of abnormal arterial vasomotion (Mangin et al.

1993; Fernández-Ortiz and Fuster 1996). Other major risk factors for CHD are among additional nonlocal factors (Table 6.1) that have been associated with endothelial dysfunction (Fernández-Ortiz and Fuster 1996; Vogel 1997; Vita et al. 1990; Seiler et al. 1993; Celermajer et al. 1994; Baron 1996). Atherosclerosis resembles chronic inflammation in several regards, and it is now recognized that cellular components of the immune system are involved in its genesis, as is discussed in Chapter 9.

Local factors also play a role in atherogenesis, because, as noted in Chapter 5, lesions develop preferentially at specific sites, for example, where arteries are poorly supported, subject to repetitive bending, dilated, or, when relatively narrow, subject to rapid and variable blood flow (O'Rourke 1995). Lesion-prone sites include sites near vessel branches and bifurcations as well as regions of arterial narrowing and curvature (Davies 1997b). Not only fluid shear stress but also transmural pressure and pulsatile stretch are important mechanical factors in the development of disease (Luscher 1994). Transmission of the shear stress signal throughout vascular cells leads to changes in structure, metabolism, and gene expression (Papadaki and Eskin 1997). One effect of morphologic changes in endothelial cells may be to increase endothelial permeability (Asakura and Karino 1990).

MONOCYTE MIGRATION

The initial lesion of atherosclerosis develops when leukocytes, specifically monocytes, cross the endothelial barrier to accumulate in the intima. The first readily discernible morphologic change is monocyte adhesion to a usually intact but activated endothelial surface (Ross 1993; Faggiotto et al. 1984). After migration into the intima, monocytes are converted into

Table 6.1. SELECTED FACTORS ASSOCIATED WITH ENDOTHELIAL DYSFUNCTION/INJURY

Hypercholesterolemia
Minimally modified or oxidized LDLs
Active and passive cigarette smoking
Hypertension
High-fat diet
Physical inactivity
Advanced glycosylated end-products in diabetes mellitus
Obesity/insulin resistance
Increasing age
Male sex
Family history of premature CHD
Circulating vasoactive amines
Immunocomplexes
Certain viral infections

macrophages, which normally are not a component of the artery wall. Macrophages contribute to the formation of fatty streaks (see Chapter 5) by imbibing large amounts of lipid to become foam cells, so-called because of their foamy cytoplasm (Davies 1998; Faruqi and DiCorleto 1993). In addition to forming a morphologic basis for foam cells, emigrated monocytes can release cytotoxic substances (e.g., hydrolytic enzymes and reactive oxygen metabolites) as well as cytokines (e.g., TNF-α), growth factors, and procoagulant substances (including tissue factor) that can lead to far-reaching metabolic and functional changes, including potential contributions to the proliferative stage of atherosclerosis development, vascular remodeling, and plaque destabilization (Lehr and Messmer 1995; Ross 1993; Raines et al. 1996; Libby 1995; Barath et al. 1990; Dollery et al. 1995; Annex et al. 1995).

Monocytes are recruited to an area of dysfunctional vascular endothelium through complex changes, such as changes in vascular permeability and alterations in expression of endothelial cell adhesion receptors, coordinated by a variety of inflammatory mediators (Jones et al. 1995) (Figure 6.1). The presence of minimally modified LDL is believed to be important to monocyte recruitment (see later). Migration of leukocytes through the vascular endothelium is a multistep process of initial contact, rolling, activation, firm adhesion, and transmigration (Jones et al. 1995; Ley 1996) (Figure 6.2). Rolling of leukocytes refers to their movement along the vessel wall at reduced velocity compared with that of other blood cells (Ley et al. 1995). Activation of a leukocyte entails effects on its adhesion, mobility, surface projections, and deformability, among other qualities (Zweifach 1995). Abnormal generalized circulatory cell activation can be found associated with risk factors for atherosclerosis even before signs of overt disease are seen (Schmid-Schönbein et al. 1997).

Activated endothelium expresses several proteins on its surface that increase its "stickiness" to blood-borne cells. Among these surface adhesion molecules are selectins, integrins, and members of the immunoglobulin superfamily (such as ICAMs and VCAMs), which are important in immunology and in atherosclerosis (Schmid-Schönbein et al. 1997). Cell adhesion molecules that mediate leukocyte rolling include E-, L-, and P-selectins and α_4 integrins. Those that mediate strong and stable adhesion include β_1 and β_2 integrins, ICAMs, and VCAM-1; β_1 and β_2 integrins and platelet–endothelial cell adhesion molecule 1 are known to be involved in transmigration (Ley 1996). The concentration of soluble ICAM-1 has been found to be elevated in the serum of patients with ischemic heart disease (Morisaki et al. 1997), and E-selectin gene polymorphisms have been associated with accelerated atherosclerosis in young patients (Wenzel et al. 1996, 1997).

In addition, a variety of stimulators (e.g., hypercholesterolemia, modified LDL, viruses, IL-1, TNF-α, reactive oxygen species) and inhibitors (e.g., glucocorticoids, IL-4, IL-8) of leukocyte adhesion to the endothelium have been described, and there is a search for clinically useful

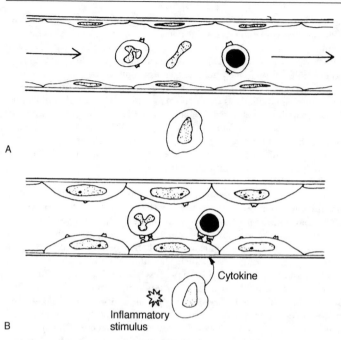

A

B

Figure 6.1. Schematic representation of events during inflammation leading to entry of leukocytes into the intima. **A.** Leukocytes pass through the lumen over a healthy endothelium. **B.** A resident extravascular cell recognizes an inflammatory stimulant and produces a mediator that diffuses to the endothelium. This mediator, such as a cytokine, induces the endothelium to thicken and express cell surface adhesion receptors for which there are ligands on leukocytes. The leukocytes adhere to endothelium and then can emigrate. (Reprinted from Munro 1993, by permission of the publisher W B Saunders Company Limited, London.)

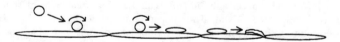

Figure 6.2. Monocytes cross the endothelial barrier to enter the intima through a multistep process of initial contact, rolling (i.e., movement at reduced velocity), firm adhesion, and transmigration. Initial contact and rolling are independent of monocyte activation and mediated largely by selectin-carbohydrate bonds. Firm adhesion and transmigration require monocyte activation and are mediated largely by integrins. (From Jones et al. 1995; used with permission.)

inhibitors of adhesion (Faruqi and DiCorleto 1993; de Prost and Hakim 1997; van de Stolpe and van der Saag 1996). OxLDL has both leukocyte chemoattractant and adhesion-promoting roles (Lehr and Messmer 1995). Hemodynamic forces such as fluid shear stress also play a role in the multistep process leading to leukocyte migration (Jones et al. 1995).

LIPID INSUDATION

The source of the cholesterol that accumulates in the artery wall is plasma lipoproteins, in particular LDL. Lipoproteins flux into and out of the artery wall as a normal function, LDL providing cholesterol and nutrients to peripheral cells. The normal entry of LDL into cells is regulated by the LDL (apo B/E) receptor, which was discovered by Brown and Goldstein, who became the 1985 Nobel Laureates in Medicine for their work in lipid metabolism. Synthesis of the LDL receptor is down-regulated when a cell has acquired sufficient cholesterol. For LDL, VLDL, and IDL, flux into the arterial wall is related directly to their plasma concentrations (Nordestgaard et al. 1992). It appears, however, that selective retention of lipoproteins rather than rate of transport across the endothelium may determine their concentration and perhaps susceptibility to modification in the artery wall (Beisiegel and St. Clair 1996). LDL enters atherosclerotic arteries faster than normal arteries, and its accumulation in the former is greater (Nordestgaard 1996). How lipoproteins come to be retained in the artery wall is not well understood, although proteoglycans are believed to play a major role (Beisiegel and St. Clair 1996). Ultimately, lipoproteins are taken up by macrophages, and the lipid-stuffed macrophages, as noted above, contribute to the formation of foam cells.

There is an apparent paradox, however, in that severe atherosclerosis develops in humans who lack functional LDL receptors in homozygous familial hypercholesterolemia. It was Brown and Goldstein (Goldstein et al. 1979) who first proposed that LDL modification is required for LDL uptake by macrophages. Oxidative modification has been the best studied of the candidate modifications of LDL enabling macrophage uptake, although others may also have importance (Steinberg 1997b). Acetylation and malondialdehyde conjugation, for example, also enable in vitro receptor-mediated macrophage uptake of LDL. Other processes that can contribute, by receptor or nonreceptor mechanisms, to macrophage uptake of LDL include phagocytosis and LDL self-aggregation, complex formation with proteoglycans, immune complex formation, and degradation by hydrolytic enzymes (Steinberg 1997b; Beisiegel and St. Clair 1996).

The oxidative modification of trapped LDL is believed to occur in two stages, the first taking place before (and promoting) monocyte recruitment and the second occurring after monocytes/macrophages contribute their great oxidative capacity (Berliner et al. 1995). OxLDL in fact comprises a spectrum of oxidatively modified particles that can differ not only structurally but functionally (Steinberg 1997b).

Minimally Modified Low-Density Lipoprotein

After LDL accumulates in the subendothelial space, its lipids can be mildly oxidized through the action of resident vascular cells, with little change in its apo B (Berliner et al. 1990, 1995; Steinberg and Witztum 1990; Diaz et al. 1997). This minimally modified LDL, which unlike unmodified LDL is proinflammatory, induces local vascular cells to produce factors (e.g., VCAM, monocyte chemotactic protein 1, and macrophage colony–stimulating factor) that stimulate recruitment of monocytes and differentiation of monocytes into macrophages in the intima (Diaz et al. 1997; Parhami et al. 1993; O'Brien et al. 1993; Nelken et al. 1991; Rosenfeld et al. 1992). Oxidized LDL may also exert direct effects on the recruitment of monocytes from the circulation (Steinberg 1997a; Quinn et al. 1988; Frostegard et al. 1991). Several major lines of evidence indicate that LDL oxidation occurs in vivo (Steinberg 1997b). LDL from subjects with risk factors such as CHD (Cominacini et al. 1993; Regnstrom et al. 1992), diabetes mellitus (Bucala et al. 1993), or smoking (Harats et al. 1989) has increased susceptibility to lipid peroxidation, as does small, dense LDL (Nigon et al. 1991) and LDL obtained from subjects in the postprandial state (McKeone et al. 1993) (see also Chapter 8). Nordestgaard (1996) proposed that some circulating LDL particles are already minimally modified and could be degraded in the intima in preference to unmodified LDL. Because the artery wall has a variety of mechanisms to prevent oxidation (e.g., suppression of lipoprotein oxidation by nitric oxide), a loss of balance between pro-oxidant and antioxidant forces is likely important in the formation of atherosclerosis (Beisiegel and St. Clair 1996).

Fully Oxidized Low-Density Lipoprotein

The second stage of LDL oxidation begins when the monocytes enter the intima and are converted into macrophages (Berliner et al. 1995). The monocytes/macrophages stimulate further peroxidation of LDL (Steinbrecher et al. 1984), including modification of the protein portion (apo B-100) so that it is more negatively charged. The protein modification leads to a loss of recognition by the LDL receptor and a shift to recognition by the macrophage scavenger receptors, the oxLDL receptor, or both (Berliner et al. 1995; Brown and Goldstein 1990; Sparrow et al. 1989), so that LDL is internalized by macrophages (Henriksen et al. 1981) (Figure 6.3). This uptake, unlike LDL uptake by means of the LDL receptor, is not subject to down-regulation, so that the macrophage can become heavily laden with lipids. Oxidized LDL has been demonstrated within macrophages in both human and rabbit atherosclerotic lesions (Yla-Herttuala et al. 1989).

Beyond the contribution of oxLDL to the formation of foam cells, around 20 potentially proatherogenic properties of oxLDL have been described, although only a few have been validated as having in vivo relevance (Steinberg 1997b). The contribution of biologically active molecules generated during the process of oxidation could be as important to atherogenesis as foam cell formation (Witztum and Hörkkö 1997). In addition to promoting, as described earlier, chemoattraction for circulating monocytes, oxLDL inhibits the motility of macrophages, which might exert a trapping effect (Steinberg 1997a; Quinn et al. 1987) (see Figure 6.3). It is also a chemoattractant for T cells and is cytotoxic to a number of cell types (Steinberg 1997a; Schwartz et al. 1991; Cathcart et al. 1985; Heinecke et al. 1984), thus promoting the release of lipids and lysosomal enzymes into the intimal extracellular space. OxLDL can rapidly impair endothelium-dependent dilation, probably through multiple mechanisms, including direct inactivation of nitric oxide (Selwyn et al. 1997). In addition, it may promote formation of thrombi (Hirose et al. 1996). A further property of oxLDL not shared by native LDL is immunogenicity (Steinberg 1997a). Autoantibodies to oxLDL are higher in patients with carotid atherosclerosis than in age-matched healthy subjects (Salonen et al. 1992), and the plasma concentration of immunoreactive oxLDL is higher in patients who have suffered acute MI compared with that in control subjects (Holvoet et al. 1995).

SMOOTH MUSCLE CELL PROLIFERATION AND CAP FORMATION

The migration and proliferation of SMCs are the principal intimal changes during the development of the fibrous plaque (Ross 1998). Some populations of SMCs in atherosclerosis appear to be locally derived, arising from clonal lineages (Murry et al. 1997) (see "Monoclonality of Smooth Muscle Cells" in Chapter 9). A variety of growth-regulatory molecules, generally not expressed in a normal artery, are up-regulated in atherosclerotic lesions; a number of these (e.g., platelet-derived growth factor, basic fibroblast growth factor, IL-1, and TNF-α) can induce SMC proliferation, chemotaxis, or both (Ross 1993). Monocytes/macrophages are a potent source of some such factors, as are SMCs themselves (Ross 1993; Berliner et al. 1995), and oxidized lipids can stimulate the secretion of IL-1 (Ku et al. 1992). In addition, fibrin, thrombin, and platelets can stimulate SMC proliferation when deposited on the vessel wall (Bini et al. 1989). Plaques contain T lymphocytes (Libby and Hansson 1991), which may modify SMC proliferation by means of production of IFN-γ (Davies 1998).

SMCs usually form a fibrous cap related to their deposition of new connective tissue matrix and the accumulation of intracellular and extracellular lipids (Ross 1998). The structure of the cap in a lesion with a lipid core is a collagen lattice, within which are lacunae containing SMCs that produce the connective tissue matrix (Davies 1998). Numerous cytokines (Libby 1995) control the balance in the plaque cap between deposition of collagen and degradation of the connective tissue matrix by a range of proteases (Davies 1998).

SMCs also transform into foam cells, although macrophages are the major cell type of foam cells (Kruth 1997), and accretion of cholesteryl ester in SMCs may be mediated by factors secreted by macrophages (Stein and Stein 1995). Induction of the scavenger receptor in SMCs may promote their transformation (Stein and Stein 1995).

The extracellular matrix of the plaque, which is in constant flux, not only provides the architectural framework that influences structural integrity, but also participates in the adhesive, proliferative, and migratory events of lesion development. For example, matrix formed during the proliferative phase may promote SMC migration and proliferation, whereas matrix formed during later remodeling may inhibit SMC proliferation and promote additional complications (Wight 1995). The active and regulated process of extracellular matrix formation does not appear to be controlled by oxLDL (Hirose et al. 1996).

LIPID CORE FORMATION

Some macrophage foam cells may exit the intima to export accumulating lipoproteins; in response to lipid uptake, macrophages can produce apo E, which can bind to HDL (Geng and Libby 1995). Other macrophages die within the lesion, releasing their contents and contributing to the formation of the highly thrombogenic lipid-rich core (Libby 1996). Hypoxia and cytotoxic peroxides have been popular explanations for this cell death (Kruth 1997), although there is now evidence that to some extent macrophage death is by apoptosis (programmed cell death) (Kruth 1997; Bjorkerud and Bjorkerud 1996; Hardwick et al. 1996; Ball et al. 1995). The trigger for apoptosis could be deprivation of a growth factor such as macrophage colony–stimulating factor, the cell line's normal growth factor, particularly in association with the TNF-α present in large amounts in cellular atherosclerotic lesions (Davies 1998). An alternative view of lipid core formation (Guyton and Klemp 1994; Wissler and the PDAY Collaborating Investigators 1994) is that some extracellular lipid is derived from

Figure 6.3. Early events in atherogenesis. Native LDL becomes trapped in the ▶ subendothelial space, where it can be oxidized by resident vascular cells such as SMCs, endothelial cells, and macrophages. OxLDL (simplified in the figure to include both minimally modified and fully oxidized LDL; see text) stimulates (+) monocyte chemotaxis (**A**) and inhibits (–) monocyte egress from the vascular wall (**B**). Monocytes differentiate into macrophages that internalize fully oxidized LDL, leading to foam cell formation (**C**). OxLDL also causes endothelial dysfunction and injury (**D**), as well as foam cell necrosis (**E**), resulting in the release of lysosomal enzymes and necrotic debris. *Broken arrows* indicate adverse effects of oxLDL. (Reprinted with permission from Diaz et al. 1997. Copyright 1997 Massachusetts Medical Society. All rights reserved. The Diaz et al. figure was adapted from Quinn et al. 1987.)

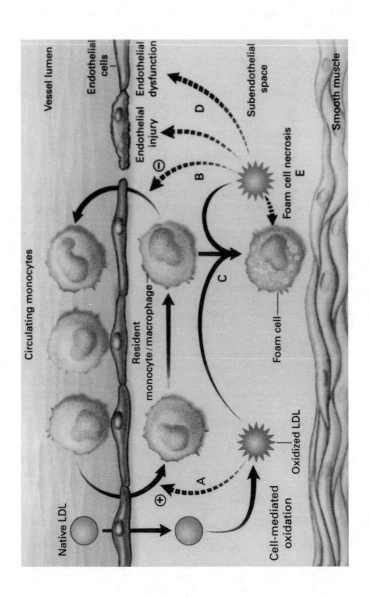

plasma LDL bound to glycosaminoglycans, collagen, or fibrinogen deep within the intima; this lipid would not have passed through macrophages (Kruth 1997; Falk et al. 1995). It is generally believed, however, that necrosis makes the greater contribution to core formation (Falk et al. 1995; Davies 1998).

In the artery wall, LDL can undergo both fusion and aggregation. These processes can lead to its increased uptake by macrophages or increased retention in lesion connective tissue matrix. As lesions calcify, cholesterol can become entombed within the mineralized calcium. Cholesterol crystals usually accumulate in advanced lesions; they can also form within macrophages (Kruth 1997).

PLAQUE VASCULARIZATION

Healthy adult coronary arteries normally lack microvasculature except for a scant plexus of vasa vasorum in the adventitia and outer media (Pels et al. 1997). Microvessels grow into the artery wall, however, when the intima thickens in the development of atherosclerosis. In monkeys fed an atherogenic diet for 17 months, blood flow to atherosclerotic intima and media increased by a factor of 5 because of neovascularization (Heistad and Armstrong 1986); with lesion regression, blood flow decreased sixfold (Williams et al. 1988). Microvessels likely play a fundamental role in atherogenesis through nourishing the growing lesion. In addition, they may act as an important source of growth factors and adhesion molecules, deliver vasoconstrictive or vasodilatory substances, provide another route for monocyte entry, or be involved in plaque hemorrhage, and inflammatory cells may enter plaque through breaches in the endothelium they create (Pels et al. 1997; O'Brien et al. 1996). Microvessels near the core base are thin walled, and red cell extravasation is common (Davies 1998). Loss of adventitial microvessels may lead to tissue hypoxia, and preservation of the neovasculature may be necessary to prevent excessive tissue scarring and possibly contracture (Pels et al. 1997).

Plaque vascularization rather than cap erosion was the source of the intraplaque thrombus without rupture found in 21% of 76 surgical specimens of carotid endarterectomies by Milei et al. (1996). Most of the lipid cores were highly vascularized, and the neovasculature was in close contact with macrophages and T cells. The authors speculated that abrupt growth of the lipid core or overproduction of oxygen free radicals may have led to the breakdown of the core vessels and hemorrhage.

PLAQUE PROGRESSION

There is a wide and poorly understood variability in how plaques evolve, and coronary artery lesion progression is typically unpredictable, sudden, and nonlinear (Falk et al. 1995). Plaque disruption is common, and a substantial percentage of plaques causing high-grade stenosis result from previous disruption. In lesions causing 0–20% stenosis on angiograms,

16% have healed disruption; with 21–50% stenosis, 19% have healed disruption; and with more than 50% stenosis, 72% show healed disruption (Davies 1996a). Thus, lesions seem to undergo cycles of disruption and repair, with periods of clinical instability representing major plaque events (Davies 1998). There is also a role in plaque progression for accelerated SMC proliferation and matrix synthesis driven by factors such as growth factors or superficial inflammation (Falk et al. 1995). It is possible that wounds are created by multiple episodes of plaque rupture, and that wound contracture contributes to vessel narrowing (Schwartz 1997).

ONSET OF ACUTE CORONARY SYNDROMES

The development of a thrombus large enough to protrude into the lumen and acutely decrease blood flow is the major factor initiating clinical symptoms of CHD (Figure 6.4). Other mechanisms are continued plaque growth until lumen size is reduced and abnormal coronary vasomotor tonal responses in subjects with coronary atherosclerosis (Davies 1998). The disordered control of tone in part reflects endothelial dysfunction, and resulting vasospasm may be localized or more generalized (Davies 1998).

A high percentage of acute coronary ischemic events appear to be triggered by external factors; for example, the frequency of MI increases during emotional stress or (especially if unaccustomed) vigorous exercise, as well as in the morning soon after waking, on Mondays, and during the winter (Falk et al. 1995; Muller et al. 1989, 1994; Willich et al. 1993; Mittleman et al. 1993). Acute risk factors have been reported in almost 50% of cases of acute MI (Robertson and Strong 1968). Although mechanisms have not been established, plaque disruption and thrombosis or local or generalized vasoconstriction may underlie the phenomenon (e.g., sympathetic activity increasing with suddenly heightened blood pressure or heart rate) (Falk et al. 1995). The morning peak in MI is blunted by beta blocker therapy, likely through blockage of the morning sympathetic surge (Willich et al. 1989).

ACUTE THROMBOSIS

Postmortem studies have shown acute thrombosis to result from erosion of a fibrous plaque rich in SMCs and proteoglycans or, more commonly, from plaque rupture (Davies 1998). Also, endothelial dysfunction could facilitate thrombus formation in the presence of other predisposing conditions, and hemorrhage of vessels within lesions could conceivably lead to thrombosis (Stary et al. 1995). Such conditions allow the attachment of passing platelets and the absorption of coagulation proteins; circulating platelets never or rarely adhere to normal endothelium in vivo (Verstraete and Fuster 1998).

A number of local and systemic factors favor thrombus formation (Fuster et al. 1996) (Table 6.2). Such factors affect both the degree and duration of thrombus formation and may thereby influence the pathologic and clinical manifestations of acute ischemic syndromes (Fuster et al.

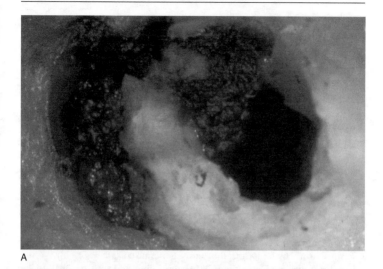

A

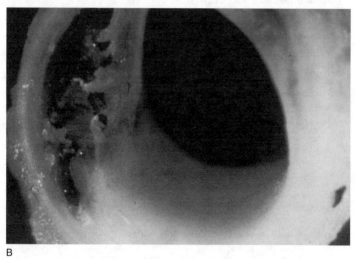

B

Figure 6.4. **A.** Plaque disruption with thrombus in the artery lumen and in the large lipid core. **B.** Intraplaque thrombus. Both fixed specimens are from human arteries. (Photographs courtesy of Michael J. Davies, MD, FRCP, FRCPath, St. George's Hospital Medical School, University of London; used with permission.)

Table 6.2. SELECTED LOCAL AND SYSTEMIC THROMBOGENIC RISK FACTORS FOR THROMBOTIC COMPLICATIONS OF PLAQUE DISRUPTION

Local factors
  Degree of plaque disruption (fissure, ulcer)
  Degree of stenosis (change in geometry)
  Tissue substrate (lipid-rich plaque)
  Surface of residual thrombus (recurrence)
  Vasoconstriction (platelets, thrombin)
Systemic factors
  Catecholamines (smoking, stress, cocaine)
  Renin-angiotensin (DD genotype)
  Plasma cholesterol, TG,* and Lp[a], as well as other metabolic states (homocysteinemia, diabetes mellitus)
  Fibrinogen (which is increased by smoking), impaired fibrinolysis (e.g., PAI-1), activated platelets, and clotting (factor VII, thrombin generation or activity)

Source: Modified (*) from Fuster et al. 1996.

1996). As regards lipid risk factors, elevated plasma cholesterol has been associated with hypercoagulability and enhanced platelet reactivity (Badimon et al. 1991); hypertriglyceridemia may be related to factor VII activation (Simpson et al. 1983; Miller et al. 1991a; Mitropoulos et al. 1989) and correlates with impaired fibrinolysis (Hamsten et al. 1985); and Lp[a] interferes with plasminogen activation and binding, among other prothrombotic effects (Loscalzo 1990) (see also Chapter 8). HDL may help prevent intracoronary thrombus formation (Kawai 1994) (see Chapter 8).

Endothelial Erosion

Loss of small areas of plaque endothelial cells exposes connective tissue to the circulating blood and leads to local platelet adhesion. Symptoms can result when larger areas of endothelial denudation or erosion give rise to thrombus formation, characteristically without hemorrhage into the plaque (Davies 1998). Indicators of inflammatory activation, such as T lymphocytes and activated macrophages, have been associated with eroded plaque (van der Wal et al. 1994; Davies 1998). Endothelial erosion accounts for at least one-fourth of significant coronary thrombi (Davies 1990) (see also Chapter 7).

Plaque Rupture

Most thrombi leading to acute coronary syndromes overlie atherosclerotic plaques that have undergone rupture (also called disruption, fissuring, cracking, tearing, or ulceration) (Falk 1983; Falk et al. 1995; Davies 1990, 1998; van der Wal et al. 1994) (Figure 6.5). In this process, the fibrous cap separating the core from the lumen may tear, break, or disintegrate, allow-

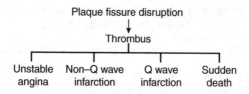

Figure 6.5. Disrupted atherosclerotic plaques are found beneath most thrombi responsible for acute coronary syndromes. (From Ambrose and Weinrauch 1996; used with permission.)

ing the flowing blood to come into contact with thrombogenic plaque contents, inducing platelet adhesion, aggregation, and activation. Thrombosis may be confined to a plaque's interior when there is a small tear that allows only limited blood entry, or the entire cap may be torn away so that core material is extruded into the lumen (Davies 1998). The likelihood of significant thrombosis within the lumen increases with reduction of blood flow and reflects the balance of systemic prothrombotic and fibrinolytic mechanisms (Davies 1998). The rough surface produced by fibrous cap disruption further stimulates thrombosis (Fernández-Ortiz et al. 1994). The plaque disruption itself is asymptomatic, and the associated plaque growth is usually clinically silent (Falk et al. 1995). According to data from autopsy studies, 9% of healthy individuals have asymptomatic disrupted coronary artery lesions; this increases to 22% in individuals who have high blood pressure or diabetes (Davies et al. 1989).

   The characteristics of plaques that are most likely to rupture have been determined from studies of necropsy and atherectomy samples of plaques that have already been disrupted (Davies et al. 1993; Moreno et al. 1994; Falk 1983). Features of rupture-prone plaques include a large lipid core, a thin cap, high macrophage densities, and reduced SMC content (Davies 1996b). The macrophages are activated and likely responsible for the destruction of the connective tissue of the cap (Libby 1994; Davies 1996b) (Figure 6.6). The likelihood of a clinical ischemic event is related to the number of rupture-prone lesions present, although even one strategically located vulnerable lesion can lead to death. Rupture can represent an interaction of various local, mechanical, and hemodynamic forces (e.g., shear stress, coronary spasm) with a reduction in the innate mechanical strength of the lesion (Davies 1995). Rupture-prone lesions are discussed in greater detail in Chapter 7. As is also discussed there,

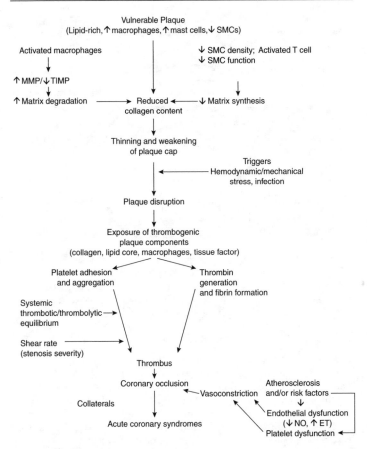

Figure 6.6. Summary of the pathophysiology of plaque rupture. Atheromatous lesions (types IV and Va) are especially prone to disruption. ET, endothelial activation; MMP, matrix-degrading metalloproteinases; NO, nitric oxide activity; TIMP, tissue inhibitors of metalloproteinases. (Reprinted from Shah 1997, with permission from Excerpta Medica Inc.)

most type IV and type Va lesions do not cause angiographic stenosis and are not symptomatic, which is consistent with compensatory vessel remodeling (Glagov et al. 1987, 1995a, 1995b). The media thins and atrophies as atherosclerosis develops in overlying intima, allowing the plaque to bulge outward, in some cases rupturing the internal elastic lamina (Davies 1996a).

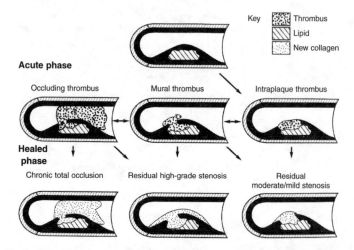

Figure 6.7. Diagram of the dynamic state of the acute thrombotic response with different stages—intraplaque, mural nonocclusive, and occlusive thrombus. The end result, after healing by SMC proliferation, ranges from chronic total occlusion to a mild increase in stenosis. (Reprinted with permission from Davies 1998.)

PLAQUE HEALING

In the healing response that follows plaque rupture, natural fibrinolysis removes thrombotic material to a variable extent, followed by SMC proliferation and the generation of new collagen (Davies 1998). Hematomas and thrombi may be incorporated into the lesion as plaque fissures reseal (Stary et al. 1995). Plaque disruptions can result in a range of changes in plaque size, from trivial to substantial (Figure 6.7), and doubtless contribute to the sudden and unpredictable progression of atherosclerosis. Residual mural thrombus predisposes vessels to recurrent occlusion (Davies et al. 1991; Ohman et al. 1993).

Suggested Reading

Berliner JA, Navab M, Fogelman AM, et al. Atherosclerosis: basic mechanisms—oxidation, inflammation and genetics. Circulation 1995;91:2488–2496.

Davies MJ. Pathology of coronary atherosclerosis. In: Alexander RW, Schlant RC, Fuster V, eds. Hurst's the heart arteries and veins, 9th ed., vol. 1. New York: McGraw-Hill, 1998:1161–1173.

Falk E, Shah PK, Fuster V. Coronary plaque disruption (review). Circulation 1995;92:657–671.

Fernández-Ortiz A, Fuster V. Pathophysiology of coronary artery disease (review). Clin Geriatr Med 1996;12:1–21.

Libby P, Geng Y-J, Sukhova GK, et al. Molecular determinants of atherosclerotic plaque vulnerability. Ann N Y Acad Sci 1997;11:134–142.

Ross R. The pathogenesis of atherosclerosis: a perspective for the 1990s
(review). Nature 1993;362:801–809.

Steinberg D, Lewis A. Conner Memorial Lecture. Oxidative modification of
LDL and atherogenesis. Circulation 1997;95:1062–1071.

Verstraete M, Fuster V. Thrombogenesis and antithrombotic therapy. In:
Alexander RW, Schlant RC, Fuster V, eds. Hurst's the heart arteries and
veins, 9th ed., vol. 1. New York: McGraw-Hill, 1998:1501–1551.

Witztum J. The oxidation hypothesis of atherosclerosis. Lancet 1994;344:
793–795.

Chapter 7

Atherosclerosis and Myocardial Infarction: A Sea Change in Concept

MOST CLINICAL EVENTS ARISE
FROM MILD OR MODERATE LESIONS

Atherosclerosis encroaches to varying degrees on the coronary artery lumen. Both histologic analyses and intravascular ultrasound studies have demonstrated that substantial atherosclerosis may be present in epicardial coronary arteries without angiographic luminal narrowing, consistent with vascular remodeling (Di Mario et al. 1994) (see later). Most plaques of histologic type IV or Va, which are rupture prone (see Chapter 5 and later in this chapter), are clinically silent and, because they do not encroach on the lumen, angiographically invisible (Glagov et al. 1987, 1995a; Davies 1998). In patients undergoing transcatheter therapy for symptomatic CHD, Mintz et al. (1995) found only 60 (6.8%) of 884 angiographically normal coronary artery reference segments to be normal by intravascular ultrasound. Compared with the target lesions, the reference segments contained proportionately more soft plaque elements and less calcific and dense fibrotic plaque.

Cross-sectional area narrowing of more than 75% on angiography (as measured from the internal elastic membrane) is considered significant. Coronary lesion length is also a factor in reduction of blood flow (Waller et al. 1992b); in 565 severe coronary stenoses, Baroldi (1966) found lesion length to be less than 5 mm in 13%, 5–20 mm in 38%, and more than 20 mm in 49%. The use of "significant" in angiography has been questioned (Hurst 1994), however, because, as reviewed by Brown et al. (1993), most ischemic clinical events, including unstable angina, acute MI, and death, arise from mild or moderate coronary lesions (Brown et al. 1986; Ambrose et al. 1988), which can undergo rapid change. In a study of patients with acute MI who received thrombolytic therapy, atherosclerosis underlying the thrombotic occlusion caused less than 50% diameter stenosis in one-third of cases and 50–60% stenosis in another one-third (Brown et al. 1986). Based on findings on preinfarct angiograms, lesions precipitating MI cause on average 50% stenosis and generally do not have visualized features suggesting the likelihood of occlusion (Brown et al. 1986; Ambrose et al. 1988; Taeymans et al. 1992). Serial angiographic studies have indicated that the more obstructive an atherosclerotic lesion, the more frequently it progresses to coronary occlusion or gives rise to MI (Alderman et al. 1993), which supports the use of lesion-specific interventions such as CABG and PTCA. But whereas a given severe lesion is more likely than a given mild or moderate lesion to lead to total occlusion, mild and moderate lesions are much more numerous in the arterial tree and, thus, more clinical events arise from them (Brown et al. 1989). Furthermore, because hemodynamically insignificant stenoses do not stimulate collateral vessel development (Danchin 1993; Cohen et al. 1989), sequelae of sudden complete occlusion at such locations can be more severe (see "Collateralization," later).

The progression of coronary atherosclerosis typically occurs in sudden increments in an individual; it is rarely slow and steady (Davies 1996a) (see Chapter 6). Often, acute occlusions occur at sites that previously appeared normal on angiograms; likewise, high-grade stenoses often appear suddenly (Davies 1996a).

RUPTURE-PRONE LESIONS

Plaque disruption has been reported to be more common than endothelial denudation in precipitating major thrombi on the order of 3 to 1 (Davies 1990), although in relatively young subjects a ratio of 1.3 to 1 has been reported (Farb et al. 1996). Burke et al. (1997) reported a ratio of 2.3 to 1 in an autopsy series of men (mean age, 47 years) who had died suddenly. Studies of necropsy and atherectomy material (Davies et al. 1993; Moreno et al. 1994; Falk 1983) have allowed delineation of the features of plaques that have broken up, that is, plaques that are rupture prone. Those features involve both morphology and degree of inflammatory activity, in particular a large lipid core, a thin cap, reduced SMC content, and high density of macrophages, which are activated (Davies 1996b) (Figure 7.1). It is the presence of type IV and type Va plaques that allows clinical events to develop (Davies 1998). Risk for ischemic coronary events depends on the number of vulnerable plaques; in most subjects—and even within one coronary artery—both stable and unstable lesions are found (Davies 1995). There is no readily discernible relation between variables of plaque component heterogeneity and degree of stenosis or plaque size, nor has a statistical relation been found between core size and cap thickness (Davies 1998; Mann and Davies 1996). Burke et al. (1997), in an autopsy study of men, found that the mean ratio of serum levels of TC to HDL-C was

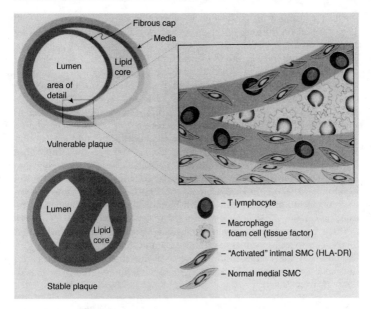

Figure 7.1. Comparison of vulnerable and stable atherosclerotic plaques. A vulnerable plaque typically has a substantial lipid core and a thin fibrous cap that separates macrophages (bearing tissue factor) from the blood. SMCs are often activated at sites of lesion disruption. In a stable plaque, in contrast, a relatively thick fibrous cap protects the lipid from contact with the blood. Because plaque growth is initially outward, the lumen is often well preserved when a vulnerable plaque is present, whereas clinical data suggest that stable plaques more often cause angiographically apparent luminal narrowing. (Reprinted with permission from Libby 1995.)

markedly elevated (8.5) in the men who died of acute thrombosis with plaque rupture but only somewhat elevated in men without acute thrombosis (5.5) and in men with thrombi overlying eroded plaques (5.0).

Large Lipid Core

The contribution of the lipid core to the overall volume of an atherosclerotic lesion varies widely, and core margins may be surrounded by macrophages or there may be no macrophages (Davies 1998). Davies et al. (1994) assessed aortic plaques (group A) from patients with no ruptured plaques, as well as ruptured and unruptured aortic plaques (groups B and C) from patients with ruptured plaques. From group A (stable plaques) to group C (unstable plaques), lipid content increased from 13% to 28% to 57%, and the contribution of the cap to plaque volume decreased from 16% to 12% to 3%. The lipid core typically occupies more than 50% of overall volume in ruptured plaques (Davies 1998).

The consistency of the atheromatous core also appears to be important, and it depends on lipid composition and temperature. Examination of postmortem specimens at room temperature shows that the core is usually soft, like toothpaste; cholesteryl esters confer a soft quality, whereas crystalline cholesterol has the opposite effect (Falk et al. 1995). The results of experiments in animals predict depletion of plaque lipid with lowering of circulating lipid concentrations (Falk et al. 1995).

Lesions rich in lipid gruel appear to be not only more vulnerable to rupture but also more thrombogenic when their contents are exposed to circulating blood. Experimentally, the lipid core is about six times more thrombogenic than the collagen-rich component of plaque (Fernández-Ortiz et al. 1994).

Thin, Weak Fibrous Cap

Fibrous tissue, the sclerotic component of a plaque, often makes up more than 70% of the lesion (Falk et al. 1995). A cap of fibromuscular tissue in which collagen and elastin occur in a woven pattern separates a lipid core from the lumen (type Va plaque); the collagen is important for tensile strength. Fibrous caps vary widely in matrix, cellularity, thickness, strength, and stiffness (Falk et al. 1995). The entire cap may be relatively thick, or there may be focal points of weakness. Caps are often thinnest at their shoulder regions, where disruption most frequently occurs (Devries et al. 1995). Thick caps have higher numbers of SMCs, the collagen-synthesizing cells in lesions, whereas relatively thin caps have fewer SMCs and contain appreciable numbers of macrophages (Davies 1998).

Activated Macrophages ("Hot" Plaque)

The fibrous cap is now recognized as a dynamic structure in which numerous cytokines control a balance of collagen synthesis and degradation (Libby 1996). Disrupted fibrous caps are typically heavily infiltrated by activated macrophage foam cells (van der Wal et al. 1994; Libby 1994) and are associated with T cell infiltration, elements indicating ongoing inflammation (Falk et al. 1995). Thus, a plaque can be viewed in inflammatory terms as "hot" or "burnt out" (Davies 1998), and plaque cap tears can be viewed as resulting when macrophage-related plaque degradation gains ascendancy over repair by collagen synthesized by SMCs. Proteolytic destruction of fibrous caps is under intense investigation (Davies 1998).

Active enzymes have been shown to be present in vulnerable plaques, as have macrophage-derived metalloproteinases such as collagenases,

gelatinases, and stromelysins (Galis et al. 1994; Libby 1996). Metalloproteinases are zinc ion– and calcium ion–dependent enzymes involved in the
degradation of components of the connective tissue matrix. Macrophages
can also degrade extracellular matrix by phagocytosis and by secreting
other proteolytic enzymes such as plasminogen activators (Matrisian 1992).

The increase in the number of macrophages in the thin or ruptured
cap is associated with a decrease in the number of SMCs (Davies et al.
1993). There is now evidence that SMCs could disappear as the result of
apoptosis (Majno and Joris 1995), a process wherein the cell is induced to
participate actively in its own destruction by synthesizing enzymes that
degrade and fragment the DNA strands within the nucleus (Davies 1997a).
It is possible that apoptosis in this instance is triggered by proximity to
macrophages (Kockx et al. 1996); TFN-α and IL-1β are produced by activated macrophages (Geng et al. 1996).

The vascular cell dysfunctions related to LDL oxidation (i.e., constriction, loss of dilation, inflammation, thrombosis) operate throughout
the development of atherosclerosis but are particularly important during
plaque rupture (Selwyn et al. 1997). Lipid lowering very quickly restores
endothelium-dependent vasomotor function (see Chapter 10).

Additional Mechanical Factors

Additional mechanical characteristics of plaque that may play a role in
rupture at focal sites of weakness include the juxtaposition of regions of
contrasting composition and high computed circumferential stresses
(Berliner et al. 1995; Glagov et al. 1997) (Table 7.1). Soft plaque sitting
on an area of calcification may be particularly important with regard to
the tissue interface of differing physical properties subjected to the pulsatile changes of arterial blood pressure (Demer et al. 1994; Berliner et
al. 1995). Farb et al. (1996) found calcification in 69% of ruptured coronary artery lesions, compared with 23% of superficial erosions leading to
coronary thrombosis. In that series of 50 consecutive cases of sudden
death due to coronary artery thrombosis, 100% and 75% of ruptured
lesions showed infiltration by macrophages and T cells, respectively,
compared with values of 50% and 32% in superficial erosions. Once disruption has occurred, the resulting rough surface within the lumen further stimulates the development of acute thrombosis (Fernández-Ortiz
et al. 1994).

Imaging Rupture-prone Lesions

Coronary angiography can visualize advanced lesions, plaque disruption,
luminal thrombosis, and calcification but not other qualitative features
(Falk et al. 1995). Imaging modalities that would distinguish in vivo the
plaques likely to rupture or progress would be of clinical value. Also needed
are noninvasive techniques that would image lesions in their earliest stages
of development (Kritz et al. 1996).

Ultrasound

In the carotid and lower extremity arteries, duplex ultrasound is useful in determining the degree of stenosis, changes in wall thickness, and the morphologic features of plaque (Vallabhajosula and Fuster 1997). The only imaging technique that appears to have clinical usefulness in distinguishing unstable lesions in coronary arteries is intravascular ultrasound, which is very invasive (Vallabhajosula and Fuster 1997). Under ideal conditions, it can measure a plaque's cap and core (Nissen et al. 1991), although calcification precludes measurement and minor technical variations in application may cause results to vary (Davies 1996b). Although a number of imaging modalities can detect calcification of coronary arteries, including electron-beam (ultrafast) computed tomography, which is noninvasive, studies have not confirmed that there is a good clinical correlation between calcium content and plaque vulnerability (Vallabhajosula and Fuster 1997).

Magnetic Resonance Imaging

In six patients undergoing carotid endarterectomy, in vivo magnetic resonance imaging (MRI) scans were shown to correlate well with the in vitro MRI values for plaque components (Toussaint et al. 1996). It was possible to discriminate lipid cores, fibrous caps, calcifications, and nor-

Table 7.1. MORPHOLOGIC CORRELATES OF PLAQUE INSTABILITY

Factors associated with disruption
  Structural
    Large lipid pools
    Focal thinning or defects of the fibrous cap
    High computed circumferential stresses at site of cap fracture
    Large plaque with marked stenosis
    Juxtaposed regions of contrasting composition
    Lumen irregularities and asymmetry
    Proximity of the necrotic core to the fibrous cap or lumen
  Cellular
    Abundant macrophage-derived foam cells
    T lymphocyte accumulation near sites of rupture
    Paucity of vascular smooth muscle cells
    Evidence for local inflammation
    T lymphocytes and macrophages
    Endothelial dysfunction (increased vasoconstriction and vascular cell adhesion)
Features implying resistance to disruption
  Uniform plaque fibrosis on cross section
  Circular, regular lumen contour
  Demarcated fibrous cap of uniform thickness (with absence of focal erosion, inflammation, and proximity of necrotic core)

Source: Adapted from Glagov et al. 1997, with permission from Elsevier Science.

mal media and adventitia and to characterize intraplaque thrombus and acute thrombosis in carotid lesions on in vivo MRI studies. However, several key technical problems remain unresolved with coronary MRI, which was made possible with the development of ultrafast sequences; after 5 years of preclinical trials, it has not been able to match traditional contrast coronary angiography in sensitivity and specificity (Duerinckx 1997).

COMPENSATORY VESSEL CHANGES

It has been known for some time that myocardial perfusion can be preserved by collateral circulation in some instances of progressive atherosclerotic obstruction of a large coronary vessel (Gregg and Patterson 1980). More recently, arterial remodeling has been recognized as another important compensatory mechanism in vessels burdened by atherosclerosis.

Collateralization

In experimental models, arterial occlusion in normal animals stimulates the formation of collateral blood channels, which help maintain tissue perfusion (Schaper 1993; White et al. 1993). However, collateral formation is often insufficient to prevent acute MI or ischemia in patients with advanced atherosclerosis (McPherson et al. 1991; Vanoverschelde et al. 1993). Like luminal expansion (see next section), angiogenesis can represent compensatory vascular changes to help maintain organ perfusion in the presence of insufficient arterial supply. The response has been described both in humans (Habib et al. 1991) and in animals (Schaper 1993). Although exercise training has been shown to promote the formation of collateral coronary vessels in animals with induced CHD, such a role for exercise in humans with CHD remains uncertain (Haidet 1995).

Compensatory angiogenesis, or collateral formation, should be differentiated from neovascularization in the atherosclerotic plaque. The latter, which is often potentiated by locally abundant growth factors and cytokines, may be viewed as an inflammatory reaction during plaque formation (Brogi et al. 1993). In contrast, compensatory collateralization is significantly impaired by hypercholesterolemia, as demonstrated in both rabbit ear (Chen and Henry 1997; Bucay et al. in press) and hindlimb (Van Belle et al. 1997) models. The etiology for the impaired compensatory vascular growth is not entirely clear. However, growth of capillary-like microtubules in human coronary and rabbit aortic explants has been demonstrated to be impaired by exposure to hypercholesterolemia or oxLDL (Chen et al. 1995, 1997). This impairment is strongly associated with a decreased availability of endogenous basic fibroblast growth factor (bFGF) and can be corrected by the administration of exogenous bFGF (Chen et al. 1995, 1997). More recent evidence shows that endothelial expression of bFGF can be inhibited by oxLDL (Chen and Henry 1997).

In animal models, gene transfer of bFGF, acidic fibroblast growth factor, and vascular endothelial growth factor (VEGF) has been shown to stimulate collateral growth in ischemic regions (Ueno et al. 1997; Tabata et al. 1997; Tsurumi et al. 1996).

The first angiogenic therapy of human atherosclerotic disease has recently been reported, suggesting regulation of blood vessel growth as a new modality (Folkman 1998a). Using intramuscular gene transfer of naked plasma DNA encoding phVEGF$_{165}$, which is an isoform of VEGF, Isner's group induced collateral neovascularization in critically ischemic limbs in nine patients in a phase 1 clinical trial (Baumgartner et al. 1998). The study was preceded by an initial report of a study in one patient (Isner et al. 1996). The increase in limb perfusion achieved in the phase 1 clinical trial was equivalent to or greater than successful surgical or percutaneous treatment (Folkman 1998b). Schumacher et al. (1998), in a randomized, controlled clinical trial, injected recombinant human bFGF close to the vessels after completion of internal mammary artery/left anterior descending coronary artery anastomosis in 20 patients with three-vessel coronary disease. At follow-up 12 weeks later, formation of capillaries was found by angiography in all cases around the injection site, and distal stenoses were bridged by neovascularization. In 20 patients in whom inactivated bFGF was injected, there was no evidence of myocardial neovascularization. Angiogenic therapy raises the question of whether pathologic angiogenesis at a remote site or plaque vascularization could be stimulated (Folkman 1998b).

The clinical value of angiographically visible collaterals is seen in such effects as an extended "time window" for the benefit of reperfusion therapy, with greater improvement in cardiac function and reduction in infarct size (Topol and Ellis 1991), reduced deterioration of left ventricular function with acute coronary occlusion (Rentrop et al. 1988), and reduced incidence of late aneurysm formation after MI (Hirai et al. 1989), as reviewed by Wilson and White (1995). Factor and Bache (1998) noted that approximately 20% of chronic total coronary occlusions are not associated with infarction in dependent myocardium according to autopsy findings (Baroldi and Scomazzoni 1967), and that preservation of myocardium in an ischemic region is quantitatively related to the degree of collateral inflow (Rivas et al. 1976). Given that most clinical CHD events arise from angiographic lesions causing only mild or moderate stenosis, it is important to note that the regular finding of angiographically well-developed coronary collateral vessels is limited to patients with more than 80% stenosis of a major coronary artery (Cohen et al. 1989). The preinfarct presence of severe stenosis—and, thus, of a developed collateral circulation (Figure 7.2)—substantially lowers risk for hemodynamically severe consequences of MI, and, conversely, more severe clinical consequences result when acute occlusion occurs at a site of previously mild stenosis (Epstein 1988; Wilson and White 1995).

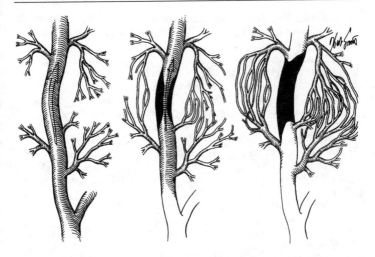

Figure 7.2. Stenosis caused by atherosclerosis can stimulate the development of collateral circulation. Angiographically well-developed coronary collaterals occur in patients with greater than 80% stenosis of a major coronary artery. More severe clinical consequences result when acute occlusion occurs at a site of previously mild stenosis (and, thus, of poor collateral development). In experiments in ears and hindlimbs of rabbits, compensatory collateralization is significantly impaired by an elevated plasma cholesterol concentration. (Reprinted with permission from DeBakey and Gotto, *The New Living Heart*, 1997.)

Vascular Remodeling

Beyond an ability to change its tone acutely, a blood vessel can alter its structure chronically in response to certain conditions. The active process of remodeling—representing a dynamic interaction of locally generated growth factors, vasoactive substances, and hemodynamic stimuli—results in a change in the vessel's geometry, whether to increase its mass (thickening the wall) or to enlarge or dilate it (not necessarily increasing the mass of the wall) (Dzau and Gibbons 1993; Gibbons and Dzau 1994). Usually, remodeling is an adaptive response to long-term changes in hemodynamic conditions (e.g., pressure, flow, shear stress); subsequently, however, it may contribute to the pathophysiology of vascular diseases and circulatory disorders (Dzau and Gibbons 1993; Gibbons and Dzau 1994). In chronic, focal de novo stenoses in the coronary and femoral arteries, pathologic vascular remodeling (a decrease in lumen diameter or chronic constriction) has been shown to contribute to lumen loss (Pasterkamp et al. 1995; Mintz et al. 1997). Mintz et al. (1997), using intravascular ultrasound, described inadequate remodeling in at least 15% of chronic, focal new coronary arterial stenoses in patients with stable angina, noting that the magnitude of remodeling appeared to be a lesion-specific response.

Remodeling as a result of changing metabolic and mechanical states occurs at all stages of atherosclerosis; during early development, SMC proliferation tends to correspond to increased vessel diameter and wall volume, whereas matrix accumulation tends to correspond to tensile strength (Glagov et al. 1995b, 1997). Both the endothelium and changes in the extracellular matrix metabolism are likely important in the process (Dzau and Gibbons 1993; Gibbons and Dzau 1994; Faxon et al. 1997). How the vessel wall responds to mechanical forces at the cellular and molecular level is under intense investigation (Glagov et al. 1995b; Giddens et al. 1993; Gibbons and Dzau 1994). In addition to the setting of atherosclerosis, vascular remodeling has been described in arterial hypertension, diabetes mellitus, angiogenesis, ischemia/reperfusion, angioplasty (see "Restenosis after Angioplasty" in Chapter 9), and other situations (Ponte et al. 1997). Some key points regarding compensatory vessel remodeling in atherosclerosis are shown in Table 7.2.

Compensatory Remodeling and Risk Factors

Frequently cited as an example of compensatory arterial remodeling (Faxon et al. 1997) are the 1958 autopsy findings in the case of Clarence DeMar, which were published (Currens and White 1961) as being of interest because of his lifetime of physical effort. DeMar, a Harvard- and Boston University–educated teacher, proofreader, and small farm manager described as disdaining officialdom, had authored the 1937 book *Marathon,* in which he had recorded his experiences as a self-trained long-distance runner; he was known as "Mr. Marathon." At his death from cancer, he had been a runner for 49 years. His coronary arteries were estimated to be two to three times the normal diameter; moderate coronary and aortic atherosclerosis was present, with luminal narrowing esti-

Table 7.2. VESSEL REMODELING IN ATHEROSCLEROSIS

Active process resulting in changes in geometry
    Can be changes in mass, dilation, or both
    Endothelium and changes in extracellular matrix likely important
Occurs at all stages of disease
Ubiquitous: coronary, carotid, peripheral, etc.
Can be compensatory, to hinder stenosis
    Appears to closely correlate with intimal area of lesion
    May fail when stenosis ≥40%
    CHD risk correlates may enhance (e.g., exercise, reduced LDL-C, reduced
        plasma TG, low-fat diet) or blunt (e.g., type 1 diabetes mellitus, smoking)
Can be pathologic

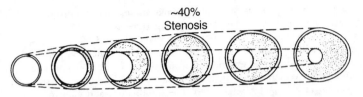

Figure 7.3. Diagram of the possible sequence of changes in arteries with atherosclerosis. Left to right: Initially, the artery enlarges as plaque progresses, but at more than 40% luminal stenosis, enlargement no longer counterbalances plaque expansion and luminal narrowing is no longer prevented. In the early stages of lesion development there may even be overcompensation. (Reprinted with permission from Glagov et al. 1987. Copyright 1987, Massachusetts Medical Society. All rights reserved.)

mated to be at most 30%, a degree of stenosis seen at several coronary sites. There was no evidence of myocardial infarct. In 1972, Mann et al. reported enlargement of coronary arteries in Masai men, enough to compensate for atherosclerosis comparable to that in contemporary American men. The Masai men consumed almost exclusively meat and milk (300 g fat daily on average) but were exceptionally physically fit, in part from extensive walking. Clinical manifestations of atherosclerosis were rare, even among the elderly. High blood pressure was unusual, blood pressure did not increase with age, and TC rarely exceeded 150 mg/dL. Experiments in monkeys with diet-generated atherosclerosis have shown increased enlargement of coronary artery diameter and decreased lumen narrowing with exercise (Kramsch et al. 1981).

In 1987, Glagov et al. galvanized interest in compensatory vascular remodeling when they reported, on the basis of histologic study of the left main coronary artery in 136 hearts obtained at autopsy, that arteries enlarge in relation to plaque area and that functionally important stenosis may be delayed until the lesion occupies 40% of the area of the internal elastic lamina (Figure 7.3). Patient age and heart weight were also factors in determining ultimate lumen diameter, although statistical regression analysis showed their contributions to be small. Ensuing pathologic and intravascular ultrasound studies of human coronary, carotid, and peripheral arteries showed the process of remodeling to be ubiquitous, with vessel enlargement apparently closely related to lesion intimal area (Faxon et al. 1997). Data from Clarkson et al. (1994), however, did not support the concept that compensation fails when stenosis reaches 40%. In their histologic study of left anterior descending coronary arteries from 100 autopsied patients and 416 nonhuman primates, they found that lumen size on average remained unaffected by atheroscle-

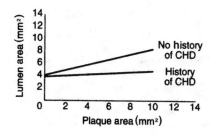

Figure 7.4. Relation between luminal area and plaque area in 100 left anterior descending coronary arteries obtained at autopsy, according to the presence or absence of a patient history of clinical manifestations of CHD. Artery compensation (increasing luminal area in response to increased plaque area) appears among the patients with no history of clinical CHD. (Reprinted with permission from Clarkson et al. 1994. Copyright 1994, American Medical Association.)

rotic plaque size. In this series, arteries with larger intimal areas had on average slightly larger lumina.

It has been reported from the cholesterol-lowering Monitored Atherosclerosis Regression Study, in which lovastatin was tested, that angiographic lesion progression in one coronary segment is associated with significant increases in segmental diameter of remote parts of the coronary tree (Shircore et al. 1995). The degree of compensatory change inversely correlated with on-trial plasma apo B and apo C-III concentrations and with blood pressure level; that is, vascular compensatory change was enhanced by decreases of LDL-C and plasma TG in the trial. The results are in accord with findings of enhanced coronary vessel remodeling with a low-fat diet and lower blood cholesterol in nonhuman primates (Kaplan et al. 1993). Adaptive remodeling has been described as blunted in patients with type 1 diabetes mellitus compared with those with type 2 diabetes or no diabetes (Kornowski et al. 1997b), and focal constriction was found to be more common than compensatory enlargement at sites of stenosis in smokers compared with nonsmokers (Weissman et al. 1997). Clarkson et al. (1994), on the other hand, did not find a relation between traditional risk factors and compensation in humans except for a previous history of clinical manifestations of CHD. Vessel compensation was better among those with no such history (Figure 7.4). They had only limited data on plasma lipids in humans, however. Intravascular ultrasound data quantitating de novo coronary lesions in patients with chronic angina suggested similar arterial remodeling in women and men (Kornowski et al. 1997a). Potential therapeutic strategies directed specifically at influencing the remodeling process may prove valuable—for example, the arrest of atherosclerosis progression through increasing endogenous vasodilators (e.g., nitric oxide) or decreasing endogenous vasoconstrictors (e.g., angiotensin II) (Gibbons and Dzau 1994).

Suggested Reading

Brown BG, Zhao X-Q, Sacco DE, Albers JJ. Lipid lowering and plaque regression: new insights into prevention of plaque disruption and clinical events in coronary disease. Circulation 1993;87:1781–1791.

Chen CH, Henry PD. Atherosclerosis as a microvascular disease: impaired angiogenesis mediated by suppressed basic fibroblast growth factor expression. Proc Assoc Am Phys 1997;109:351–361.

Davies MJ. The contribution of thrombosis to the clinical expression of coronary atherosclerosis. Thromb Res 1996;82:1–32.

Faxon DP, Coats W, Currier J. Remodeling of the coronary artery after vascular injury (review). Prog Cardiovasc Dis 1997;40:129–140.

Folkman J. Angiogenic therapy of the human heart (editorial). Circulation 1998;97:628–629.

Folkman J. Therapeutic angiogenesis in ischemic limbs (editorial). Circulation 1998;97:1108–1110.

Gibbons GH, Dzau VJ. The emerging concept of vascular remodeling (review). N Engl J Med 1994;330:1431–1438.

Glagov S, Bassiouny HS, Giddens DP, Zarins CK. Pathobiology of plaque modeling and complication (review). Surg Clin North Am 1995;75:545–556.

Libby P. Molecular bases of the acute coronary syndromes. Circulation 1995;91:2844–2850.

Selwyn AP, Kinlay S, Libby P, Ganz P. Atherogenic lipids, vascular dysfunction, and clinical signs of ischemic heart disease (editorial). Circulation 1997;95:5–7.

Vallabhajosula S, Fuster F. Atherosclerosis: imaging techniques and the evolving role of nuclear medicine (review). J Nucl Med 1997;38:1788–1796.

Chapter 8

Mechanisms of Atherosclerosis Beyond Low-Density Lipoprotein

A principal role for LDL and its derivatives is considered central to the initiation and progression of atherosclerosis described in Chapter 6, although precise mechanisms remain unknown. The role for cholesterol in CHD is supported by observational epidemiologic studies, findings of CHD in familial forms of hypercholesterolemia, laboratory and animal studies, and clinical trials of cholesterol-lowering therapy, including the superb reductions in morbidity and mortality rates in trials of HMG-CoA reductase inhibitors (Grundy 1997). Most people with elevated TC have elevated LDL-C, and LDL is considered the predominant atherogenic lipoprotein. Strong evidence supports the initiation and promotion of atherosclerosis by LDL at every stage (Grundy 1997).

Nevertheless, there is great variability in the clinical expression of CHD at any given LDL-C concentration. How the other major lipoprotein classes—that is, HDL and the TGRLs (and remnants of the latter)—and selected factors may participate in the process of atherothrombosis is described here. Many of the mechanisms of the risk factors are shared or overlapping. Also, in many instances, it is not established which among related factors may be a consequence or marker and which a cause, or what the relative contributions of factors with shared origins are.

HIGH-DENSITY LIPOPROTEIN

HDL particles are considered antiatherogenic. A strong inverse relation between HDL-C concentration and risk for CHD is well established by observational epidemiology (Gordon et al. 1989; Assmann et al. 1996; Jacobs et al. 1990; Goldbourt et al. 1997; Hausmann et al. 1996). It is likely that several mechanisms contribute to a defense by HDL particles against atherosclerosis, and that there is variation depending on the stage

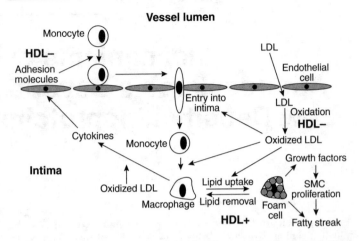

Figure 8.1. Points at which HDL might affect the early development of atherosclerosis. HDL+ indicates that the process is enhanced by HDL; HDL− indicates an inhibition by HDL. (Reprinted from Barter and Rye 1996; with permission from Elsevier Science.)

of disease (Andersson 1997). Much of the effect appears to occur early in the process of the formation of lesions (Figure 8.1).

Like other lipoprotein classes, HDL particles form a heterogeneous population, and cardioprotectivity could vary by subpopulation. Gradient gel electrophoresis has been used to define five subclasses: HDL_{2b}, HDL_{2a}, HDL_{3a}, HDL_{3b}, and HDL_{3c}, in decreasing order of particle size (Blanche et al. 1981; Nichols et al. 1986). The HDL_2:HDL_3 ratio appears to be a reliable indicator of the efficiency of postprandial lipolysis, which evidence suggests is related to CHD risk (Kirchmair et al. 1995), but measurement of HDL_2 and HDL_3 cholesterol may offer no advantage over measuring total HDL-C for CHD prediction (Wilson 1995). It is not yet recommended that clinicians extend measurement of HDL-C to include the determination of HDL subclasses (von Eckardstein et al. 1994). Regarding protein-defined subpopulations, most studies have shown CHD to be associated with decreased concentrations of Lp A-I (i.e., HDL particles containing apo A-I but not apo A-II, whereas both of the major proteins of HDL are present in Lp A-I:A-II) (Roheim and Asztalos 1995).

Another view holds that the inverse relation between HDL and risk for CHD may in fact reflect a positive relation between the TGRLs (see next section) and CHD (for review, see Patsch and Gotto 1995). Studies of subjects in the postprandial state suggest that metabolism of the TGRLs is a major determinant of HDL-C concentration. In two clinical studies, markers of postprandial TG metabolism were at least as accurate as HDL-C in identifying subjects with angiographic CHD versus controls (Patsch et al. 1992; Groot et al. 1991).

Reverse Cholesterol Transport

The cardioprotective effect of HDL has heretofore chiefly been attributed to its role in reverse cholesterol transport, in which cholesterol is mobilized from the periphery for delivery to the liver for catabolism (Pieters et al. 1994; Glomset 1968). Cholesterol cannot be degraded in peripheral tissue, including the artery wall; reverse cholesterol transport provides a pathway for the transfer of cholesterol to the liver, where it is degraded. Evidence to support the antiatherogenicity of reverse cholesterol transport is weak, however (Bruce and Tall 1995). In vitro, HDL particles promote the efflux of cholesterol from cholesterol-laden cells (Fielding and Fielding 1995) and reduce cholesterol content in foam cells (Miyazaki et al. 1992). The preferred acceptor of cell cholesterol is the minor subpopulation of small, pre-β-migrating particles, which contain apo A-I (Barter and Rye 1996; Castro and Fielding 1988).

Another mechanism leading to cholesterol efflux is suggested by the binding of HDL to specific surface sites referred to as HDL receptors (Roheim and Asztalos 1995). The binding leads to the translocation of intracellular cholesterol to the plasma membrane (Oram et al. 1983; Graham and Oram 1987). From the peripheral cells, the transferred free cholesterol is transported through the lymph system to the thoracic duct and then to the systemic circulation. The cholesterol after esterification by LCAT is transferred from HDL to LDL and finally to VLDL; the VLDL is taken up by the liver by means of LDL receptors.

Other Mechanisms

According to a growing body of evidence, the cardioprotective effect may be secondary to one or more HDL functions that are not related to cholesterol transport, as has been well reviewed by Barter and Rye (1996). An antioxidant function and a capacity to inhibit monocyte adhesion may be of major importance. Other functions reported include protection of erythrocytes against the generation of procoagulant activity, amelioration of the abnormal vasoconstriction that is a feature of early atherosclerosis, reduction of epidermal growth factor–induced DNA synthesis in vascular SMCs, stimulation of endothelial cell prostacyclin synthesis, and binding of prostacyclin and thus prolongation of its half-life (Barter and Rye 1996). The stabilization of prostacyclin may be a function of apo A-I (Kawai 1994). Amelioration of the inflammatory cascade has been suggested by inhibition of the membrane attack complex of complement (Hamilton et al. 1993).

TRIGLYCERIDE-RICH LIPOPROTEINS AND THEIR REMNANTS

An increasing body of evidence indicates that the metabolism of TGRLs is a strong predictor of CHD and is linked to atherosclerosis, although the relation appears to be both statistically and biologically more complex than the relation between plasma cholesterol and CHD risk (Patsch and Gotto 1995; Davignon and Cohn 1996; Hokanson and Austin 1996; Criqui et al. 1993; The International Committee 1991). The accumulating evidence includes results showing that specific TGRLs and markers of TGRL metabolism are key predictors of angiographic or ultrasonographic lesion progression (Hodis and Mack 1995)—for example, IDL mass concentration in the NHLBI Type II trial (Krauss et al. 1987), apo C-III in CLAS (Blankenhorn et al. 1990), and IDL in MARS (Hodis et al. 1997) (see Table 10.1 for angiographic trials). The combination of elevated plasma TG with low HDL-C may confer a particularly high risk for CHD (Assmann and Schulte 1992; Castelli 1992; Manninen et al. 1992). Usual estimates of LDL-C include IDL-C (which typically accounts for 10–15% of the value), which is considered acceptable because of the probable atherogenicity of IDL (Grundy 1997).

The strength of fasting TG concentration as a predictor is believed to lie in its reflection of the presence of atherogenic remnants of the TGRLs (Davignon and Cohn 1996; Patsch and Gotto 1995). Type III hyperlipidemia (familial dysbetalipoproteinemia), a disorder in which atherosclerosis can be extensive and xanthomas are seen, provides the most dramatic demonstration of the atherogenic potential of remnant lipoproteins. In type III hyperlipidemia, there is delayed remnant removal (and, thus, extended residence in the circulation) because of impaired uptake by the remnant receptor (related to apo E isoform) as well as impaired conversion of IDL to LDL and overproduction of VLDL (Davignon and Cohn 1996). It is believed that a second factor (e.g., diabetes mellitus) is required to promote the disorder.

Patsch and colleagues (Miesenböck et al. 1993) developed the concept of the syndrome of impaired TG tolerance, an atherogenic lipoprotein profile encompassing TG intolerance, elevated plasma IDL, reduced HDL_2, and a preponderance of small LDL and HDL. The derangement may be metabolically linked to the so-called insulin resistance syndrome (see later). Determinants of postprandial lipemia are shown in Figure 8.2. Others (Grundy 1997) would dispute the use of "atherogenic" with a lipid profile that does not include increased LDL-C, because a relatively low prevalence of CHD can be shown in populations without elevated LDL-C even if other risk factors are common (Grundy et al. 1990).

The mechanism whereby TGRLs and their remnants promote atherosclerosis is not understood, although a number of hypotheses exist. It is likely that differences in atherogenicity exist among the TGRLs, because they are a heterogeneous population, varying in origin, structure, and interactions with cell receptors (Karpe and Hamsten 1995). The interac-

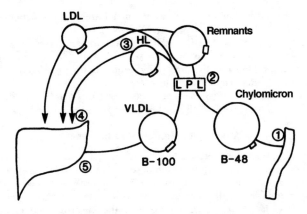

Figure 8.2.   The main determinants of the magnitude and duration of postprandial lipemia. (1) Intestinal fat absorption; (2) lipolysis of TGs in TGRLs by LPL; (3) hepatic lipase activity, which is thought to be involved in formation of LDL and remnant removal; (4) remnant removal; and (5) hepatic production of TGRLs during the postprandial state. (Reprinted with permission from Patsch and Gotto 1995.)

tion of cholesteryl ester–enriched VLDL and chylomicron remnants with cells of the artery wall, leading to cholesterol deposition, is one plausible mechanism (Patsch and Gotto 1995). The severity of atherosclerosis in human coronary arteries correlates with apo B insudation in the artery wall (Zhang et al. 1993). Macrophages are transformed into cells with foam cell–like characteristics when incubated with chylomicron remnants or VLDL remnants (Mahley and Innerarity 1983). Unlike LDL, hypertriglyceridemic VLDL particles do not require modification for uptake by macrophages (Sehayek and Eisenberg 1990).

Lipoprotein Size and Arterial Penetrance

The size of VLDL particles and chylomicrons is important because macromolecule size is a determinant of arterial wall influx (Roheim and Asztalos 1995). It appears that chylomicrons and VLDL the size of chylomicrons do not enter the intima (Nordestgaard 1996). It is not surprising that the plasma elevations of chylomicrons (which are particles 3–30 times larger than LDL particles) in familial chylomicronemia are not generally associated with atherosclerosis, although the considerably smaller chylomicron remnants should be able to enter the artery wall (Ebenbichler et al. 1995). A study by Rapp et al. (1994) demonstrated TG-containing lipoproteins the size of VLDL in the extracellular lipid in lesions. These results suggest that VLDL can cross the endothelial barrier. However, other authors (Chung et al. 1994) have proposed that the particles are surface remnants, because the material found is biochemically similar to products of LPL-mediated lipolysis of TGRLs.

It is possible that VLDL and IDL, as well as Lp[a] (see later), are selectively retained in the intima (Nordestgaard 1996). It has been observed in rabbits that the rates of movement of lipoproteins both into and out of the arterial wall decrease with increasing particle size (Nordestgaard et al. 1995). This observation suggests that lipoprotein diffusion within the arterial wall may be limited by a sieving mechanism.

Atherogenic Remnant Hypothesis

Zilversmit (1995) has updated his hypothesis that atherosclerosis results from the postprandial accumulation of remnants of TGRLs. Postprandial lipoproteins might cause atherosclerosis either through becoming a lesion component or through metabolic processes involved in their formation (Goldberg 1996). A key event in the Zilversmit model is the attachment of TGRLs to the arterial endothelium. Their lipolysis by LPL requires this interaction with the artery or capillary wall, where LPL is located. When LPL hydrolyzes their TG, they decrease in size to the extent that they might enter the artery wall. Furthermore, the release of fatty acids during lipolysis might cause endothelial injury and initiate thrombotic events (Zilversmit 1995). Zilversmit (1979) observed that LPL activity is increased in atherosclerotic areas of arteries.

In individuals with elevated VLDL or chylomicron remnants, as well as in those with increased LDL, arterial uptake of free and esterified cholesterol is increased. Because lipoprotein arterial influx proceeds in both the postprandial and fasting states, risk for CHD in an individual who consumes a high-fat and -cholesterol diet might be higher than is indicated by lipoprotein determinations made during the fasting state (Zilversmit 1995). Impaired chylomicron clearance occurs in subjects with both mild hypertriglyceridemia and reduced HDL-C (Ooi et al. 1992), and the postprandial state increases LDL susceptibility to oxidation (McKeone et al. 1993). Karpe et al. (1994), in a case-control study, related delayed clearance of chylomicron remnants to angiographic progression of coronary atherosclerosis.

Oxidation

Like LDL, VLDL particles are cytotoxic when oxidized (Hessler et al. 1983). Oxidative resistance of VLDL and LDL has been shown to be enhanced by both fibrate therapy (Vazquez et al. 1996) and statin therapy (Salonen et al. 1995a). In normocholesterolemic subjects, a high-fat meal, probably through the accumulation of TGRLs, provoked a decrease in brachial artery vasodilation. Because the effect was reversed by pretreatment with antioxidant vitamins, the authors suggested that postprandial TGRLs may impair endothelial function in an oxidative fashion similar to hypercholesterolemia (Plotnick et al. 1997).

Atherothrombosis

Hypertriglyceridemia may also have a role in atherothrombosis; this is perhaps related to factor VII activation (Simpson et al. 1983; Miller et al. 1991a; Mitropoulos et al. 1989). Also, plasma TG correlates with impaired fibrinolysis (Hamsten et al. 1985), a relation attributed to an effect of TGRLs on PAI-1 concentration (Patsch and Gotto 1995). In the observational Atherosclerosis Risk in Communities (ARIC) study, elevations of apo B were higher than elevations of LDL-C in subjects with symptomatic CHD, although the lipid profiles of subjects with asymptomatic carotid disease and those with symptomatic CHD were otherwise similar (Sharrett et al. 1994). Because the ratio of apo B to LDL-C is inversely related to LDL size (see next section), the metabolism of the TGRLs and its effect on LDL and HDL structure may be particularly important in late stages of CHD (Patsch and Gotto 1995).

SMALL, DENSE LOW-DENSITY LIPOPROTEIN

Small, dense LDL and its immediate precursor, IDL, have been associated in cross-sectional studies with increased risk for CHD by clinical and angiographic indices (Austin et al. 1988; Lamarche et al. 1997; Coresh et al. 1993; Hodis et al. 1997; Mack et al. 1996; Steiner et al. 1987). In prospective studies, however, it has not been established that LDL particle size has a predictive value beyond that of TC, HDL-C, TC:HDL-C ratio, or plasma TG (Coresh and Kwiterovich 1996; Stampfer et al. 1996; Gardner et al. 1996). The association of LDL size with risk could simply reflect metabolic processes of importance in atherogenesis. On the other hand, laboratory findings indicating increased susceptibility to oxidation or decreased LDL receptor binding have fueled speculation that small LDL particles have an independent, causal role in the development of atherosclerosis.

Reflection of Metabolic State

The formation of small, dense LDL is believed to be closely related to metabolism of TGRLs (Campos et al. 1992; Deckelbaum et al. 1984) (Figure 8.3). Thus, the atherogenicity of dense LDL may be related to the broader metabolic defect of impaired TG tolerance (Ebenbichler et al. 1995) or the insulin resistance syndrome (Austin et al. 1994; Austin and Edwards 1996). A preponderance of small LDL particles, called LDL phenotype B, is associated with a more atherogenic lipoprotein profile than is a preponderance of larger LDL (type A phenotype), including higher plasma concentrations of TG, VLDL, IDL, and apo B and lower concentrations of HDL-C and apo A-I (Austin et al. 1990; Krauss 1994). Small, dense LDL or LDL phenotype B has been statistically related not only to CHD but also to conditions associated with CHD, for example, obesity, insulin resistance, and diabetes mellitus (Slyper 1994). Hyperapobetal-

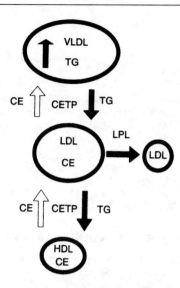

Figure 8.3. Possible mechanism for small, dense LDL formation. With increased VLDL in the circulation, increased net transfer of cholesteryl esters (CEs) by CETP leads to decreased HDL-C. In the same mechanism, the VLDL will replace the transferred CEs, and LDL will become enriched in TGs. This TG-rich LDL is subjected to the action of LPL, resulting in an LDL particle that is depleted in CEs and enriched in protein (apo B-100). (Reprinted with permission from Roheim and Asztalos 1995.)

ipoproteinemia (hyper–apo B), a familial lipoprotein disorder strongly associated with CHD, is characterized by an increase in small, dense LDL (Kwiterovich et al. 1991). An increased prevalence of small, dense LDL occurs as well in FCH (Austin 1991) and familial dyslipidemic hypertension (Hunt et al. 1989).

Direct Effects

Small lipoproteins may bind more readily to proteoglycans and enter the artery wall more easily (Rajman et al. 1994; Packard 1994; Anber et al. 1997). Dense LDL particles from normolipidemic subjects have reduced binding affinity for the LDL receptor compared with more buoyant LDL particles (Nigon et al. 1991). In vivo, smaller LDL particles are cleared from the circulation more slowly than larger LDL particles in both normal subjects and those with hyper–apo B (Teng et al. 1986). With a longer residence in plasma, there may be prolonged exposure to free radical oxidation and easier particle uptake by means of mechanisms not mediated by the LDL receptor (Rajman et al. 1994). Furthermore, denser LDL particles are more susceptible to oxidation in vitro than more buoyant LDL particles (Packard 1994; Nigon et al. 1991).

LIPOPROTEIN [a]

A number of case-control and cross-sectional studies, most of them retrospective, have shown a strong positive association between CHD risk and the plasma concentration of Lp[a] (Maher and Brown 1995; Howard and Pizzo 1993), a lipoprotein identical to LDL except for the addition of apo[a]. The physiologic function of Lp[a] is not known.

Prothrombotic Mechanisms

Given the extensive sequence homology between apo[a] and plasminogen (Eaton et al. 1987; McLean et al. 1987), it has been suggested that much of the atherogenic potential of Lp[a] derives from interference in normal pathways of thrombolysis, to predispose patients to acute thrombotic complications. Prothrombotic effects of Lp[a] include interference with the activation of plasminogen and with its binding to endothelial cells, monocytes, fibrin, and thrombospondin; interference with the binding of tissue plasminogen activator to fibrin; and stimulation of the synthesis of PAI-1 (reviewed by Stein and Rosenson 1997; Chapmann et al. 1994; Loscalzo 1990).

Other Mechanisms

Other hypotheses include a role for Lp[a] in cholesterol delivery to the injured vessel wall and stimulation of vascular cell proliferation (Hajjar and Nachman 1996). Pathologic and laboratory evidence includes observations that Lp[a] binds lipoproteins containing apo B, avidly binds to arterial proteoglycans and fibronectin, accumulates in atherosclerotic lesions, stimulates SMC proliferation, and promotes cholesterol accumulation in cells (reviewed by Maher and Brown 1995). With oxidation or modification by malondialdehyde, Lp[a] becomes a ligand, both in vitro and in vivo, for the scavenger receptor (De Rijke et al. 1992; Haberland et al. 1992; Naruszewicze et al. 1994), and macrophage foam cells may express a distinct Lp[a] clearance receptor (Keesler et al. 1994). Vascular lesions induced by a lipid-rich diet were increased 30 times in area in transgenic mice expressing human apo[a] compared with control mice (Lawn et al. 1992). Thus, Lp[a] might interfere with the normal degradation of cholesterol by way of the LDL receptor or itself be targeted to early atherosclerotic lesions, possibly through the macrophage scavenger receptor (Hajjar and Nachman 1996).

The interaction of Lp[a] with the vascular endothelial barrier has been reviewed by Nordestgaard (1996). Lp[a] appears to enter the intima at about the same rate as LDL but may be retained there to a greater extent, particularly at sites of injury.

Possible Risk Dependence on Low-Density Lipoprotein

Recent post hoc analyses of angiographic clinical trial data have suggested that a concomitantly high LDL-C concentration is required for Lp[a] to exert its most adverse effects. In FATS (see Table 10.1), Lp[a] concentration was a dominant predictor of baseline angiographic CHD severity, its progression, and the clinical event rate in men with elevated LDL-C but lost its predictive value in patients in whom LDL-C was substantially reduced (Maher et al. 1995). In FHRS, lowering both Lp[a] and LDL-C achieved no greater angiographic benefit than lowering LDL-C alone (Thompson et al. 1995). Maher and Brown (1995) analyzed the results of a number of case-control studies and found the odds ratio for developing CHD in patients with high (>30 mg/dL) or low (<10 mg/dL) Lp[a] to be a strong function of concomitant LDL-C concentration. It had previously been shown that transgenic mice expressing human apo[a] developed vascular lesions only when fed a lipid-rich diet, not when fed normal chow (Lawn et al. 1992). In a case-control study (Armstrong et al. 1986), the odds ratio for having substantial angiographic CHD in patients with high (>30 mg/dL) versus low (≤5 mg/dL) Lp[a] concentrations increased from 1.67 to 6.0 as concomitant LDL-C increased.

Maher and Brown (1995) have suggested several possible mechanisms for these findings, including Lp[a] and LDL aggregate formation (which would prolong their intimal residence time), the propensity of both particles to bind arterial wall proteoglycans, and entrapment in the artery intima of LDL by proteoglycan-bound Lp[a] particles with free apo[a] chains. The last speculation arises because the apo B component of Lp[a] binds proteoglycans more avidly than its apo[a] component.

SMOKING

Smoking doubles to quadruples the risk for CHD events (Lakier 1992), and the risk is synergistically compounded by hypertension, hypercholesterolemia, glucose intolerance, or diabetes (Lakier 1992). The pathophysiologic mechanisms underlying contributions of smoking to CHD are complex and incompletely understood. It is believed that cigarette smoke plays a role not only in the development of atherosclerosis but also as an initiator or accelerator of coronary events such as MI, angina pectoris, sudden cardiac death, and arrhythmias regardless of the extent of coronary atherosclerosis (Rigotti and Pasternak 1996; Tresch and Aronow 1996). The presence and extent of atherosclerosis in all vascular beds are quantitatively related to smoking (McBride 1992; Rigotti and Pasternak 1996). Smoking appears to accelerate the atherogenic process in both dose-dependent and duration-dependent manners, in particular in the medium-sized and large vascular beds (McGill 1988; Rigotti and Pasternak 1996).

Effects on atherogenesis may be mediated at least in part by the promotion of platelet aggregation and fibrinolytic activity and by a rise in shear stress from increased heart rate and blood pressure (McBride 1992). Increases in plasma fibrinogen reflect the number of cigarettes smoked (Eliasson et al. 1995) and have been described by cross-sectional data in passive smokers (Iso et al. 1996). Smoking just two cigarettes increases platelet activation more than 100 times (Pittilo et al. 1984). In an autopsy study in men, Burke et al. (1997) found that cigarette smoking was a risk factor in 75% of men with acute thrombosis in a coronary artery, compared with 22% of men with stable plaque (see Chapter 7 for a discussion of stable and unstable plaque).

Smoking elicits acute insulin resistance and smokers exhibit several other characteristics of the insulin resistance syndrome, including increases in blood pressure, fibrinogen, PAI-1 activity, and serum glucose (Eliasson et al. 1994, 1997; Facchini et al. 1992; Porkka and Ehnholm 1996).

Lipid Effects

Meta-analysis by Craig et al. (1989) of 54 published studies showed plasma TC, LDL-C, TG, and VLDL-C concentrations to be significantly higher and HDL-C and apo A-I to be significantly lower in smokers than in nonsmokers (Figure 8.4). A dose-response relation was seen between smoking (light, moderate, or heavy) and concentration for all these variables. In addition, concentrations of FFAs are higher in smokers (McBride 1992). The increase in sympathetic nervous system activity caused by smoking leads to increases in circulating catecholamines (Cryer et al. 1976), which in turn increase lipolysis. Enhanced lipolysis leads to elevated plasma FFA and enhanced hepatic extraction, and hence increased VLDL secretion. Significantly decreased HDL-C has been demonstrated in adults and in dyslipidemic and healthy children and adolescents exposed to second-hand cigarette smoke (Feldman et al. 1991; Moffatt et al. 1995; Moskowitz et al. 1990; Neufeld et al. 1997). Smokers may have higher postheparin hepatic lipase activity (Eliasson et al. 1997).

Smoking is also associated with increased proportions of small, dense LDL particles (Eliasson et al. 1997). Axelsen et al. (1995) found that, compared with nonsmokers, smokers had 50% higher postprandial increases in serum TG without a difference in effect on fasting TG ($N = 22$), which suggests that smokers may have impaired lipolytic removal capacity (Porkka and Ehnholm 1996). Decreased plasma clearance of chylomicrons and chylomicron remnants has been shown in rats exposed to smoke (Pan et al. 1997). The metabolic disturbances of FCH resemble those induced by smoking, and environmental factors such as smoking influence the phenotype in both FCH and nonfamilial combined hyperlipidemia (Porkka and Ehnholm 1996). In addition, smoking appears to modify LDL particles oxidatively and to make them more susceptible to oxidation by other agents (Harats et al. 1989; Rigotti and Pasternak 1996).

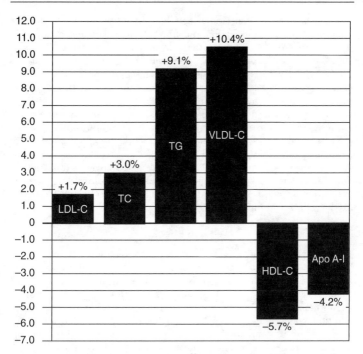

Figure 8.4. Effects of smoking on lipid concentrations, from a pooled analysis of 54 published studies (all values *P* <.001 vs. nonsmokers). Effects in heavy smokers only were TC, +4.5%; LDL-C, +11.0%; TG, +18.0%; VLDL-C, +39.0%; HDL-C, –8.9%; and apo A-I, –5.7%. Increased TG and decreased HDL-C are aspects of the insulin resistance syndrome, a syndrome that may play an important role in the high risk for death from CVD among smokers. (Data from Craig et al. 1989.)

Nicotine

Current data suggest that nicotine is less important than the effects of carbon monoxide or the prothrombotic effects of smoking in contributing to acute cardiovascular events. Animal and mechanistic studies suggest that nicotine may play a role in the development of atherosclerosis, but relevance in humans has not been shown (Benowitz 1997).

The major cardiovascular effect of nicotine is sympathetic neural stimulation. The carotid chemoreceptor appears to be very sensitive to nicotine even at low concentrations. Nicotine stimulates catecholamine release from the adrenals and stimulates direct release or enhances release of catecholamines from vascular nerve endings (Benowitz and Gourlay 1997).

The hemodynamic effects of cigarette smoking may be mediated by nicotine. Nicotine delivered intravenously or through spray or gum raises blood pressure as much as 5–10 mm Hg and speeds the heart rate as much as 10–15 beats per minute, which are responses similar to those seen with cigarette smoking. Transdermal nicotine appears to have lesser hemodynamic effects (Benowitz and Gourlay 1997). Nicotine increases cardiac output by increasing myocardial contractility and heart rate. Even low-dose nicotine can constrict coronary arteries in humans (Benowitz and Gourlay 1997). Individuals with unstable coronary disease may be at risk for larger MIs because of the effects of nicotine on the coronary circulation (McKenzie et al. 1985). Nicotine's enhancement of the release of acetylcholine, serotonin, nitric oxide, calcitonin growth-related peptide, and vasopressin may contribute to effects on blood vessels (Benowitz and Gourlay 1997).

Dietary Risk

Smokers versus nonsmokers have been found to have lower intakes of some nutrients, such as vitamin C, vitamin E, beta-carotene, folic acid, thiamine, calcium, magnesium, and fiber (Bolton-Smith et al. 1991; Cade and Margetts 1991; D'Avanzo et al. 1997; English et al. 1997; Koo 1997; Larkin et al. 1990; Subar et al. 1990); a lower ratio of polyunsaturated to saturated fat (Cade and Margetts 1991); and higher cholesterol intake (Larkin et al. 1990). Baseline data from the Multiple Risk Factor Intervention Trial (MRFIT) showed fat intake to relate directly to cigarette smoking (Tillotson et al. 1997). In addition, there is a significant relation between smoking and excessive alcohol use (English et al. 1997). Plasma concentrations of the antioxidants vitamins C and E and beta-carotene are also lower in smokers (Bolton-Smith et al. 1991; Preston 1991). Smokers appear to require more vitamin C daily than nonsmokers, by at least 60 mg/day and up to 140 mg/day to prevent hypovitaminosis (Weber et al. 1996b). The U.S. recommended dietary allowance for ascorbic acid in smokers is 100 mg/day, compared with 60 mg/day for nonsmokers.

HYPERTENSION

The strong and independent positive relation between SBP and DBP levels and cardiovascular risk is continuous, graded, and etiologically significant (National Institutes of Health 1997). In MRFIT follow-up data, the relative risk for CHD events progressively increased from 1.0 (reference) in those with SBP of less than 120 mm Hg and DBP of less than 80 mm Hg (optimal) to 3.23 in those with an isolated increase of DBP to 100 mm Hg or higher, to 4.19 in those with an isolated increase of SBP to 160 mm Hg or higher, and to 4.57 in those with SBP of 160 mm Hg or higher plus DBP of 100 mm Hg or higher (Stamler et al. 1993a). Meta-analysis of nine prospective observational studies showed the risk for

CHD events and stroke to be increased 5 and 10 times, respectively, with an increase in DBP from 76 to 105 mm Hg (MacMahon et al. 1990). Hypertensive patients frequently have atherosclerosis of the epicardial coronary arteries (World Health Organization 1996). There may be a particularly important role for the cardiovascular angiotensin-generating system in the occurrence of both hypertension and MI; candidate genes investigated that could be responsible for both conditions include the ACE, angiotensinogen, and angiotensin receptor genes (Rakugi et al. 1996). It has been estimated that approximately 50% of the variance in human blood pressure can be explained by about five genes; however, phenotypic expression of essential hypertension is modulated by environmental factors (Frohlich and Re 1998).

How hypertension participates in the development of atherosclerosis is still poorly understood. Atherosclerosis is rare in low-pressure areas in the vascular tree unless those areas are exposed to systemic pressure (e.g., absence in veins unless veins are used in coronary artery bypass grafting or arteriovenous shunts; pulmonary artery atheroma when the artery's pressure is elevated) (Srikanthan and Dunn 1997). Possible mechanisms described for the relation between hypertension and atherosclerosis are complex. Insulin resistance has been suggested to link glucose intolerance, hypertension, and dyslipidemia with accelerated atherosclerosis (Reaven 1988, 1995; Ferrannini et al. 1987; Kaplan 1989) (see Figure 8.5). Endothelial dysfunction, including increased permeability, and an increase of mechanical stress on blood vessels have been reported to be induced by hypertension, and their contribution to atherosclerosis progression has been investigated (Rakugi et al. 1996). Autonomic nervous imbalance may also play an important role in hypertension and MI. Vascular endothelial dysfunction in hypertension is viewed as likely a consequence rather than a cause of hypertension (Vanhoutte 1996; Noll et al. 1997).

Hypertension Syndrome

Weber (1994) emphasizes that the key to understanding the role of hypertension in CHD risk is a realization that hypertension rarely exists as isolated high blood pressure. Some of the metabolic and cardiovascular abnormalities that cluster with hypertension include insulin resistance, dyslipidemias (which act synergistically with hypertension to increase CHD risk), truncal obesity, microalbuminuria, increased activity of coagulation factors, reduced arterial compliance, and hypertrophy and altered diastolic function of the left ventricle (Weber 1994). Many of the components appear to be inherited. Plasma cholesterol is significantly higher in normotensive offspring of hypertensive parents than in controls without a family history of hypertension (Neutel et al. 1992). It has been reported that 40% of individuals with high blood pressure have unequivocal plasma lipid abnormalities, and another 40% have borderline plasma lipid changes (Joint National Committee 1993). The disorder originally described in

Utah families as familial dyslipidemic hypertension entails elevated plasma TG, low HDL-C, and/or elevated LDL-C concentrations (Hunt et al. 1989). Blood pressure levels correlate among family members, attributable to a common genetic background or shared environmental factors (National Institutes of Health 1997).

DIABETES MELLITUS

Diabetes mellitus increases risk for CHD 2 to 4 times (Garcia et al. 1974; Assmann and Schulte 1988; Stamler et al. 1993b), and atherosclerosis is rapidly progressive. Macrovascular complications are encountered more often in type 2 than in type 1 diabetes. The high prevalence and rapid progression result from multiple causes, as reviewed by Schneider and Sobel (1997) and Bierman (1992). Although multiple risk factors such as hypertension, dyslipidemia, and visceral obesity are common in adults with type 2 diabetes, they do not account for all the increased risk in diabetes. At 12-year follow-up in MRFIT (Stamler et al. 1993b), the absolute risk for cardiovascular death was much higher for diabetic than nondiabetic men at every age and risk factor level, and risk increased more steeply in the diabetic men as risk factor levels increased.

Associations with insulin resistance, including dyslipidemia (typically increased plasma TG, decreased HDL-C, and a higher proportion of small, dense LDL), changes in fibrinolytic and coagulation factors, and possible direct deleterious effects of insulin are described in "Insulin Resistance Syndrome," later. It is unknown which, if any, of the risk factors that have been described as clustering in association with insulin resistance increase the CVD rate in type 2 diabetes. Concentrations of postprandial lipoproteins are increased in type 2 diabetes. Increased supplies of FFAs and glucose contribute to overproduction of VLDL; the increased FFAs, which inhibit lipolysis, and reduced LPL activity further impair lipolysis of postprandial lipoproteins (De Man et al. 1996). In addition, clearance of remnants of TGRLs is delayed in diabetes; evidence supports a relative hepatic removal defect secondary to impaired remnant-receptor interaction and increased competition with VLDL remnants (De Man et al. 1996). Increased procoagulant activity, decreased anticoagulant activity, increased platelet aggregation, and decreased fibrinolytic activity in diabetes are in sum likely to predispose to atherothrombosis (Schneider and Sobel 1997); among changes described are increased PAI-1 (McGill et al. 1994; Vague et al. 1986), factor VIII (both antigen and coagulant activity), fibrinogen (Kannel et al. 1990; Pasi et al. 1990), and platelet aggregability and hypercoagulability (Hamet et al. 1985).

Potential mechanisms related to hyperglycemia (Schneider and Sobel 1997) include toxic effects on endothelial cells that can lead to glycosylation of proteins through nonenzymatic linkage of glucose to proteins (glycation) and production of advanced glycation end-products (AGEs) (Brownlee 1994); reduced endothelium-mediated vascular reactivity and activated protein kinase C (Tesfamariam et al. 1991); and enhanced production of collagen IV and fibronectin by endothelial cells (Cagliero et al. 1991). AGEs accumulated in the artery wall increase binding of nonglycated LDL (Vlassara 1994) and promote monocyte chemotaxis, production of growth factors and cytokines, and SMC proliferation (Vlassara 1994; Brownlee 1994). Foam cell formation and platelet aggregation are stimulated by glycation of apo B (Lyons et al. 1993). Moreover, in diabetes, LDL particles are more prone to oxidation (Bucala et al. 1993; Lyons et al. 1993; Vlassara 1994) and Lp[a] concentrations have been described as increased (Ramirez et al. 1992).

INSULIN RESISTANCE SYNDROME

Hyperinsulinemia and Insulin Resistance

Whether hyperinsulinemia is a risk factor for CHD is controversial. There is no consensus that it contributes significantly to risk in the same way as hypercholesterolemia, smoking, or hypertension (Laakso 1996); in a continuing debate, strong arguments both for (Stout 1996) and against (Jarrett 1994) are made on the basis of fairly limited data. No study has shown a relation between insulin concentration and clinical CHD in women (Haffner 1997). Prospective data are not available on the relation between CHD and insulin resistance (i.e., a decrease in the effect of insulin to stimulate glucose uptake normally at a given insulin concentration) (Laakso 1996; Haffner 1997). Whether or to what degree the epidemiologic data available regarding hyperinsulinemia illuminate risk associations with insulin resistance is unclear; fasting and postglucose insulin concentrations correlate with insulin sensitivity determined by the euglycemic clamp technique, which is expensive and limited by patient acceptance, but the correlation does not exceed 0.60–0.70 (Laakso 1993). Increased insulin generally reflects insulin resistance in nondiabetic subjects, and fasting (but not postglucose) insulin may still be a reasonable surrogate in type 2 diabetes (Haffner 1997). Prospective studies have consistently shown insulin resistance and hyperinsulinemia to be strong predictors of type 2 diabetes mellitus (Haffner 1997), although there is a strong view that a primary or secondary defect in beta cells is also required to cause type 2 diabetes (Chisholm et al. 1991, 1997).

Direct mechanisms by which insulin could participate in the development of atherosclerosis (Stout 1990) have been described, including mitogenic properties (Sowers et al. 1993), particularly on vascular SMCs, and inhibition of endogenous fibrinolysis. Insulin has been shown to prevent regression of diet-induced lesions in animals (Stout 1990). These physiologic observations may not be considered as strong an argument as in the case of some other factors and often were made in experiments using supraphysiologic concentrations of insulin (Laakso 1996). Baron

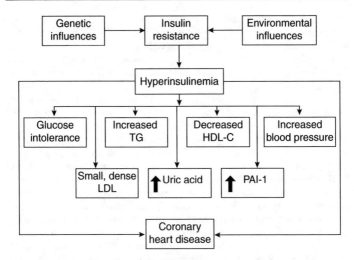

Figure 8.5. Insulin resistance syndrome. Schematic description of proposed relation between resistance to insulin-mediated glucose disposal, compensatory hyperinsulinemia, multiple consequences, and CHD. (Redrawn with permission from Reaven 1995. The American Physiological Society.)

(1996) assembled data to suggest that obesity/insulin resistance is associated with endothelial dysfunction.

Clustering of Risk Factors

Although controversy surrounds roles for hyperinsulinemia and insulin resistance per se in CHD risk, there is some consensus that insulin resistance and a variety of CHD risk factors tend to cluster in individuals. Reaven, in 1988, described this clustering as syndrome X and proposed insulin resistance as the fundamental defect; the syndrome is now commonly referred to as insulin resistance syndrome to highlight that proposed etiology (Haffner et al. 1992). (The metabolic syndrome X is distinct from the cardiologic syndrome X of symptoms and electrocardiographic evidence of CHD in the absence of significant angiographic coronary stenosis.) Reaven's initial description of the insulin resistance syndrome included resistance to insulin-stimulated glucose uptake, glucose intolerance, compensatory hyperinsulinemia, increased plasma TG activity representing VLDL TG, decreased HDL-C, and hypertension. To these basic components have been added other metabolic abnormalities, including smaller, denser LDL particles, hyperuricemia, microalbuminuria, and increased circulating concentrations of fibrinogen and PAI-1

(Reaven 1993, 1995; Laakso 1996). Reaven's hypothesis is that insulin resistance plays a role in the development of these changes, and the cluster of abnormalities increases risk for CHD, as illustrated in Figure 8.5. It must be emphasized, however, that no causal relation has been established between insulin resistance and any of these problems (Chisholm et al. 1997).

Other factors have been proposed as the "hub of the wheel," for example, visceral obesity (Hopkins et al. 1996) (see "Visceral Obesity," later). Other clusters that may represent the same syndrome or closely related disorders include not only visceral fat syndrome but also familial dyslipidemic hypertension, atherogenic lipoprotein phenotype, impaired TG tolerance, metabolic syndrome, the deadly quartet, hyper–apo B, and FCH (Hopkins et al. 1996; Sniderman et al. 1998). Reaven (1995) rejects terms that make reference to environmental factors (e.g., the deadly quartet comprises upper-body obesity, glucose intolerance, hypertriglyceridemia, and hypertension), not because he discounts the increased frequency with obesity, a sedentary lifestyle, or smoking, but because all the clinical features of the syndrome as he has defined it can be independent of these factors. Regardless of whether insulin resistance itself predisposes to CHD or gives rise to the other components of the syndrome, many of the clustered components are themselves risk factors for atherosclerosis, thrombosis, or both.

VISCERAL OBESITY

Recent analyses and evidence have increasingly supported a causal role for obesity in CHD. In particular, a strong link has been reported for deposition of adipose tissue in the abdomen (Garrison et al. 1996). Although intra-abdominal fat accounts for less than 20% of body fat, it is a major determinant of fasting and postprandial lipid availability because of its physiologic (lipolytic rate and insulin resistance) and anatomic (portal drainage) properties (Carey 1998). Risk for type 2 diabetes and CVD may relate closely to the inheritance of central obesity and susceptibility to lipotoxicity (Carey 1998). Carey (1998) has reviewed evidence that the phenotypic expression of adult obesity can be identified in children aged 6–10 years, with increases in abdominal fat probably beginning then as well. Also as reviewed by Carey, visceral obesity and the clustering of risk factors seen in insulin resistance syndrome may be fully expressed by adolescence (Caprio et al. 1996), and young adult men with increased visceral fat, although apparently healthy, may have cardiac pathology (Kortelainen 1996; Kortelainen and Sarkioja 1997).

Precise measurement of body fat by magnetic resonance imaging, computed tomography (CT), and other techniques has shown a powerful relation between central abdominal fat and insulin resistance, stronger than the moderate links seen with BMI or waist:hip ratio

(Chisholm et al. 1997). Chisholm et al. (1997) noted that Matsuzawa and colleagues (Yamashita et al. 1996; Matsuzawa et al. 1990), by using such techniques, demonstrated striking differences in intra-abdominal fat between sumo wrestlers active in competition and retired sumo wrestlers, with concomitant changes in insulin sensitivity and lipid concentrations. In men who were not overweight according to BMI, visceral fat area determined by CT was significantly higher in subjects with CHD (Nakamura et al. 1994), and the amount of visceral fat according to ultrasound examination significantly correlated with fasting insulin and with ultrasound-determined carotid intimal–medial thickness (Yamamoto et al. 1997). Estimation by sagittal abdominal diameter may offer a reasonably good alternative to measurement of intra-abdominal fat by CT (Hopkins et al. 1996).

Metabolic Profile

Increased visceral fat correlates strongly with an adverse metabolic profile, including hyperinsulinemia, decreased glucose tolerance, dyslipidemia, and increased blood pressure (Peiris et al. 1989). Insulin hypersecretion and insulin resistance are established features of obesity (Ferrannini et al. 1997). Abdominal fat influences insulin sensitivity even in healthy nonobese people (Carey 1998; Carey et al. 1996; Park et al. 1991). The lipoprotein abnormalities are characteristically increased VLDL, IDL, and small, dense LDL with elevated apo B, and decreased HDL_{2b}, that is, the patterns seen in FCH, type 2 diabetes, and the insulin resistance syndrome (Kissebah 1996; Peeples et al. 1989; Terry et al. 1989; Austin et al. 1992). In obese individuals, increases in VLDL and apo B are common; increases in VLDL-TG and apo B turnover are proportional, leading to increased VLDL secretion. In individuals with hypertriglyceridemia, a defect in VLDL-TG removal is also present. The pronounced hyperinsulinemia in individuals with upper-body obesity supports the VLDL overproduction and increased LDL turnover (Kissebah 1996).

A number of authors, such as Matsuzawa et al. (1995) and Hopkins et al. (1996), consider visceral obesity the main mediator in the metabolic syndrome. Carmelli et al. (1994) examined the clustering of hypertension, diabetes, and obesity by applying multivariate genetic methods analogous to path analysis and found an underlying latent factor to mediate the best model. Hopkins et al. (1996) note that the latent factor could conceivably be the "thrifty genotype," postulated as early as 1962, in which rapid accumulation of fat, in particular visceral fat, would occur in times of plentiful food.

Recent research indicates that adipocytes regulate energy metabolism through endocrine and paracrine mechanisms (Hwang et al. 1997). They secrete biologically active molecules, including TNF-α, which interferes with insulin signaling, and leptin, which regulates energy intake and expenditure (Hotamisligil et al. 1996; Zhang et al. 1994). Overexpression of TNF-α has been reported in obese subjects, and adipocytokines may have important roles in the development of both metabolic diseases and vascular changes (Matsuzawa 1997). TNF-α has received much attention because of its potential to cause features of insulin resistance (Hopkins et al. 1996).

Cortisol secretion is increased in subjects with central obesity, probably because of increased activity of the hypothalamic-pituitary-adrenal axis (Björntorp 1995). A high waist-to-hip ratio is correlated with decreased production of sex steroids (e.g., testosterone in men) and decreased secretion of growth hormone, and visceral fat decreases when hormone levels are normalized. A mild hyperandrogenism is often present in women with visceral obesity (Björntorp 1996). The combined effect of the abnormalities may be lipid accumulation. Smoking, alcohol, psychosocial stress, and anxiety may contribute to the endocrine abnormalities that promote visceral fat deposition (Björntorp 1995). The endocrine perturbations appear to lead to centralization of body fat in visceral depots because of the high density of steroid hormone receptors (Björntorp 1996); that is, the metabolic derangements are perpetuated (Kopelman and Albon 1997). Hemostatic and hemorheologic parameters reported to be disadvantageously affected by abdominal obesity include higher fibrinogen, factor VII, PAI-1, blood and plasma viscosity, and erythrocyte aggregability and lower erythrocyte deformability compared with peripheral obesity or absence of obesity (Solerte et al. 1997; Avellone et al. 1994).

ESTROGEN

Premenopausal women have a low incidence of vascular events (Lerner and Kannel 1986), and meta-analysis of observational epidemiologic data shows that postmenopausal estrogen supplementation in women reduces the risk for CHD by 35% (Grady et al. 1992) to 44% (Stampfer and Colditz 1991). Data on estrogen replacement are conflicting regarding stroke (in particular subarachnoid hemorrhage) (Paganini-Hill 1995) but do support a significant reduction in all-cause mortality rate (Schairer et al. 1997; Ettinger et al. 1996). However, data from large, randomized prospective trials are required to substantiate the benefit of estrogen replacement in lowering risk for CHD; such trials under way include a trial that is part of the Women's Health Initiative of the U.S. National Institutes of Health. The first such data available, from HERS (Hulley et al. 1998), showed increased CHD events in the first year of estrogen-progestin therapy in women with CHD, with decreased event rates in years 4 and 5 (see Chapter 18).

The apparent cardioprotective role for estrogen has prompted intensive investigation of possible antiatherogenic mechanisms. Evidence suggests at least two major mechanisms: a beneficial effect on the plasma lipid profile and direct effects on the vascular wall (Nathan and Chaudhuri 1997; Vischer 1997; Chae et al. 1997; Subbiah 1998; Wild 1996).

Lipid Effects

Estrogen appears to regulate lipoprotein metabolism at multiple regulatory points, as does progesterone (Kushwaha 1992). It is well established, including by prospective data from the large Postmenopausal Estrogen/Progestin Interventions (PEPI) trial, that oral estrogens usually increase HDL-C and decrease LDL-C (Barrett-Connor et al. 1997; PEPI Writing Group 1995; Nabulsi et al. 1993; Kushwaha 1992; Walsh et al. 1991; Miller et al. 1991b), by about 10–15% in either case. Other beneficial lipid effects include increasing plasma apo A-I, decreasing plasma apo B concentrations (Walsh et al. 1991), and decreasing Lp[a] activity (Darling et al. 1997; Taskinen et al. 1996; Nabulsi et al. 1993; Soma et al. 1993). In addition, however, oral estrogens may significantly increase plasma TG and, perhaps through that mechanism, reduce the size of LDL particles (Wakatsuki et al. 1997; Kushwaha 1992). It has been argued that the TG increase is possibly without atherogenic consequences because it appears to be through the production of large, TG-rich VLDL with reduced cholesterol content (Walsh et al. 1991; Appelbaum-Bowden et al. 1989), although that distinction does not militate against risk for pancreatitis from very high plasma TG.

The lipid changes appear to occur with an increased rate of removal of chylomicron remnants by the liver, increased VLDL secretion by the liver, increased hepatic uptake of VLDL remnants, increased uptake of LDL by the up-regulated LDL receptor, increased synthesis of apo A-I, and increased bile acid secretion to remove cholesterol from the body (Wild 1996).

Nonlipid Effects

Beyond its effects on plasma lipid concentrations, estrogen may act at several steps to prevent atherosclerosis, as has been well reviewed by Nathan and Chaudhuri (1997). Among described effects are direct inhibition of SMC proliferation (Farhat et al. 1996), inhibition of endothelial cell expression of adhesion molecules (Caulin-Glaser et al. 1996; Wild 1996), reduced accumulation of cholesteryl esters in macrophages (St. Clair 1997), alteration of vasoreactivity, and promotion of vasodilation (Nathan and Chaudhuri 1997; Gilligan et al. 1994; Volterrani et al. 1995; Krasinski et al. 1997). A beneficial effect through coagulation components has been suggested (Wild 1996), and estrogen has been shown to decrease fibrinogen concentration significantly (PEPI Writing Group 1995). Other studies, however, have shown estrogen to have procoagulant effects (Caine et al. 1992), and recent studies have reported increased early risk for venous thromboembolism with hormone replacement (Suissa et al. 1997). Additional suggested mechanisms for benefit include a role as an antioxidant (Chae et al. 1997; Subbiah 1998), an ability to protect against DNA damage (Subbiah 1998), and improvement in insulin sensitivity (Chae et al. 1997).

Suggested Reading

Austin MA, Edwards KL. Small, dense low density lipoproteins, the insulin resistance syndrome and non-insulin-dependent diabetes (review). Curr Opin Lipidol 1996;7:167–171.

Barter PJ, Rye K-A. High density lipoproteins and coronary heart disease (review). Atherosclerosis 1996;121:1–12.

Benowitz NL, Gourlay SG. Cardiovascular toxicity of nicotine: implications for nicotine replacement therapy. J Am Coll Cardiol 1997;29:1422–1431.

Bierman EL. Atherogenesis in diabetes. Arterioscler Thromb 1992;12: 647–656.

Coresh J, Kwiterovich PO Jr. Small, dense low-density lipoprotein particles and coronary heart disease risk: a clear association with uncertain implications (editorial). JAMA 1996;276:914–915.

Davignon J, Cohn JS. Triglycerides: a risk factor for coronary heart disease (review). Atherosclerosis 1996;124(suppl):S57–S64.

Ebenbichler CF, Kirchmair R, Egger C, Patsch JR. Postprandial state and atherosclerosis (review). Curr Opin Lipidol 1995;6:286–290.

Hajjar KA, Nachman RL. The role of lipoprotein(a) in atherogenesis and thrombosis. Annu Rev Med 1996;47:423–442.

Hopkins PN, Hunt SC, Wu LL, et al. Hypertension, dyslipidemia, and insulin resistance: links in a chain or spokes on a wheel? Curr Opin Lipidol 1996; 7:241–253.

Jarrett RJ. Why is insulin *not* a risk factor for coronary heart disease? Diabetologia 1994;37:945–947.

Kissebah AH. Intra-abdominal fat: is it a major factor in developing diabetes and coronary artery disease? Diabetes Res Clin Pract 1996;30(suppl): S25–S30.

Krauss RM. Heterogeneity of plasma low-density lipoproteins and atherosclerosis risk. Curr Opin Lipidol 1994;5:339–349.

Maher VMG, Brown BG. Lipoprotein (a) and coronary heart disease. Curr Opin Lipidol 1995;6:229–235.

McBride PE. The health consequences of smoking. Med Clin North Am 1992; 76:333–353.

Nathan L, Chaudhuri G. Estrogens and atherosclerosis (review). Annu Rev Pharmacol Toxicol 1997;37:477–515.

Patsch W, Gotto AM Jr. High-density lipoprotein cholesterol, plasma triglyceride, and coronary heart disease: pathophysiology and management (review). Adv Pharmacol 1995;32:375–427.

Rakugi H, Yu H, Kamitani A, et al. Links between hypertension and myocardial infarction (review). Am Heart J 1996;132:213–221.

Reaven GM. Pathophysiology of insulin resistance in human disease (review). Physiol Rev 1995;75:473–486.

Rigotti NA, Pasternak RC. Cigarette smoking and coronary heart disease: risks and management. Cardiol Clin 1996;14:51–68.

Schneider DJ, Sobel BE. Determinants of coronary vascular disease in patients with type II diabetes mellitus and their therapeutic implications (review). Clin Cardiol 1997;20:433–440.

Slyper AH. Low-density lipoprotein density and atherosclerosis: unraveling the connection. JAMA 1994;272:305–308.

Stein JH, Rosensen RS. Lipoprotein Lp(a) excess and coronary heart disease (review). Arch Intern Med 1997;157:1170–1176.

Tresch DD, Aronow WS. Smoking and coronary artery disease. Clin Geriatr Med 1996;12:23–32.

Weber MA. Coronary heart disease and hypertension. Am J Hypertens 1994;7:146S–153S.

Zilversmit DB. Atherogenic nature of triglycerides, postprandial lipidemia, and triglyceride-rich lipoproteins. Clin Chem 1995;41:153–158.

Chapter 9

Other Hypotheses, Allograft Coronary Heart Disease, and Restenosis

Although the overall cascade of events outlined in Chapter 6 represents the prevalent view of atherogenesis, some investigators would weight potential factors differently. Here, we briefly review more controversial hypotheses, which propose that atherosclerosis is chiefly an autoimmune or monoclonal response or which assign a central role to infectious agents. Also highlighted in this chapter are two important processes that are pathophysiologically distinct from de novo atherosclerosis and that narrow coronary arteries: allograft CHD, in which the immune response appears to be of major significance, and restenosis occuring after angioplasty.

ROLES FOR IMMUNOLOGIC MEDIATION

The idea that cellular components of the immune system are involved in atherosclerosis was recognized fairly recently, and an increasing amount of evidence supports such an idea (for a detailed review see Hansson 1997; Libby and Hansson 1991; George et al. 1996; Witztum and Palinski 1996). Atherosclerosis has several similarities with chronic inflammation, characterized by monocyte and T cell infiltration, immunoglobulin–complement deposition, and lipid accumulation (Metzler and Xu 1997). The pathways are extremely complex. The fairly profound humoral- and cell-mediated responses suggested by data obtained to date may modulate the atherogenic process in both positive and negative ways (Witztum and Hörkkö 1997). Studies in animal models have yielded evidence for both protective and pathologic effects: For example, studies in Watanabe and cholesterol-fed rabbits show that immunization with oxLDL significantly reduces atherosclerotic lesion formation (Palinski et al. 1995; Ameli et al. 1996), and immunization with a heat shock protein elicits atherosclerosis in normocholesterolemic rabbits (Xu et al. 1992, 1993a; see later). Such studies support in a very preliminary fashion the hypothesis that immunomodulation/immunoprevention might provide a useful therapeutic approach in atherosclerotic diseases.

A variety of immune factors have been found in human atherosclerotic lesions, among them adhesion molecules (ICAM-1, VCAM-1), CD3, CD40, CD40L, the T cell subsets CD4+ and CD8+, immunoglobulin G (IgG), IFN-γ, interleukins (IL-1, IL-10, IL-12, IL-2R/CD25), leukocyte function–associated molecule #1, major histocompatibility complex (MHC) class II, monocyte chemoattractant protein 1, inducible nitric oxide synthase, T cell antigen receptor, TGF-β, TNF-α, and very late antigen 1 (Hansson 1997). IgG is produced by plasma cells, and the other factors are produced variously by endothelial cells, SMCs, macrophages, and T cells. Functions vary; among them are antigen recognition, adhesion, recognition of MHCs, antigen presentation, T cell activation, costimulation, proinflammation, and anti-inflammation. T cells and macrophages are found in a ratio of about 1 to 8 in human fatty streaks (Munro et al. 1987), and advanced human plaques include SMCs, macrophages, and T cells (Hansson 1997). Cytokines secreted by activated T cells may control macrophage activation, metalloproteinase secretion, and scavenger receptor expression, and cytokines secreted by T cells and macrophages induce endothelial activation and modulate SMC proliferation, apoptosis (programmed cell death), and production of nitric oxide (an important mediator of inflammation) (Hansson 1997).

Molecular genetic characterization of T cell clones originating in atherosclerotic lesions showed the cells to be heterogeneous with regard to antigen receptor gene organization, indicating that they are derived from multiple progenitors and respond to different antigenic epitopes (Hansson 1994; Stemme et al. 1991). Thus, a fairly large immune repertoire would be expected in atherosclerosis, with T cells specific for a variety of antigenic epitopes, some of which might be generated by oxidation (and/or within heat shock proteins). A speculative interpretation by Hansson of how immunologic factors interact in the induction of atherosclerosis is shown in Figure 9.1.

POSSIBLE INITIATORS OF AUTOIMMUNITY

The inflammatory process in the early stages of lesion development may represent the initiating event, leading to the production of cytokines by local cells, or it may represent a defense. Two candidates have emerged as principal antigenic targets against which an immune reaction may be triggered: oxidized lipoproteins, in particular oxLDL, and heat shock protein (hsp) 60/65. These could serve as primary initiators of an autoimmune response, or they could contribute to enhanced atherogenesis in the presence of pre-existing risk factors (George et al. 1996).

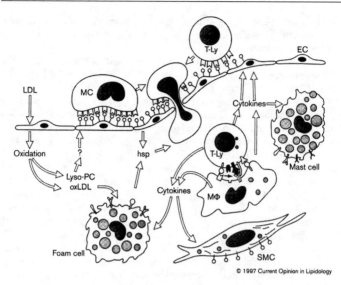

© 1997 Current Opinion in Lipidology

Figure 9.1. Hypothetical scheme depicting immunologic mechanisms in the induction of atherosclerosis. LDL leaks into the arterial intima, where it is oxidized. Lysophosphatidylcholine (Lyso-PC) and other components of oxLDL activate endothelial cells (ECs), which respond by expressing adhesion molecules that promote the recruitment of monocytes (MCs) and T lymphocytes (T-Ly) from the blood. MCs differentiate into macrophages (MΦ) and produce cytokines, oxygen radicals, and heat shock proteins (hsp) in response to oxLDL. An inflammatory reaction (i.e., an innate immune response) has developed. Antigenic components of oxLDL and hsp are taken up by MΦ and presented to antigen-specific T-Ly, which respond by releasing cytokines. Th1 cytokines activate MΦ, leading to radical production and protease secretion but also to down-regulation of scavenger receptors, inhibiting foam cell formation. Th1 cytokines act on SMCs to inhibit proliferation and the production of alpha-actin and collagen, on ECs to up-regulate adhesion to molecules, and on MΦ, SMCs, and ECs to induce nitric oxide production. Th2 cytokines activate mast cells, resulting in protease release, and also B cells, leading to anti-oxLDL antibodies. (Reprinted with permission from Hansson 1997.)

Oxidized Lipoproteins

Only recently did it emerge that oxidative modification renders LDL immunogenic through the formation of a large number of neoepitopes on the modified LDL (Palinski et al. 1990). Both T cell and B cell epitopes that elicit adaptive immune responses are found on oxLDL. Moreover, innate immunity is promoted or induced by lipid compounds, including lysophosphatidylcholine, that are generated during oxidation

(Hansson 1997). Lysophosphatidylcholine is strongly proinflammatory and induces endothelial cells to express VCAM-1 (Kume et al. 1992), which promotes monocyte adhesion (Gerszten et al. 1996); it also can activate and enhance the proliferation of monocyte-derived macrophages (Sakai et al. 1996).

Dahlén proposed that an autoimmune process might especially occur in people with inherited elevated plasma Lp[a] and certain HLA class II genotypes, triggered by a concurrent infection by, for example, *Chlamydia pneumoniae* (Dahlén 1994; Dahlén and Stenlund 1997). Because Lp[a] and LDL are subject to modifications such as oxidation in arterial wall lesions, modified antigenic sites might elicit a T cell–mediated immune response to both apo [a] and apo B-100. That Lp[a] may be involved in immuno-logic mechanisms is suggested by its association with diabetes mellitus, rheumatoid arthritis, and renal diseases (Dahlén 1994).

Heat Shock Proteins

Because vascular cells produce high levels of stress proteins to protect against damage during hemodynamic stress and to maintain vascular homeostasis, it has been posited that an immune reaction to heat shock proteins could contribute to atherogenesis (Xu and Wick 1996; Wick et al. 1995a, 1995b). Involvement of heat shock proteins in atherogenesis is controversial, however, and many more data would be needed to support such a role. In atherosclerosis, the 60/65-kDa and 70-kDa heat shock proteins have been the most widely investigated (hsp 60 is the human homologue of bacterial hsp 65) (Roma and Catapano 1996). Their roles may be different: On review, Roma and Catapano (1996) concluded that it seems most likely hsp 60 is acting as an autoantigen, whereas hsp 70 is involved in cytoprotection.

A link between hsp 60/65 and atherosclerosis was initially suggested by work in the early 1990s by Wick's group, which demonstrated that pro-nounced aortic atherosclerosis developed in normocholesterolemic rabbits immunized with mycobacterial hsp 65 (Xu et al. 1992, 1993a). Subse-quently, high concentrations of anti–hsp 65 antibodies were found to be associated with the presence of human carotid luminal narrowing (Xu et al. 1993b) and the presence of CHD (but not acute MI) (Hoppichler et al. 1996).

On the basis of such findings, Wick, Xu, and colleagues postulated an *immunologic hypothesis* of atherogenesis, whereby the first stages of the dis-ease—the formation of reversible lesions containing lymphocytes, mono-cytes, and SMCs—arise from an immune reaction to hsp 60/65, followed by the formation of foam cells in the presence of hypercholesterolemia (Kleindienst et al. 1995; Xu and Wick 1996). The expression of the heat shock protein is itself a response to injury to a stress factor such as hyper-tension, oxLDL, or a viral infection. Thus, the immunologic hypothesis provides an integrative model for the response to injury and oxLDL models. It remains to be clarified whether the immune system through cellular or humoral components is responsible for initiating the reaction or whether sensitization to hsp 60/65 results from, for example, viral infection or autologous contact with the protein (Kleindienst et al. 1995).

MONOCLONALITY OF SMOOTH MUSCLE CELLS

The monoclonal hypothesis of atherogenesis, which suggests that a single progenitor cell gives rise to proliferative cells in an atherosclerotic lesion, was proposed by Benditt and Benditt in 1973. The original description of aortic plaque monoclonality and interim confirmatory studies, using a glucose-6-phosphate dehydrogenase (G6PD, an X-linked enzyme) assay, found that 75–90% of aortic atherosclerotic plaques contained a single pattern of X inactivation, whereas samples of adjacent, uninvolved aorta all had a mixed pattern (Schwartz et al. 1995). It was speculated that plaque cells were mutated, for example, by a virus or chemical mutagen, so that plaque would be analogous to a benign neoplasm. Indeed, as discussed later, circumstantial evidence exists to support a role for infection in the pathogenesis of atherosclerosis. Which cell type formed the monoclonal population could not be determined by the G6PD assay, although SMCs were considered a likely candidate.

Recently, Murry et al. (1997), by using a polymerase chain reaction–based assay, were able to show that SMCs constitute the monoclonal population, and they extended evidence for monoclonality to coronary artery lesions (finding a single pattern of X inactivation in 3 of 4 aortic plaques and 9 of 11 coronary plaques). An unexpected finding was that normal arteries can have large patches in which X inactivation is skewed in the same direction. This finding raises the possibility that plaque monoclonality may arise through expansion of a pre-existing clone of cells rather than through generation of a new clone by mutation or selection (i.e., selection of a pre-existing, unique lineage of SMCs in vascular injury). The initial clone would have been established during normal development of the vessel wall, and any stimulus for proliferation within that patch (e.g., subendothelial inflammatory infiltrate) would cause patch expansion (Murry et al. 1997). An increasing amount of evidence indicates that SMCs within the artery wall are a heterogeneous mix of discrete lineages (Schwartz et al. 1995). The alternatives to monoclonality as a normal part of intimal development—benign transformation of plaque SMCs or existence of a proliferative subset—imply that plaque SMCs have unique properties (Schwartz et al. 1995).

ROLE OF INFECTION

A focus on the possibility of an infectious etiology in human atherosclerosis did not begin until the 1970s, when the Fabricants, Minick, and their associates were able to produce atherosclerosis-like lesions in the coronary arteries and aortas of germ-free chickens experimentally infected with an avian herpesvirus (Fabricant et al. 1978; Minick et al. 1979). Also in the 1970s, Benditt and Benditt (1973) suggested that viral infection could lead to the clonal expansion postulated in their monoclonal hypothesis of atherosclerosis (see "Monoclonality of Smooth Muscle Cells," earlier). Since then, a large body of evidence has been generated that implicates a number of microbial agents in the pathogenesis of atherosclerotic disease. Such potential risk factors are of interest because known risk factors do not account for all cases of CHD; for example, in the Framingham cohort, 20% of MIs occurred in people with TC of less than 200 mg/dL (Wong et al. 1991; Kannel 1995). Proof of an infectious etiology could have far-reaching consequences in the prevention and treatment of the disease.

Associations reported with human CHD include some gram-negative bacteria (Cook and Lip 1996), herpesviruses (Melnick et al. 1993; Visser and Vercellotti 1993), and clinical markers of chronic dental infection (Mattila 1993; Mattila et al. 1995). Most of the published studies relate to cytomegalovirus (CMV), *Helicobacter pylori,* and *Chlamydia pneumoniae.* Most are seroepidemiologic studies based on antibody measurements, although some report evidence of the pathogen in atherosclerotic lesions and nonatheromatous blood vessels, as reviewed by Danesh et al. (1997). CMV has also been associated with post–cardiac transplant vasculopathy and postangioplasty restenosis.

Possible Mechanisms

A variety of possible causative mechanisms, acting chronically (e.g., to promote plaque development) or acutely (e.g., to precipitate plaque rupture) have been suggested to explain the reported associations between infections and CHD (Figure 9.2) (Danesh et al. 1997). Some involve direct effects of pathogens on the artery wall, but most involve indirect effects mediated in the circulation through chronic inflammation, cross-reactive antibodies, or changes in established or proposed CHD risk factors, such as plasma lipoproteins (Niemala et al. 1996), coagulation proteins (Patel et al. 1995), oxidative metabolites (Patel et al. 1995), and homocysteine (Sung and Sanderson 1996) (Danesh et al. 1997).

Thrombosis

Recent febrile illness is significantly associated with the occurrence of MI (Spodick et al. 1984), and viral infection can result in acute coronary arteritis (Burch and Shewey 1976) (Ellis 1997). Thromboembolic complications, including MI and stroke, are common in bacteremic patients with and without endocarditis (Valtonen et al. 1993). An acute change in the overall bulk of plaque is unlikely, but lesions could somehow become more able to support thrombosis and vasospasm (Vallance et al. 1997), and indeed the shift from stable to unstable angina appears to be associated with a systemic inflammatory response (Liuzzo et al. 1994; Crea et al. 1997). Activation of the coagulation system may be the most important among numerous mechanisms (Valtonen et al. 1993); chronic infections can increase hypercoagulability through, for example, elevation of circulating fibrinogen concentrations (Gupta and Camm 1997; Lip and Beevers 1997). Infectious disease (e.g., influenza) has been proposed as a factor in the demonstrated higher risk for cardiovascular death in winter; among other proposed influences are temperature changes, hours of daylight, and diet (Vallance et al. 1997).

Infection and Plasma Lipids

Various studies have shown reduced HDL-C and TC during the acute phase of infection, with the reductions remaining during convalescence (reviewed by Pesonen et al. 1993). Sammalkorpi et al. (1988) found significantly decreased LDL-C in addition to decreased HDL-C. In 54 hospitalized patients who developed sepsis, Alvarez and Ramos (1986) found decreased serum concentrations of apo A and apo B and increased serum TG in addition to decreased HDL-C and TC. Niemala et al. (1996) assessed *H. pylori* seropositivity in a case-control study of 232 subjects with and without angiographic CHD and found significantly higher serum TG

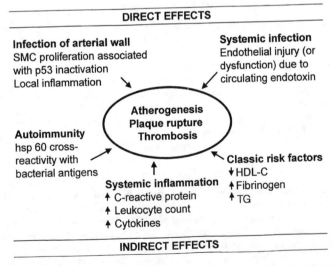

Figure 9.2. Postulated mechanisms to link infections and vascular disease. (Redrawn with permission from Danesh et al. 1997, published by The Lancet Ltd.)

among the seropositive control subjects, with a similar but nonsignificant trend in case subjects. HDL-C concentrations tended to be lower in both *H. pylori*–positive case and control subjects. Sung and Sanderson (1996) have suggested that hyperhomocysteinemia and *H. pylori* infection could be linked in the pathogenesis of atherosclerosis through a deficiency in vitamins, including folate, caused by chronic gastritis.

Perspectives

Danesh et al. (1997) reviewed observational epidemiologic and clinical studies published in any language before January 1997 that reported an association between CMV, *H. pylori*, or *C. pneumoniae* and human CHD. They found that a limited number of patients with classic atherosclerotic CHD have been studied with regard to CMV. They could account for the apparent association of *H. pylori* with CHD by residual confounding from risk factors. A stronger association was found between CHD and *C. pneumoniae* (which has also been shown in case-control studies to be associated with atherosclerotic carotid disease and stroke [Cook and Lip 1996; Gupta and Camm 1997, Cook et al. 1998]). But the sequence of infection and disease is uncertain (Danesh et al. 1997); for example, macrophages may ingest particles of the pathogen in the lung or elsewhere before migrating to atherosclerotic lesions, or *C. pneumoniae* infection might actively induce immune activation, cytokine release, endothelial damage, and thrombogenesis (Lip and Beevers 1997; Gupta and Camm 1997).

Similarly, other reviewers have concluded that the evidence for infectious causation of CHD is only circumstantial, and in some cases extremely weak (Ellis 1997). The high prevalence of most of the pathogens studied may make establishment of a link through retrospective studies impossible (Ellis 1997). About one-half of adults in developed countries have antibodies to CMV, *H. pylori*, and *C. pneumoniae*, although the presence of serum antibodies does not necessarily indicate the presence of active infection at any site (Danesh et al. 1997). Moreover, individuals with a greater infectious or inflammatory burden may be at increased risk for CHD simply because they are older or have poor health habits or reduced access to care, and inflammation and infection are more common among smokers (Ridker 1998). A likely formulation is that an infectious agent will be neither a necessary nor a sufficient factor for the development of atherosclerosis, but that it will constitute a risk factor added to known risk factors (Epstein et al. 1996).

Two pilot interventional studies of antibiotic treatment as a secondary prevention measure in CHD have been published. Gurfinkel et al. (1997) found reduced CHD events 6 months after giving the antichlamydial macrolide antibiotic roxithromycin (which supposedly has anti-inflammatory properties) versus placebo for 1 month to 202 patients. Gupta et al. (1997) found a decreased risk for cardiovascular events with azithromycin therapy in patients seropositive for *C. pneumoniae.* Large-scale trials are needed to confirm these preliminary observations.

ALLOGRAFT CORONARY HEART DISEASE

The immune response appears to be of major significance in the unique and usually accelerated form of CHD that involves the coronary endothelium at the recipient-allograft interface after heart transplantation. It is hypothesized that the initial endothelial injury results from the patient's immune response to the allograft. Allograft CHD, also called cardiac allograft vasculopathy, is the single most important factor limiting long-term (>1-year) survival after heart transplantation (Hosenpud et al. 1997). Patients in whom allograft CHD develops are at a fivefold greater risk for MI, terminal heart failure, and sudden death (Uretsky et al. 1987), and in most patients the allograft CHD will remain silent before such an event because of the absence of afferent innervation (Valantine and Schroeder 1997).

In contrast to common atherosclerosis, cardiac allograft vasculopathy is not limited to the coronary vessels; it may also involve the venous structures and great vessels within the transplant (Ventura et al. 1995; Billingham 1989, 1992). Lesion localization is diffuse and distal rather than focal and proximal (Ventura et al. 1995). Lesions may involve the artery in a concentric rather than eccentric fashion: The classic allograft lesion consists of progressive concentric myointimal proliferation that appears as intimal thickening, with subsequent increases in lipid deposits and calcification, ultimately leading to occlusion of the lumen (Ventura et al. 1995; Billingham 1992). However, abnormalities of a wide variety have been described, including lesions closely resembling common atherosclerosis (Weis and von Scheidt 1997; Pucci et al. 1990).

Pathogenesis

Experimental models suggest that immunologic mechanisms operating in a setting of nonimmunologic risk factors constitute the key stimuli that result in the progressive myointimal hyperplasia of allograft CHD (Weis and von Scheidt 1997). Assessing transplanted carotid arteries in a mouse model, Shi et al. (1996) found an acquired immune response to be essential to development of the concentric neointimal proliferation and luminal narrowing characteristic of allograft atherosclerosis. Libby's group has proposed a model that links a cellular immune response akin to delayed-type hypersensitivity to leukocyte recruitment and altered vascular cell function through a cytokine cascade (Libby and Tanaka 1994; Libby et al. 1992). In support of the model, they cite the expression of class II histocompatibility antigens by coronary artery endothelium and the accumulation of leukocytes in transplanted coronary arteries (Libby and Tanaka 1994).

Major risk factors are common after cardiac transplantation: hyperlipidemia, reduced HDL-C, glucose intolerance, and insulin resistance are found in 50–80% of patients (Kemna et al. 1994) (see also next). Renal transplantation promotes the development of common CHD, presumably through the accentuation by immunosuppressant drugs of known risk factors such as hyperlipidemia, hypertension, and hyperglycemia (Braun and Marwick 1994). Human CMV has also been associated with cardiac allograft vasculopathy, but whether or how it may be involved pathogenically is not established (Weis and von Scheidt 1997). Another suggested mechanism is ischemic injury of endothelium between harvest and reimplantation of the heart (Libby and Tanaka 1994).

Hyperlipidemia

In our series of 100 patients, 64% had LDL-C of at least 130 mg/dL, 85% had LDL-C of at least 100 mg/dL, and 41% had plasma TG of at least 200 mg/dL 6 months after postoperative dietary instruction (Ballantyne et al. 1992). Posttransplantation hyperlipidemia appears to be related to multiple factors, including type of immunosuppressive therapy, weight gain, and history of hyperlipidemia. Both cyclosporine and prednisone can cause hyperlipidemia (Kobashigawa and Kasiske 1997; Ballantyne et al. 1997); insulin resistance is induced by corticosteroids (Valantine and Schroeder 1997). Interrelations are complex: Dyslipidemia may adversely affect inflammation and rejection in the allograft, and inflammation, infection, and trauma often alter lipoprotein metabolism (Nieminen et al. 1993) through the effects of cytokines such as TNF-α, the interleukins, and the interferons.

Lipid-lowering therapy with HMG-CoA reductase inhibitors (statins) has been shown in randomized, controlled trials to reduce transplant vasculopathy and to increase survival after heart transplantation (Kobashigawa et al. 1995; Wenke et al. 1997). Whether the potential of statins to prevent allograft CHD is the result of lipid lowering, possible immunomodulating properties, or both is not known. In a trial conducted by Kobashigawa et al., the possiblity of a direct effect on lymphocyte function was raised by the reduced natural killer cell cytotoxicity of circulating lymphocytes in a subset of the pravastatin group. In vitro studies have shown pravastatin to inhibit natural killer cell cytotoxicity and to act synergistically with cyclosporine to inhibit cytotoxic lymphocyte activity; other statins inhibit T cell proliferation and monocyte chemotaxis in vitro (Katznelson and Kobashigawa 1995). Alternatively, increased immunosuppression could arise through the increased proportion of free cyclosporine in plasma with decreased plasma cholesterol levels (Valantine and Schroeder 1997; Ballantyne et al. 1997).

When used at higher dosages with cyclosporine, the statins may cause elevation in liver function tests and increased risk for myositis (Southworth and Mauro 1997; Valantine and Schroeder 1997; Ballantyne et al. 1992). The statin should therefore be prescribed at the smallest effective dosage and increased slowly. Other classes of lipid-lowering drugs are of limited utility after heart transplantation: nicotinic acid because high percentages of patients are unable to tolerate it; bile acid resins because of interference

Table 9.1. COMPARISON OF DE NOVO ATHEROSCLEROSIS AND RESTENOSIS

Parameter	Atherosclerosis	Restenosis
Endothelial pathophysiology	Dysfunctional	Acute disruption
Severity of injury	Mild to moderate	Severe
Course of injury	Chronic	Acute
Time course of response	Years to decades	Hours to months
Arterial remodeling	Vessel tends to enlarge	Vessel contraction or reduced enlargement
Immunologic reaction	Present	Present
SMC replication	Present	Present; perhaps indolent
Response to growth factors	Present	Present
Cellular elements	Present	Present
Extracellular elements	Foam cells, fibrous material	SMCs, neointima
Clinical sequelae	Angina, MI	Recurrent angina
Relation to plasma lipid concentrations	Definite	Probably none, except perhaps Lp[a]

Source: Modified from Weintraub and Pederson 1996, with permission from Excerpta Medica, Inc.

with absorption of lipid-soluble drugs such as cyclosporine and the potential to increase plasma TG; and gemfibrozil because of modest or variable effects on the LDL-C concentration (Ballantyne et al. 1997). Fish oils may effectively lower elevated plasma TG and have been shown to confer benefit in allograft rejection after renal transplantation (van der Heide et al. 1993).

RESTENOSIS AFTER ANGIOPLASTY

Ever since its development by Andreas Gruentzig in the late 1970s, PTCA has been hindered by the problem of restenosis, which occurs in 30–60% of cases despite a successful procedure (Bauters and Isner 1997; Hong et al. 1997). Angiographic series have shown that restenosis occurs largely within the first 6 months after PTCA; it can occur as early as the first 24 hours in some cases, from subacute vascular recoil (Hong et al. 1997). Unlike the situation in the distinct process of de novo atherosclerosis (Table 9.1), no reliable, effective pharmacologic therapy has been found despite the testing of a variety of agents in more than 40 large clinical trials (Topol 1997). Only coronary stenting has proved to affect the natural history, but stents, too, have been plagued by restenosis (Topol 1997) and much of their success may result from improved immediate postdilation results (Libby and Tanaka 1997). Intracoronary irradiation has shown some promise (Teirstein et al. 1997; Weinberger and Simon 1997).

Pathogenesis

Initially, on the basis of animal studies, excessive neointimal hyperplasia as a response to injury was thought to be the major mechanism of restenosis (Hong et al. 1997). More recent studies, including preclinical and clinical investigations and those using intravascular ultrasound, suggest multiple mechanisms—perhaps variable both interindividually and intraindividually—including not only SMC proliferation but also elaboration of extracellular matrix, thrombosis, and vascular remodeling (Bauters and Isner 1997). It may be that the intimal thickening in human lesions results primarily from excess matrix accumulation rather than the SMC replication seen in animal models (Libby and Tanaka 1997). Human lesions differ in important ways from animal model lesions, in particular in that abundant SMCs and leukocytes are already present, and some data describe only indolent SMC proliferation in human restenosis (Libby and Tanaka 1997).

Chronic geometric remodeling of the treatment site leading to vessel wall constriction may be the most important factor in general in restenosis (Faxon et al. 1997; Hong et al. 1997).

Risk Factors

Variables associated with restenosis after a first PTCA include male sex, multivessel disease, brief duration of angina, the vessel dilated (left anterior descending > left circumflex > right coronary), and suboptimal initial results (residual stenosis >35–44%). Those associated with a second or subsequent angioplasty include male sex, continued smoking, diabetes mellitus, multivessel disease, and early recurrence (<4–5 months) (Anderson et al. 1995a).

Lipids

In general, it would appear that plasma lipid concentrations are not related to risk for restenosis, reflecting the different pathophysiologic processes of restenosis and de novo atherosclerosis (Weintraub and Pederson 1996; Violaris et al. 1994). Several small studies have described an association of elevated Lp[a] with coronary or femoropopliteal restenosis (Horie et al. 1997; Maca et al. 1996; Yamamoto et al. 1995; Hearn et al. 1992; Shimizu et al. 1991), although a role remains controversial and not all studies support the relation (Bussiere et al. 1996). Research into the isoforms of Lp[a] has been recommended (Bussiere et al. 1996). Concentrations at which the relation has been described range from more than 19 mg/dL (Hearn et al. 1992) to a nonsignificant trend at more than 250 mg/dL (Bussiere et al. 1996). When LDL apheresis was performed in 66 men and women 2 days before and 5 days after PTCA, the restenosis rate 2–9 months later was significantly reduced when the Lp[a] concentration was reduced at least 50% (21% vs. 50%) (Daida et al. 1994). Efficacy with this approach was enhanced by the addition of pravastatin and nicotinic acid therapy (restenosis rate of 12% at 5 months) (Yamaguchi et al. 1994). Nicotinic acid is the sole approved lipid-lowering drug that can lower Lp[a] (Stein and Rosensen 1997).

Trials of HMG-CoA inhibitors and fish oil supplementation to prevent restenosis have yielded inconclusive results (Lefkovits and Topol 1997). Interest in the statins has reflected their reported effects beyond lipid lowering (e.g., restoration of endothelial function and reduction of platelet aggregation; see Chapter 10); omega-3 fatty acids have been considered antiatherogenic through a variety of mechanisms (e.g., anti-inflammatory properties, decreases in platelet aggregation, direct inhibition of neointimal proliferation) (Lefkovits and Topol 1997). Nevertheless, lipid-lowering therapy according to clinical guidelines for secondary prevention is clearly appropriate after angioplasty to reduce the risk for atherosclerosis systemically.

Probucol has shown promise against restenosis. In a double-blind trial, Tardif et al. (1997) randomized 317 patients to receive 500 mg probucol alone, probucol plus antioxidant multivitamins (C, E, and beta-carotene), multivitamins alone, or placebo twice daily for 4 weeks before and 6 months after PTCA. At 6 months, respective restenosis rates per segment were 21%, 29%, 40%, and 39% ($P = .003$ for probucol vs. no probucol), and rates of repeated angioplasty were 11%, 16%, 24%, and 27% ($P = .009$). The mechanism of the benefit might be related to probucol's strong antioxidant effects, although that hypothesis is complicated by the lack of benefit of the multivitamins. Regarding this apparent paradox, Sirtori and Franceschini (1997) proposed a possible role for HDL: although HDL-C decreased 41% in the trial (a typical effect of probucol), the decrease may not have been adverse, perhaps representing increased formation of small HDL, which is more effective than large HDL in removing tissue cholesterol. Still, it must be borne in mind that restenosis does not appear to be a lipid-driven process.

Four small trials of less rigorous design had previously shown a benefit from probucol (Yokoi et al. 1997; Watanabe et al. 1996; Lee et al. 1996; Setsuda et al. 1993). It appears that adequate pretreatment is needed because probucol accumulation in tissue appears to be slow (Reaven et al. 1992). In a trial of probucol plus lovastatin in which no benefit was demonstrated (O'Keefe et al. 1996), treatment was started between 48 and 24 hours after angioplasty.

Suggested Reading

Ballantyne CM, El Masri B, Morrisett JD, Torre-Amione G. Pathophysiology and treatment of lipid perturbation after cardiac transplantation. Curr Opin Cardiol 1997;12:153–160.

Bauters C, Isner JM. The biology of restenosis (review). Prog Cardiovasc Dis 1997;40:107–116.

Danesh J, Collins R, Peto R. Chronic infections and coronary heart disease: is there a link? (review) Lancet 1997;350:430–436.

Ellis RW. Infection and coronary heart disease (review). J Med Microbiol 1997; 46:535–539.

George J, Harats D, Gilburd B, Shoenfeld Y. Emerging cross-regulatory roles of immunity and autoimmunity in atherosclerosis. Immunol Res 1996;15: 315–322.

Hansson GK. Cell-mediated immunity in atherosclerosis. Curr Opin Lipidol 1997;8:301–311.

Hong MK, Mehran R, Mintz GS, Leon MB. Restenosis after coronary angio-plasty. Curr Prob Cardiol 1997;22:1–36.

Kobashigawa JA, Kasiske BL. Hyperlipidemia in solid organ transplantation. Transplantation 1997;63:331–338.

Murry CE, Gipaya CT, Bartosek T et al. Monoclonality of smooth muscle cells in human atherosclerosis. Am J Pathol 1997;151:697–705.

Ventura HO, Mehra MR, Smart FW, Stapleton DD. Cardiac allograft vascu-lopathy: current concepts. Am Heart J 1995;129:791–798.

Weis M, von Scheidt W. Cardiac allograft vasculopathy: a review. Circulation 1997;96:2069–2077.

Chapter 10

Lesion Regression and Stabilization

REGRESSION TRIALS

As David Blankenhorn noted in his 1992 AHA Duff Memorial Lecture (Blankenhorn and Hodis 1994), the general view in 1977 was still that human atherosclerosis was irreversible, unaffected by any influence less drastic than wartime starvation (Malmros 1950), and the only clinical management accepted was surgery. This view was changed in the mid-1980s when long-term randomized trials of lipid lowering in which lesions were monitored by imaging modalities began to be published. The era of these "regression trials" was ushered in with data from the NHLBI Type II Coronary Intervention Study in 1984 and the CLAS in 1987.

Coronary Angiography Trials

Major studies using coronary angiography have shown that intensive lipid modification by a variety of interventions retards the progression of atherosclerotic lesions and in a small subset of patients leads to their regression (Table 10.1). The patients in the trials were both men and women with CHD, some of whom had a history of angina pectoris, MI, CABG, or PTCA, and many with multiple risk factors for CHD. The trials included a wide range of LDL-C concentrations at enrollment, and all except BECAIT and LOCAT (see later) focused therapy on lowering cholesterol. The decrease in LDL-C varied substantially, and large increases in HDL-C concentrations were achieved with regimens that included nicotinic acid or a fibrate. As determined typically by digitized or computer-assisted QCA, coronary lesion progression occurred more often in control patients and lesion regression occurred more often in treated patients, effects seen in both native vessels and bypass grafts. Many trials have also significantly reduced the formation of new lesions (Figure 10.1). Vos et al. (1993) pooled the results of NHLBI II, CLAS, the FATS, POSCH, UCSF-SCOR, and STARS with interventions of diet, drug therapy, or ileal bypass surgery and trial

Table 10.1. MAJOR RANDOMIZED LIPID-MODIFYING TRIALS ASSESSING CORONARY ATHEROSCLEROSIS BY ANGIOGRAPHY

Trial (publication date)[a]	Subjects analyzed[b]	Trial period (years)	Mean baseline LDL-C in treatment group (mg/dL)	Intervention[c]	Percentage lipid response vs. baseline value LDL-C	HDL-C	Percentage of patients in whom coronary lesions progressed/regressed (Rx/control)[d]	Statistically significant angiographic results with treatment 1° end-point	2° end-point	Clinical events (Rx/control)[e]
Testing lifestyle intervention without drug therapy										
Lifestyle Heart Trial (July 1990)	36 M/5 F	1	152	VLF diet and other lifestyle	−7	−3	Q 18/53 82/42	+	+	1/0
STARS (Mar 1992)	74 M	3.2	193	Diet alone	−16	0	Q 15/46 38/4	+	+	3/10 ✓
			203	Ch[f]	−36	−4	Q 12/46 33/4	+	+	1/10 ✓
Heidelberg Trial (July 1992)	92 M	1	164	Diet and intensive exercise	−8	+3	Q 23/48 32/17	+ (1°/2° not stated)		5/4

Continued

Table 10.1. *Continued*

Trial (publication date)[a]	Subjects analyzed[b]	Mean baseline LDL-C in treatment group (mg/dL)	Trial period (years)	Intervention[c]	Percentage lipid response vs. baseline value LDL-C	HDL-C	Percentage of patients in whom coronary lesions progressed/regressed (Rx/control)[d]	Statistically significant angiographic results with treatment 1° endpoint	2° endpoint	Clinical events (Rx/control)[e]
Testing single-agent pharmacotherapy										
NHLBI II (Feb 1984)	94 M/ 22 F	242	5	Ch	−26	+8	V 25/35 3/2	+	+	8/11
MARS (Nov 1993)	225 M/ 22 F	151	2.2	L	−38	+9	Q 29/41 23/12 V 47/65 23/11	Q−	V+	22/31
CCAIT (Mar 1994)	245 M/ 54 F	173	2	L	−29	+7	Q 33/50 10/7	+	+	15/20
MAAS (Sept 1994)	308 M/ 37 F	169	4	S	−31	+7	Q 23/32 19/12	+	+	30/36
REGRESS (May 1995)	663 M	166	2	P	−25	+9	Q 56/69 16/7	+	+	10/17 ✓
PLAC I (Nov 1995)	248 M/ 72 F	164	3	P	−28	+7	Q 26/35 12/12	−	+	7/18 ✓

Trial (date)										
BECAIT (Mar 1996)	81 M	5	180 (med)	B	-4	+9	Q 74/85 21/13	+	-	3/11 ✓
Post-CABG[g] (Jan 1997)	1256 (~94% M) (angio)	4.3	155	L (±Ch) Aggressive vs. moderate	-37–40 vs. -13–15	—	Q 27 vs. 39 (% of grafts)	+	+	85 vs. 103
LCAS (Aug 1997)	283 M/ 57 F	2.5	146	F (±Ch)	-24	+9	Q 29/39 15/8	+	+	31/41
LOCAT (Oct 1997)	372 M	2.7	139	G	-5	+21	Q —	-	+	7/7
Testing combination-agent pharmacotherapy										
CLAS I (June 1987)	162 M	2	171	N + C	-43	+37	V 39/61 16/4	+	+	14/18
FATS (Nov 1990)	120 M	2.5	190	N + C	-32	+43	Q 25/46 39/11	+	+	2/10 ✓
			196	C + L	-46	+15	Q 21/46 32/11	+	+	3/10 ✓
UCSF-SCOR (Dec 1990)	31 M/41 F	2	283	N/C/L	-39	+25	Q 20/41 33/13	+	+	0/1
CLAS II (Dec 1990)	103 M	4	See CLAS I	N + C	-40 18/6	+37	V 48/85	+	+	18/22

Continued

Table 10.1. Continued

Trial (publication date)[a]	Subjects analyzed[b]	Trial period (years)	Mean baseline LDL-C in treatment group (mg/dL)	Intervention[c]	Percentage lipid response vs. baseline value		Percentage of patients in whom coronary lesions progressed/regressed (Rx/control)[d]	Statistically significant angiographic results with treatment		Clinical events (Rx/control)[e]
					LDL-C	HDL-C		1° end-point	2° end-point	
HARP (Oct 1994)	70 M/ 9 F	2.5	140	P, N, Ch ± G	−38	+13	Q 33/38 13/15	−	−	6/10
Testing other interventions										
POSCH (Oct 1990)	578 M/ 56 F	5[h]	179	Partial ileal bypass	−42	+5	V 38/65 13/5	NA	+	82/125
SCRIP (Mar 1994)	216 M/ 30 F	4	157	Intensive lifestyle ± C/N/G/L/ Pro	−23	+12	Q 50/50 20/10	+	+	6/13 ✓
FHRS (Apr 1995)	28 M/ 11 F	2.1	309 vs. 284	LDL apheresis + S vs. S + resin	−53 vs. −44	No Δ vs. +4	Q 10 vs. 21 21 vs. 21	−	−	1 vs. 3
LAARS (May 1996)	40 M	2	301 vs. 304	LDL apheresis + S (± resin) vs. S (± resin)	−63 vs −47	+18 vs. +14	Q 45 vs. 55 10 vs. 55	−	−	7 vs. 5

*BECAIT, Bezafibrate Coronary Atherosclerosis Intervention Trial (Ericsson et al. Lancet 1996;347:849–853); CCAIT, Canadian Coronary Atherosclerosis Intervention Trial (Waters et al. Circulation 1994;89:959–968); CLAS I, Cholesterol Lowering Atherosclerosis Study I (Blankenhorn et al. JAMA 1987;257:3233–3240); CLAS II, Cholesterol Lowering Atherosclerosis Study II (Cashin-Hemphill et al. JAMA 1990;264:3013–3017); FATS, Familial Atherosclerosis Treatment Study (Brown et al. N Engl J Med 1990;323:1289–1298); FHRS, Familial Hypercholesterolemia Regression Study (Thompson et al. Lancet 1995;345:811–816); HARP, Harvard Atherosclerosis Reversibility Project (Sacks et al. Lancet 1994;344:1182–1186); Heidelberg Trial (Schuler et al. Circulation 1992;86:1–11); LAARS, LDL-Apheresis Atherosclerosis Regression Study (Kroon et al. Circulation 1996;93:1826–1835); LCAS, Lipoprotein and Coronary Atherosclerosis Study (Herd et al. Am J Cardiol 1997;80:278–286); Lifestyle Heart Trial (Ornish et al. Lancet 1990;336:129–133); LOCAT, Lopid coronary Angiography Trial (Frick, et al. Circulation 1997;96:2167–2143); MAAS, Multicentre Anti-Atheroma Study (MAAS Investigators Lancet 1994;344:633–638); MARS, Monitored Atherosclerosis Regression Study (Blankenhorn et al. Ann Intern Med 1993;119:969–976); NHLBI II, National Heart, Lung, and Blood Institute Type II Coronary Intervention Study (Brensike et al. Circulation 1984;69:313–324, Levy et al. Circulation 1984;69:325–337); PLAC I, Pravastatin Limitation of Atherosclerosis in the Coronary Arteries (Pitt et al. J Am Coll Cardiol 1995;26:1133–1139); POSCH, Program on the Surgical Control of the Hyperlipidemias (Buchwald et al. N Engl J Med 1990;323:946–955); Post-CABG, Post Coronary Artery Bypass Graft Trial (Post Coronary Artery Bypass Graft Trial Investigators N Engl J Med 1997;336:153–162); REGRESS, Regression Growth Evaluation Statin Study (Jukema et al. Circulation 1995;91:2528–2540); SCRIP, Stanford Coronary Risk Intervention Project (Haskell et al. Circulation 1994;89:975–990); STARS, St. Thomas' Atherosclerosis Regression Study (Watts et al. Lancet 1992;339:563–569); UCSF-SCOR, University of California, San Francisco, Arteriosclerosis Specialized Center of Research Intervention Trial (Kane et al. JAMA 1990;264:3007–3012).

bM, male; F, female.

cAll interventions included diet. B, bezafibrate; C, colestipol; Ch, cholestyramine; F, fluvastatin; G, gemfibrozil; L, lovastatin; N, nicotinic acid; P, pravastatin; Pro, probucol; S, simvastatin; VLF, very low fat. In UCSF-SCOR, the drugs were used in various binary and ternary combinations. In SCRIP, drug therapy consisted of single agents and drug combinations, including triple-drug therapy in some cases; 90% of patients in the intervention group and 23% of patients in the usual-care group were receiving lipid-lowering pharmacotherapy at 4-year follow-up.

dQ, assessment by quantitative coronary angiography; V, viewer estimation. Note, however, that typically the primary endpoint was an index of stenosis.

eEvents variably defined among trials; generally, coronary death, MI, and new, increased, or unstable angina are included in this table. In those checked, the difference was statistically significant.

fSTARS was designed as a test of diet; the intervention of diet plus cholestyramine was used to determine the effect of a greater reduction in cholesterol concentration.

gPost-CABG in a 2 × 2 factorial design also tested low-dose warfarin vs. placebo. Warfarin did not reduce the progression of atherosclerosis.

hFollow-up in the POSCH was 9.7 years (intervention was surgery). Mean follow-up rather than trial period (intervention was surgery). Mean follow-up in the POSCH was 9.7 years; 5-year results are provided because at that time point angiographic and lipid data were available for a high proportion of participants.

iProgression was arrested, but apheresis plus pharmacotherapy showed no advantage over pharmacotherapy alone.

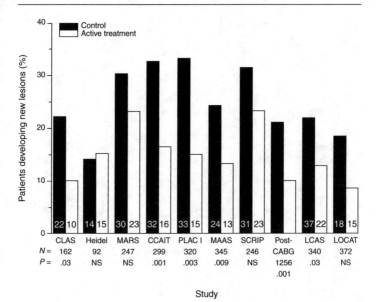

Figure 10.1. Occurrence of new lesions in lipid-lowering angiographic trials. In Post-CABG, the 21% and 10% values are in grafts per patient for moderate versus aggressive treatment. For full trial names and references, see Table 10.1. (Updated [with data from Post-CABG, LCAS, and LOCAT] from Waters 1996.)

periods of 2–5 years and found an overall relative risk for progression of 0.62 (95% CI 0.54–0.72) and an overall relative risk for regression of 2.13 (95% CI 1.53–2.98) with intervention. Rossouw (1995) found similar results in meta-analysis of 14 angiographic trials: Odds for disease progression decreased by 49% and odds for regression increased by 219%, with overall favorable angiographic effects for all classes of drugs. It should be noted that meta-analysis of the regression trials is discouraged by some because of the variety of interventions, subject selection criteria, durations, and endpoints used (Brown et al. 1993).

Typically, the primary endpoint in these trials was an index of stenosis; POSCH was exceptional in having a clinical primary endpoint. All the trials except one showed a statistically significant improvement in the primary and/or secondary angiographic endpoints (see Table 10.1). The small HARP trial remains the sole major angiographic trial that did not find an angiographic benefit with lipid-lowering therapy. HARP assessed patients with CHD and normal or only mildly elevated cholesterol (TC 180–250 mg/dL).

However, in patients with comparable mean baseline LDL-C (146 mg/dL vs. 140 mg/dL in HARP), LCAS did show significant lesion benefit, including in a subset of patients with baseline LDL-C less than 130 mg/dL. Also, in the carotid ultrasound substudy of the 4-year Long-term Intervention with Pravastatin in Ischemic Disease (LIPID) trial, in which mean baseline TC and LDL-C in the active intervention group were only 218 and 150 mg/dL, pravastatin therapy significantly reduced development of atherosclerosis compared with placebo (MacMahon et al. 1998). The effect of treatment on common carotid artery wall thickness was similar in groups classified by cholesterol tertile (mean entry TC and LDL-C of 186, 220, and 255 mg/dL and 124, 151, and 182 mg/dL).

Regression may occur in several ways, including depletion of plaque lipid, depletion of connective tissue, or both; lysis of fully occlusive thrombi or of mural thrombi, as is commonly seen in the course of unstable clinical syndromes; and remodeling of underlying vascular architecture or relaxation of vasomotor tone (Brown et al. 1993). Although the slow, natural course of atherosclerosis allows for some compensatory vessel remodeling (see Chapter 7), the compensatory change with therapeutic intervention probably does not occur at the same rate as the action of the intervention, so that the regression and slowed progression reported in the lipid-lowering trials likely represent actual improvements in disease (Gotto 1995).

The absolute changes in stenosis in the coronary angiography trials were small, however. In FATS, for example, the minimum lumen diameter of lesions in the control group narrowed by a per-patient average of 0.050 mm over 2.5 years, whereas lesions in the treated group improved by 0.024 mm (P <.01) (Brown et al. 1993). The general angiographic results found by Brown et al. in their 1993 review of nine lipid-lowering trials were improvements in stenosis of 1–2% in intervention groups and about a 3% progression of stenosis in control groups.

In the Post-CABG trial, which assessed the effects of lipid lowering on saphenous vein grafts, the patients who had LDL-C lowered to a range of 93–97 mg/dL by aggressive treatment did significantly better than those who achieved LDL-C in the range of 132–136 mg/dL with moderate treatment. At the end of the study, 27% of patients in the aggressive treatment group had lesion progression in grafts, compared with 39% of patients receiving moderate treatment. Also, aggressive lipid reduction was associated with a 29% lower rate of revascularization procedures.

Clinical Event Reduction

Even though the degree of atherosclerotic lesion change in angiographic trials has been small, reductions in CHD events have been surprisingly great, larger than the improvement that would have been predicted on

Table 10.2. POOLED CLINICAL EVENT RESULTS IN FOUR PRAVA-STATIN REGRESSION STUDIES: PLAC I, PLAC II, KAPS, AND REGRESS

| Clinical endpoint | Number of events | | | |
	Pravastatin ($N = 955$)	Placebo ($N = 936$)	Risk reduction (%)	Log-rank P value
Nonfatal or fatal MI	21	46	62.3	0.001
Nonfatal MI or CHD death	29	52	51.4	0.006
All-cause mortality	15	23	45.6	0.168
Nonfatal MI or all-cause mortality	34	61	53.0	0.003
Nonfatal MI, all-cause mortality, stroke, or PTCA/CABG	115	160	30.0	0.002

Source: Data from Byington et al. 1995.

the basis of measurements of stenosis. Although the trials generally were not designed to assess clinical endpoints, clinical events, despite the short follow-up periods, were reduced up to 89%. Reductions were significant in FATS, POSCH, STARS, SCRIP, PLAC I, REGRESS, and BECAIT, trials encompassing patients with both moderately and severely elevated LDL-C levels at baseline. Significant event decreases were also reported from the carotid ultrasound trials Pravastatin, Lipids, and Atherosclerosis in the Carotid Arteries (PLAC II) and Asymptomatic Carotid Artery Progression Study (ACAPS) (mean baseline LDL-C of 167 and 156 mg/dL in the treatment groups) (see later). Pooling of results from 14 angiographic trials showed a highly significant reduction in cardiovascular events on the order of 47% (Rossouw 1995). The results were consistent and significant for all classes of intervention except lifestyle, with which there was no reduction in events.

As seen in Table 10.2, when clinical endpoint results were pooled from the angiographic trials PLAC I and REGRESS and the ultrasound studies PLAC II and the Kuopio Atherosclerosis Prevention Study (KAPS), nonfatal plus fatal MI was reduced 62% ($P = .001$) (Byington et al. 1995). All-cause mortality was reduced 46%. All four trials were double-blind, placebo-controlled tests of pravastatin 40 mg/day as monotherapy for 2 or 3 years. The effect on coronary events was evident in men and women, patients above and below 65 years of age, and patients without a history of hypertension or MI. All the patients in these trials had mildly or moderately elevated cholesterol, and overall LDL-C was reduced 28% with pravastatin. The meta-analysis of the four pravastatin trials was prospectively planned.

Tests of Low-Density Lipoprotein Apheresis

In the FHRS, LDL apheresis combined with simvastatin was less beneficial than simvastatin plus colestipol in influencing coronary atherosclerosis in patients with familial hypercholesterolemia. In LAARS, there
were no differences according to treatment with apheresis plus medication or medication alone in mean coronary segment diameter or minimal
obstruction diameter. However, more minor lesions disappeared in
the apheresis group (Kroon et al. 1996) and regional myocardial perfusion improved in the apheresis group but not the medication group
(Aengevaeren et al. 1996).

Trials Targeting Non–Low-Density Lipoprotein Lipid Fractions

Recent trials have begun to assess the effects on atherosclerotic lesions
of lipid modification not aimed predominantly at LDL-C concentrations. Bezafibrate, which substantially lowers VLDL-C and plasma TG,
was selected for BECAIT not only because of its effects on lipid metabolism but also for effects on glucose metabolism and hemostatic function. In BECAIT, 92 young male survivors of MI were enrolled (<45
years of age at MI). Bezafibrate had no effect on LDL-C, but it
decreased TG 31%, VLDL-C 35%, VLDL-TG 37%, and plasma fibrinogen 12% and increased HDL-C 9%. Its use was associated with significantly slowed progression of focal coronary atherosclerosis as well as a
significantly reduced coronary event rate compared with placebo. Separate post hoc subset analysis showed that bezafibrate had a preferential
effect in slowing the progression of lesions causing less than 50% stenosis at baseline (Ericsson et al. 1997). In LOCAT, 395 men who had
undergone CABG and whose predominant lipid abnormality was
reduced HDL-C (≤42.5 mg/dL, with LDL-C ≤174 mg/dL) were randomized to gemfibrozil or placebo. Gemfibrozil therapy reduced lesion
progression in native coronary vessels by several criteria and reduced
the proportion of patients with new lesions in bypass grafts, favorable
angiographic results comparable with those achieved using statins in
patients with higher LDL-C (Havel 1997).

Findings in Women

Coronary angiography trials that have included a sufficient proportion of
women to enable subset analysis report angiographic benefit similar to that
found in men. A comparison of 162 coronary angiography film pairs in
POSCH women, between baseline examination and 3, 5, 7, and 10 years,
consistently showed less lesion progression in the surgery group (Buchwald
et al. 1992b). In CCAIT, the benefit in angiographic endpoints was not significantly different between the 54 women and 245 men who completed
the trial (Waters et al. 1995). In UCSF-SCOR, conducted in patients with
heterozygous FH (mean LDL-C, 283 mg/dL), the primary endpoint of

change in mean percent area stenosis for coronary lesions was significantly different between the multidrug treatment and control groups (regression vs. progression on average); on subset analysis, this difference was significant in women but not in men (Kane et al. 1990).

Prognostic Value of Lesion Changes

Graded correlations have been described between the rate of coronary lesion progression and risk for future coronary events. Waters et al. (1993), in follow-up data from the Montreal Heart Institute Nicardipine Trial, found that coronary angiographic progression was as strong a predictor of future coronary events as ejection fraction or number of diseased vessels. In POSCH, which clearly showed a reduction in CHD events, changes between coronary angiograms from baseline to 3-year follow-up were significantly associated with subsequent clinical events. With lesion progression at 3-year follow-up, rates of nonfatal CHD events, CHD mortality, and all-cause mortality were all approximately doubled by the time of follow-up at a mean 6.7 years later (Buchwald et al. 1992a). POSCH was unique not only in its intervention—bypass of the terminal 200 cm or distal one-third of the small intestine, the segment where bile acid absorption occurs—but also in its large size and long follow-up. At 7-year follow-up of CLAS, both consensus panel and QCA endpoints of CHD progression predicted clinical coronary events, as did formation of new lesions in bypass grafts (Azen et al. 1996).

Correlates of Lesion Change

Analyses of predictors of angiographic or ultrasound lesion change have yielded different results. In some reports, cholesterol concentration correlated with progression, but in others no such relation was found (Waters 1996). Waters (1996), in analyzing the results of several LDL-lowering trials, inferred that (1) worsening percent diameter stenosis occurs in groups in which LDL-C does not decrease or decreases less than 10%; (2) treatment groups with a mean angiographic change in the direction of regression show substantial reduction in LDL-C; and (3) the amount of regression that can be achieved with LDL-C reduction appears to be limited. Recently, however, as discussed previously, BECAIT and LOCAT, in which fibrate therapy was used, reported significant angiographic improvement with little or no decrease in LDL-C.

There is increasing evidence from angiographic and ultrasound studies that TGRLs and their remnants are important risk factors in the progression of atherosclerotic disease (Hodis and Mack 1995; Phillips et al. 1993). The MARS identified TGRLs and their remnants as being the most important risk factors in progression of coronary and carotid lesions (Hodis et al. 1994, 1997; Mack et al. 1996). Multivariate regression analysis of CLAS I data showed the predominant risk factor predicting the probability of global progression of coronary lesions to be non-HDL-C in the placebo-treated subjects (a positive correlation) and the content of apo C-III in HDL in the drug-treated subjects (an inverse correlation) (Blankenhorn et al. 1990). Increased apo C-III in HDL is indicative of rapid metabolism of TGRLs.

Trials Assessing Carotid and Femoral Disease

The angiographic benefit of pharmacologic lipid lowering has been confirmed by B-mode ultrasound monitoring of carotid disease. Carotid atherosclerosis is a marker for both CHD risk (Chambless et al. 1997; Howard et al. 1996; Salonen and Salonen 1991; Burke et al. 1995) and the risks for stroke and ischemic CVD (Craven et al. 1990; O'Leary et al. 1992). Significant benefit in carotid artery thickness was demonstrated in CLAS, a trial of colestipol and nicotinic acid in men who had undergone CABG (Mack et al. 1993); in PLAC II, in patients with carotid disease and a history of MI or coronary stenosis (Crouse et al. 1995); in KAPS using pravastatin for primary prevention of both carotid and femoral atherosclerotic lesions in men (Salonen et al. 1995b); in ACAPS using lovastatin in men and women with moderately elevated LDL-C (Furberg et al. 1994); in the Carotid Atherosclerosis Italian Ultrasound Study (CAIUS) testing pravastatin in asymptomatic, moderately hypercholesterolemic men and women (Mercuri et al. 1996); and, as noted above, in a substudy of LIPID, a trial of pravastatin in men and women with a history of MI or unstable angina but with average or below-average cholesterol concentrations (MacMahon et al. 1998). Each of these trials except for LIPID and CLAS lasted 3 years; active treatment period assessment in the LIPID substudy extended 4 years, and the CLAS results in the carotid arteries were reported for 1- and 4-year follow-ups. Active treatment in the PLAC II was also associated with a reduction in fatal and nonfatal coronary events (Crouse et al. 1995) and in the ACAPS appeared to reduce the risk for major cardiovascular events and all-cause mortality rate (Furberg et al. 1994). The 3.5-year Risk Intervention Study (RIS), however, found no carotid ultrasound benefit with a comprehensive risk factor modification program emphasizing nonpharmacologic intervention in high-risk hypertensive patients (Suurküla et al. 1996); the authors speculated that a greater reduction in risk factors may have been required.

Ultrasound and angiographic findings in the femoral bed have been inconsistent and largely disappointing. The therapy effect in CLAS in femoral arteries as evaluated by angiography was significant but less marked than in coronary native vessels and bypass grafts (Blankenhorn et al. 1991). In KAPS there was no significant effect in the femoral bed according to ultrasound monitoring (Salonen et al. 1995b). In the 3-year Probucol Quantitative Regression Swedish Trial (PQRST), which assessed effects on femoral atherosclerosis, the addition of probucol to cholestyramine and diet did not lead to any angiographic improvement over cholestyramine and diet alone, although in the latter group there was statistically significant evidence of improvement (Walldius et al. 1994). Peripheral atherosclerosis is associated with prevalence and clinical symptoms of CHD (Bergstrand et al. 1994; Valentine et al. 1994) and is predictive of long-term mortality in patients with stable CHD (Eagle et al. 1994). Intermittent claudication is predictive of long-term cerebrovascular disease mortality (Bowlin et al. 1997, in a study in men).

LESION STABILIZATION

As outlined above, there is an apparent discrepancy between the small changes in stenosis and the large improvements in coronary event rates in the regression trials. Furthermore, whereas years are usually required for angiographic improvement, benefit in coronary event rates has been reported from statin clinical endpoint trials within 6 months to 1 year (see Chapter 12). Given this angiographic-clinical paradox and emerging laboratory and animal data, it has been hypothesized that lipid-modifying therapy may achieve its clinical benefit at least in part and perhaps to a major degree through pathophysiologic mechanisms other than effects on stenosis (Brown 1993; Brown et al. 1993; Gotto 1995; Shah 1996; Kinlay et al. 1996; Müller-Wieland et al. 1997). Beneficial effects on plaque biology unrelated to major changes in stenosis have been loosely termed "lesion stabilization" and encompass a reduced propensity to plaque rupture/thrombosis and improvement in abnormal vasomotor function (Shah 1996) (Table 10.3).

Lipid lowering has been shown in experimental models to affect many of the cellular processes (described in Chapters 6 and 7) that predispose to plaque disruption and thrombosis. Its effects include improvement of endothelial function (see later), depletion of cholesteryl ester levels (Armstrong et al. 1970; Clarkson et al. 1981; Small et al. 1984), a reduction of inflammatory cells within plaque (Padgett et al. 1992), loss of vasa vasorum (Williams et al. 1988), and an increase in collagen matrix (Small et al. 1984; Wissler and Vesselinovitch 1990) (reviewed by Shah 1996 and Kinlay et al. 1996). Like effects have been reported with the administration of HDL to experimental animals (Badimon et al. 1990; Shah 1996). Lipid lowering can also lead to the hydrolysis of (liquid) cholesteryl ester to (solid-phase crystalline) cholesterol monohydrate, which also promotes plaque stiffness and stability (Loree et al. 1994; Small 1988). It has been shown to reduce macrophage infiltration, as have antioxidants and apo A-I Milano (Ameli et al. 1994; Ferns et al. 1992), and to have beneficial effects on platelets, coagulation, fibrinolysis, and blood viscosity (Shah 1996). A reduction in cytokine production might occur through reducing concentrations of oxidized or modified lipoproteins in particular.

Effects on vascular reactivity (see later), rheologic/thrombotic effects (decreased blood viscosity, red cell wall rigidity, platelet aggregation, and fibrinogen), local cellular actions, modulation of immune function, and

Table 10.3. POTENTIAL APPROACHES TO PREVENTION OF ADVERSE CONSEQUENCES OF CORONARY ATHEROSCLEROSIS

Prevention of atherosclerosis and its progression and facilitation of regression
Plaque stabilization
   Reduced vulnerability to rupture
      Reduced lipid core or modification of its composition
      Reduced macrophage density or matrix-degrading activity
      Increased SMC density and matrix synthesis
   Elimination of extrinsic triggers to plaque rupture
   Reduced plaque thrombogenicity
      Reduced lipid core
      Reduced macrophage density and tissue factor content/activity
   Improved endothelial function
      Restoration of normal vasodilator function
      Reduced prothrombotic phenotype
      Reduced proinflammatory phenotype
      In each case:
         Reduced lipid core
         Reduced lipid concentrations
         Reduced lipid peroxidation
Improved systemic thrombotic-thrombolytic equilibrium
Promotion of collateral recruitment

Source: Adapted with permission from Shah 1996.

reduced oxidation potential are among the mechanisms with possible therapeutic benefit for which evidence is available for the HMG-CoA reductase inhibitors (reviewed by Vaughan et al. 1996, Corsini et al. 1996, Kinlay et al. 1996, and Dujovne 1997). Many of these effects have occurred within 3 months of the beginning of statin therapy (Dujovne 1997). In vitro data suggest that these drugs affect cholesterol metabolism of macrophages and vascular SMCs and might also interfere with other intracellular signaling pathways of potential mitogenic or growth factor significance (Müller-Wieland et al. 1997). Fibrate effects include well-defined effects on hemostatic variables, including reduction of circulating fibrinogen concentration (Havel 1997). Such effects may be specific or modified through a reduction of LDL-C or other lipid modifications. The possibility of nonlipid effects in the West of Scotland Coronary Prevention Study (WOSCOPS) has been raised by its investigators on the basis of the results of applying a Framingham risk prediction model to the data: Whereas risk for a CHD event was accurately predicted in the placebo group, risk reduction in the pravastatin group was significantly underestimated. The predicted risk reduction was 24%; the observed reduction was 35% (predicted: 5.7 in 100; observed: 4.5 in 100) (West of Scotland Coronary Prevention Study Group 1998).

Improvement in Endothelial Function

As discussed in Chapter 6, endothelial function is impaired in athero-sclerotic arteries, a dysfunction that predisposes to vasoconstriction, thrombosis, and inflammatory cell recruitment. Restoration of normal endothelial function may play a role of central importance in reduction of clinical events. Impaired endothelial function is associated with risk factors for CHD, including dyslipidemias such as increased LDL-C, dense LDL, and oxLDL and decreased HDL-C, and is independent of the presence of atherosclerosis on angiography or ultrasound (Reddy et al. 1994; Zeiher et al. 1991, 1994; Leung et al. 1993; Egashira et al. 1994; Anderson et al. 1995b; Kinlay et al. 1996). Other studies have shown altered vascular responses to platelets as well as increased thromboxane formation in hypercholesterolemic subjects (Davi et al. 1992; Kaul et al. 1993). With risk factor modification, endothelial function improves rapidly, even in the presence of atherosclerosis (Benzuly et al. 1994).

At least 12 clinical studies have demonstrated improved endothelial function with cholesterol lowering in patients with and without CHD and with marked or borderline hypercholesterolemia (Vogel 1997) (Table 10.4). The improvement has been demonstrated within 2–4 weeks of the initiation of therapy (Stroes et al. 1995; Vogel et al. 1996; O'Driscoll et al. 1997). Endothelial function in such studies is commonly assessed by (1) QCA, measuring changes after infusion of acetylcholine; (2) ultrasound, measuring changes in brachial artery diameter after induction of hyperemia with blood pressure cuff occlusion; and (3) venous plethysmography, measuring forearm blood flow after intra-arterial infusion of a cholinergic stimulus such as methacholine (Vogel 1997). Other interventions may have like effects (Vogel 1997); for example, smoking cessation (Celermajer et al. 1993), regular exercise (Hornig et al. 1996), and lowering of blood pressure (Luscher et al. 1987; Panza et al. 1993a, 1993b) have been associated with improvement in endothelial function, as has, variably, vitamin C supplementation (Levine et al. 1996). Vitamin C improves endothelium-dependent vasodilation in subjects who smoke and decreases the expression of monocyte adhesion molecules (Heitzer et al. 1996; Weber et al. 1996a; Reilly et al. 1996). Probucol, a lipid-altering agent that is a powerful antioxidant, improved acetylcholine-induced coronary vasodilation beyond the beneficial effect of cholesterol lowering alone in patients with CHD (Anderson et al. 1995b). Oxidative stress appears to be an important factor in endothelial dysfunction (Shah 1997); the association of decreased HDL-C with endothelial dysfunction may reflect the antioxidant properties of HDL (Kuhn et al. 1991). In normocholesterolemic subjects, a single high-fat meal (50 g fat) decreased flow-mediated brachial artery vasodilation for up to 4 hours; the effect was reversed by pretreatment with combined vitamins C and E (Vogel et al. 1997; Plotnick et al. 1997). Experimentally, atherosclerotic plaques have also been modified by some dietary fatty acids,

Table 10.4. CLINICAL TRIALS DEMONSTRATING IMPROVEMENT IN ENDOTHELIAL FUNCTION WITH CHOLESTEROL LOWERING

Study	CHD	Mean TC (mg/dL)	Circulation	Treatment	Duration (mos)
Egashira et al. 1994	Y	272	CA	Pravastatin	6
Seiler et al. 1995	Y	300	CA	Bezafibrate	7
Treasure et al. 1995	Y	226	CA	Lovastatin	5
Anderson et al. 1995b	Y	209	CA	Lovastatin/ cholestyramine	12
Eichstadt et al. 1995*	Y	284	CA	Fluvastatin	3
Tamai et al. 1997*	Y	195	FBF	LDL apheresis	Single session
Muramatsu et al. 1997*	NR	263	CA + peripheral	Pravastatin	6
Leung et al. 1993	N	239	CA	Cholestyramine	6
Stroes et al. 1995	N	354	FBF	Simvastatin/ cholestyramine	3
Vogel et al. 1996	N	200	BA	Simvastatin	3
Megnien et al. 1996*	N	289	BA	Pravastatin	3
O'Driscoll et al. 1997*	Y/N	255	FBF	Simvastatin	3

BA, brachial artery; CA, coronary arteries; FBF, forearm blood flow; NR, not reported.
Source: Updated (*) from Vogel 1997. Copyrighted and reprinted with permission of Clinical Cardiology Publishing Company, Inc., and/or the Foundation for Advances in Medicine and Science, Inc., Mahwah, NJ 07430-0832.

avoidance of psychosocial stress, ACE inhibition, and estrogen replacement (Falk et al. 1995).

Improvement of myocardial perfusion capacity has been demonstrated with positron emission tomography after 90 days of cholesterol-lowering treatment in hypercholesterolemic patients with angina (Gould et al. 1994), as well as after 5 years of risk factor modification in the Lifestyle Heart Trial (very low fat vegetarian diet, mild to moderate exercise, and group support vs. usual care; see Table 10.1) (Gould et al. 1995). The improvement is considered likely to involve not only partial anatomic regression of localized coronary artery stenosis but also improved endothelium-mediated coronary artery and arteriolar vasodilation (Gould 1994).

TRIGGER REDUCTION

Although stabilization of atherosclerotic lesions is required to eliminate or reduce their vulnerability to rupture, reducing trigger activities may also help prevent or at least delay disruption (Falk et al. 1995). Candidate triggers include smoking and, in the physically unfit, sudden vigorous exertion (see "Onset of Acute Coronary Syndromes" in Chapter 6). CHD event risk from cigarette smoking is rapidly reversible with smoking cessation (see Chapter 11), implicating acute triggering in the risk. ACE inhibitors, beta-blockers, and heart rate–reducing calcium antagonists may also modify triggering mechanisms (reviewed by Falk et al. 1995).

Suggested Reading

Blankenhorn DH, Hodis HN. Arterial imaging and atherosclerosis reversal. George Lyman Duff Memorial Lecture. Arterioscler Thromb 1994;14: 177–192.

Brown BG. Lipid-lowering therapy for the stabilization of the vulnerable atherosclerotic plaque (review). Curr Opin Lipidol 1993;4:305–309.

Buchwald H, Matts JP, Fitch LL, et al. for the Program on the Surgical Control of the Hyperlipidemias (POSCH) Group. Changes in sequential coronary arteriograms and subsequent coronary events. JAMA 1992;268:1429–1433.

Gotto AM Jr. Lipid lowering, regression, and coronary events: a review of the Interdisciplinary Council on Lipids and Cardiovascular Risk Intervention, Seventh Council Meeting. Circulation 1995;92:646–656.

Gould KL. Reversal of coronary atherosclerosis: clinical promise as the basis for noninvasive management of coronary artery disease (review). Circulation 1994;90:1558–1570.

Kinlay S, Selwyn AP, Delagrange D, et al. Biological mechanisms for the clinical success of lipid-lowering in coronary artery disease and the use of surrogate end-points. Curr Opin Lipidol 1996;7:389–397.

Shah PK. Pathophysiology of plaque rupture and the concept of plaque stabilization (review). Cardiol Clin 1996;14:17–29.

Vaughan CJ, Murphy MB, Buckley BM. Statins do more than just lower cholesterol (review). Lancet 1996;348:1079–1082.

Vogel RA. Coronary risk factors, endothelial function, and atherosclerosis: a review. Clin Cardiol 1997;20:426–432.

REFERENCES

Aengevaeren WRM et al. J Am Coll Cardiol 1996;28:1696–1704.

Alderman EL et al. J Am Coll Cardiol 1993;22:1141–1154.

Alvarez C, Ramos A. Clin Chem 1986;32:142–145.

Ambrose JA, Weinrauch M. Arch Intern Med 1996;156:1382–1388.

Ambrose JA et al. J Am Coll Cardiol 1988;12:56–62.

Ameli S et al. Circulation 1994;90:1935–1941.

Ameli S et al. Arterioscler Thromb Vasc Biol 1996;16:1074–1079.

Anber V et al. Arterioscler Thromb Vasc Biol 1997;17:2507–2514.

Anderson HV et al. In: Willerson JT, Cohn JN, eds. Cardiovascular medicine. New York: Churchill Livingstone, 1995a:617–651.

Anderson TJ et al. N Engl J Med 1995b;332:488–493.

Anderson TJ et al. Circulation 1996;93:1647–1650.

Andersson L-O. Curr Opin Lipidol 1997;8:225–228.

Annex BH et al. Circulation 1995;91:619–622.

Applebaum-Bowden D et al. J Lipid Res 1989;30:1895–1906.

Armstrong ML et al. Circ Res 1970;27:59–67.

Armstrong VW et al. Atherosclerosis 1986;62:249–257.

Asakura T, Karino T. Cir Res 1990;66:1045–1066.

Assmann G, Schulte H. Am Heart J 1988;116:1713–1724.

Assmann G, Schulte H. Am J Cardiol 1992;70:733–737.

Assmann G et al. Atherosclerosis 1996;124(suppl):S11–S20.

Austin MA. Diabetes Metab Rev 1991;7:173–177.

Austin MA, Edwards KL. Curr Opin Lipidol 1996;7:167–171.

Austin MA et al. JAMA 1988;260:1917–1921.

Austin MA et al. Circulation 1990;82:495–506.

Austin MA et al. Atherosclerosis 1992;92:67–77.

Austin MA et al. Curr Opin Lipidol 1994;5:395–403.

Avellone G et al. Thromb Res 1994;75:223–231.

Axelsen M et al. J Intern Med 1995;237:449–455.

Azen SP et al. Circulation 1996;93:34–41.

Badimon JJ et al. J Clin Invest 1990;85:1234–1241.

Badimon JJ et al. Arterioscler Thromb 1991;11:395–402.

Ball RY et al. Atherosclerosis 1995;114:45–54.

Ballantyne CM et al. J Am Coll Cardiol 1992;19:1315–1321.

Ballantyne CM et al. Curr Opin Cardiol 1997;12:153–160.

Barath P et al. Am J Pathol 1990;137:503–509.

Baroldi G. Am Heart J 1966;71:826–836.

Baroldi G, Scomazzoni G. Coronary circulation in the normal and the pathologic heart. Washington, DC: Department of the Army, 1967:217–228.

Baron AD. J Invest Med 1996;44:406–412.

Barrett-Connor E et al. Maturitas 1997;27:261–274.

Barter PJ, Rye K-A. Atherosclerosis 1996;121:1–12.

Baumgartner I et al. Circulation 1998;97:1114–1123.

Bauters C, Isner JM. Prog Cardiovasc Dis 1997;40:107–116.

Beisiegel U, St. Clair RW. Curr Opin Lipidol 1996;7:265–268.

Benditt EP, Benditt JM. Proc Natl Acad Sci U S A 1973;70:1753–1756.

Benowitz NL. Prev Med 1997;26:412–417.

Benowitz NL, Gourlay SG. J Am Coll Cardiol 1997;29:1422–1431.

Benzuly KH et al. Circulation 1994;89:1810–1818.

Bergstrand L et al. J Intern Med 1994;236:367–375.

Berliner JA et al. J Clin Invest 1990;85:1260–1266.

Berliner JA et al. Circulation 1995;91:2488–2496.

Bierman EL. Arterioscler Thromb 1992;12:647–656.

Billingham ME. Transplant Proc 1989;21:3665–3666.

Billingham ME. J Heart Lung Transplant 1992;11:S38–S44.

Bini A et al. Arteriosclerosis 1989;9:109–121.

Bjorkerud S, Bjorkerud B. Am J Pathol 1996;149:367–380.

Björntorp P. Metabolism 1995;44(suppl 3):21–23.

Björntorp P. Ciba Found Symp 1996;201:68–80.

Blanche PJ et al. Biochim Biophys Acta 1981;665:408–419.

Blankenhorn DH, Hodis HN. Arterioscler Thromb 1994;14:177–192.

Blankenhorn DH et al. JAMA 1987;257:3233–40. Corrigenda appear in JAMA 1988;259:2698.

Blankenhorn DH et al. Circulation 1990;81:470–476.

Blankenhorn DH et al. Circulation 1991;83:438–447.

Blankenhorn DH et al. Ann Intern Med 1993;119:969–976.

Bolton-Smith C et al. Br J Nutr 1991;65:337–346.

Bostrom K et al. J Clin Invest 1993;91:1800–1809.

Bowlin SJ et al. Ann Epidemiol 1997;7:180–187.

Braun WE, Marwick TH. Cleve Clin J Med 1994;61:370–385.

Brensike JF et al. Circulation 1984;69:313–324.

Brogi E et al. J Clin Invest 1993;92:2408–2418.

Brown BG. Curr Opin Lipidol 1993;4:305–309.

Brown BG et al. Circulation 1986;73:653–661.

Brown BG et al. Arteriosclerosis 1989;9(suppl I):181–190.

Brown BG et al. Circulation 1993;87:1781–1791.

Brown G et al. N Engl J Med 1990;323:1289–1298.

Brown MS, Goldstein JL. Nature 1990;343:508–509.

Brownlee M. Diabetes 1994;43:836–841.

Bruce C, Tall AR. Curr Opin Lipidol 1995;6:306–311.

Bucala R et al. Proc Natl Acad Sci U S A 1993;90:6434–6438.

Bucay M et al. Atherosclerosis (in press).

Buchwald H et al. N Engl J Med 1990;323:946–955.

Buchwald H et al. Ann Surg 1992a;216:389–400.

Buchwald H et al. JAMA 1992b;268:1429–1433.
Buja LM. In: Willerson JT, Cohn JN, eds. Cardiovascular medicine. New York: Churchill Livingstone, 1995:1090–1099.
Burch GE, Shewey LL. Am Heart J 1976;92:11–14.
Burke AP et al. N Engl J Med 1997;336:1276–1282.
Burke GL et al. Stroke 1995;26:386–391.
Bussiere JL et al. Arch Mal Coeur Vaiss 1996;89:425–429.
Byington RP et al. Circulation 1995;92:2419–2425.
Cade JE, Margetts BM. J Epidemiol Community Health 1991;45:270–272.
Cagliero E et al. Diabetes 1991;40:102–110.
Campos H et al. Arterioscler Thromb 1992;12:187–195.
Caprio S et al. Am J Clin Nutr 1996;64:12–17.
Carey DGP. Curr Opin Lipidol 1998;9:35–40.
Carey DG et al. Diabetes 1996;45:633–638.
Carmelli D et al. Am J Hum Genet 1994;55:566–573.
Cashin-Hemphill L et al. JAMA 1990;264:3013–3016.
Castelli WP. Am J Cardiol 1992;70(suppl):3H–9H.
Castro GR, Fielding CJ. Biochemistry 1988;27:25–29.
Cathcart MK et al. J Leukoc Biol 1985;38:341–350.
Caulin-Glaser T et al. J Clin Invest 1996;98:36–42.
Celermajer DS et al. Circulation 1993;88:2149–2155.
Celermajer DS et al. J Am Coll Cardiol 1994;24:1468–1474.
Chae CU et al. Thromb Haemost 1997;78:770–780.
Chambless LE et al. Am J Epidemiol 1997;146:483–494.
Chapmann MJ et al. Atherosclerosis 1994;110(suppl):S69–S75.
Chen CH, Henry PD. Proc Assoc Am Phys 1997;109:351–361.
Chen CH et al. Atherosclerosis 1995;116:261–268.
Chen CH et al. Arterioscler Thromb Vasc Biol 1997;17:1303–1312.
Chisholm DJ et al. In: Alberti KGMM, Krall LP, eds. The diabetes annual. Amsterdam: Elsevier Science, 1991:276–285.
Chisholm DJ et al. Clin Exp Pharmacol Physiol 1997;24:782–784.
Chung BH et al. Arterioscler Thromb 1994;14:622–635.
Clarkson TB et al. Exp Mol Pathol 1981;34:345–368.
Clarkson TB et al. JAMA 1994;271:289–294.
Cohen M et al. J Am Coll Cardiol 1989;13:297–303.
Cominacini L et al. Atherosclerosis 1993;99:63–70.
Cook PJ, Lip GY. QJM 1996b;89:727–735.
Cook PJ et al. Stroke 1998;29:404–410.
Coresh J, Kwiterovich PO Jr. JAMA 1996;276:914–915.
Coresh J et al. J Lipid Res 1993;34:1687–1697.
Corsini A et al. Cardiology 1996;87:458–468.
Cottet J, Lenoir M. Bull Acad Natl Med 1992;176:1385–1390.

Craig WY et al. BMJ 1989;298:784–788.
Craven TE et al. Circulation 1990;82:1230–1242.
Crea F et al. Am J Cardiol 1997;80(5A):10E–16E.
Criqui MH et al. N Engl J Med 1993;328:1220–1225.
Crouse JR III et al. Am J Cardiol 1995;75:455–459.
Cryer PE et al. N Engl J Med 1976;295:573–577.
Currens JH, White PD. N Engl J Med 1961;265:988–993.
Dahlén GH. Eur J Immunogenet 1994;21:301–312.
Dahlén GH, Stenlund H. Clin Genet 1997;52:272–280.
Daida H et al. Am J Cardiol 1994;73:1037–1040.
Danchin N. Lancet 1993;342:224–225.
Danesh J et al. Lancet 1997;350:430–436.
Darling GM et al. N Engl J Med 1997;337:595–601.
D'Avanzo B et al. Nutr Cancer 1997;28:46–51.
Davi G et al. Circulation 1992;85:1792–1798.
Davies MJ. Circulation 1990;82(3 suppl): II-38–II-46.
Davies MJ. Eur Heart J 1995;16(suppl L):3–7.
Davies MJ. Thromb Res 1996a;82:1–32.
Davies MJ. Lancet 1996b;347:1422–1423.
Davies MJ. Heart 1997a;77:498–501.
Davies MJ. In: Alexander RW, Schlant RC, Fuster V, eds. Hurst's the heart arteries and veins, ed. 9, vol. 1. New York: McGraw-Hill, 1998:1161–1173.
Davies MJ, Woolf N. Br Heart J 1993;69(suppl):S3–S11.
Davies MJ et al. Eur Heart J 1989;10:203–208.
Davies MJ et al. Br Heart J 1993;69:377–381.
Davies MJ et al. Basic Res Cardiol 1994;89 (suppl 1):33–39.
Davies PF. Atherosclerosis 1997b;131 (suppl):S15–S17.
Davies SW et al. J Am Coll Cardiol 1991;18:669–674.
Davignon J, Cohn JS. Atherosclerosis 1996;124(suppl):S57–S64.
DeBakey ME, Gotto AM Jr. The new living heart. Holbrook, MA: Adams, 1997.
DeBakey ME et al. Ann Surg 1985;201:115–131.
Deckelbaum RJ et al. Arterioscler Thromb 1984;4:225–231.
De Man FHAF et al. Eur J Clin Invest 1996;26:89–108
Demer LL et al. Trends Cardiovasc Med 1994;4:45–49.
de Prost D, Hakim J. Atherosclerosis 1997;131(suppl):S19–S21.
de Rijke YB et al. J Lipid Res 1992;33:1315–1325.
Devries S et al. J Am Coll Cardiol 1995;25:76–82.
Diaz MN et al. N Engl J Med 1997;337:408–415.
Di Mario C et al. J Cardiovasc Pharmacol 1994;24(suppl 3):S5–S15.
Dollery CM et al. Circ Res 1995;77:863–868.
Duerinckx AJ. Int J Card Imaging 1997;13:191–197.
Dujovne CA. Curr Opin Lipidol 1997;8:362–368.
Dyce MC et al. Circulation 1996;88(suppl I):I-466–I-471.
Dzau VJ, Gibbons GH. J Cardiovasc Pharmacol 1993;21(suppl 1):S1–S5.
Eagle KA et al. J Am Coll Cardiol 1994;23:1091–1095.

Eaton DL et al. Proc Natl Acad Sci U S A 1987;84:3224–3228.

Ebenbichler CF et al. Curr Opin Lipidol 1995;6:286–290.

Egashira K et al. Circulation 1994;89:2519–2524.

Eliasson B et al. Arterioscler Thromb 1994;14:1946–1950.

Eliasson B et al. Atherosclerosis 1997;129:79–88.

Eliasson M et al. Atherosclerosis 1995;113:41–53.

Ellis RW. J Med Microbiol 1997;46:535–539.

English RM et al. Aust N Z J Public Health 1997;21:141–146.

Epstein SE. Am J Cardiol 1988;61:866–868.

Epstein SE et al. Lancet 1996;348:s13–s17.

Ericsson CG et al. Lancet 1996;347:849–853.

Ericsson CG et al. Am J Cardiol 1997;80:1125–1129.

Ettinger B et al. Obstet Gynecol 1996;87:6–12.

Fabricant CG et al. J Exp Med 1978;148:335–340.

Facchini FS et al. Lancet 1992;339:1128–1130.

Factor SM, Bache RJ. In: Alexander RW, Schlant RC, Fuster V, eds. Hurst's the heart arteries and veins, ed. 9. New York: McGraw-Hill, 1998:1241–1262.

Faggiotto A et al. Arteriosclerosis 1984;4:323–340.

Falk E. Br Heart J 1983;50:127–131.

Falk E et al. Circulation 1995;92:657–671.

Farb A et al. Circulation 1996;93:1354–1363.

Farhat MY et al. FASEB J 1996;10:615–624.

Faruqi RM, DiCorleto PE. Br Heart J 1993;69(suppl):S19–S29.

Faxon DP et al. Prog Cardiovasc Dis 1997;40:129–140.

Feldman J et al. Pediatrics 1991;88:259–264.

Fernández-Ortiz A, Fuster V. Clin Geriatr Med 1996;12:1–21.

Fernández-Ortiz A et al. J Am Coll Cardiol 1994;23:1562–1569.

Ferns GAA et al. Proc Natl Acad Sci U S A 1992;89:11312–11316.

Ferrannini E et al. N Engl J Med 1987;317:350–357.

Ferrannini E et al. J Clin Invest 1997;100:1166–1173.

Fielding CJ, Fielding PE. J Lipid Res 1995;36:211–228.

Folkman J. Circulation 1998a;97:628–629.

Folkman J. Circulation 1998b;97:1108–1110.

Frick MH et al. Circulation 1997;96:2137–2143.

Frohlich ED, Re RN. In: Alexander RW, Schlant RC, Fuster V, eds. Hurst's the heart arteries and veins, ed. 9, vol. 1. New York: McGraw-Hill, 1998:1635–1650.

Frostegard J et al. Atherosclerosis 1991;90:119–126.

Furberg CD et al. Circulation 1994;90:1679–1687.

Fuster V et al. N Engl J Med 1992;326:242–250.

Fuster V et al. Lancet 1996;348:s7–s10.

Galis ZS et al. J Clin Invest 1994;94:2493–2503.

Garcia MJ et al. Diabetes 1974;23:105–111.

Gardner CD et al. JAMA 1996;276:875–881.

Garrison RJ et al. Curr Opin Lipidol 1996;7:199–202.

Geng YJ et al. Arterioscler Thromb Vasc Biol 1996;16:19–27.

Geng Y-L, Libby P. Am J Pathol 1995;147:251–266.

George J et al. Immunol Res 1996;15:315–322.

Gerszten RE et al. Circ Res 1996;79:1205–1215.

Gibbons GH, Dzau VJ. N Engl J Med 1994;330:1431–1438.

Gibson CM et al. Arterioscler Thromb 1993;13:310–315.

Giddens DP et al. J Biomech Eng 1993;115:588–593.

Gilligan DM et al. Circulation 1994;90:786–791.

Glagov S et al. N Engl J Med 1987;316:1371–1375.

Glagov S et al. J Vasc Invest 1995a;1:2–14.

Glagov S et al. Surg Clin North Am 1995b;75:545–556.

Glagov S et al. Atherosclerosis 1997;131(suppl):S13–S14.

Glomset JA. J Lipid Res 1968;9:155–167.

Goldberg IJ. J Lipid Res 1996;37:693–707.

Goldbourt U et al. Arterioscler Thromb Vasc Biol 1997;17:107–113.

Goldstein JL et al. Proc Natl Acad Sci U S A 1979;76:333–337.

Gordon DJ et al. Circulation 1989;79:8–15.

Gotto AM Jr. Circulation 1995;92:646–656.

Gould KL. Circulation 1994;90:1558–1570.

Gould KL et al. Circulation 1994;89:1530–1538.

Gould KL et al. JAMA 1995;274:894–901.

Grady D et al. Ann Intern Med 1992;117:1016–1037.

Graham A et al. FEBS Lett 1993;330:181–185.

Graham DL, Oram JF. J Biol Chem 1987;262:7439–7442.

Gregg DE, Patterson RE. N Engl J Med 1980;303:1404–1406.

Groot PH et al. Arterioscler Thromb 1991;11:653–662.

Grundy SM. Circulation 1997;95:1–4.

Grundy SM et al. Eur Heart J 1990;11:462–471.

Gupta S, Camm AJ. BMJ 1997;514:1778–1779.

Gupta S et al. J Am Coll Cardiol 1997;29 (suppl A):209A.

Gurfinkel E et al. Lancet 1997;350:404–407.

Guyton JR, Klemp KF. Arterioscler Thromb 1994;14:1305–1314.

Haberland ME et al. J Biol Chem 1992;267:4143–4151.

Habib GB et al. Circulation 1991;83:739–746.

Haffner SM. Ann N Y Acad Sci 1997;827:1–12.

Haffner SM et al. Diabetes 1992;41:715–722.

Haidet GC. In: Willerson JT, Cohn JN, eds. Cardiovascular medicine. New York: Churchill Livingstone, 1995:702–740.

Hajjar KA, Nachman RL. Annu Rev Med 1996;47:423–442.

Hamet P et al. Hypertension 1985;7(suppl II):II-135–II-142.

Hamilton KK et al. J Biol Chem 1993;268:3632–3638.

Hamsten A et al. N Engl J Med 1985;313:1557–1563.

Hansson GK. Arteriosclerosis 1994;89(suppl 1):41–46.

Hansson GK. Curr Opin Lipidol 1997;8:301–311.

Harats D et al. Atherosclerosis 1989;79:245–252.

Hardwick SJ et al. J Pathol 1996;179:294–302.

Haskell WL et al. The Stanford Coronary Risk Intervention Project (SCRIP). Circulation 1994;89:975–990.

Hausmann D et al. J Am Coll Cardiol 1996;27:1562–1570.

Havel RJ. Circulation 1997;96:2113–2114.

Hearn JA et al. Am J Cardiol 1992;69:736–739.

Hegele RA. Crit Rev Clin Lab Sci 1997;34:343–367.

Heinecke JW et al. J Clin Invest 1984;74:1890–1894.

Heistad DH, Armstrong ML. Arteriosclerosis 1986;6:326–331.

Heitzer T et al. Circulation 1996;94:6–9.

Henriksen T et al. Proc Natl Acad Sci U S A 1981;78:6499–6503.

Herd JA et al. Am J Cardiol 1997;80:278–286.

Hessler JR et al. Arteriosclerosis 1983;3:215–222.

Hirai T et al. Circulation 1989;79:791–796.

Hirose N et al. Keio J Med 1996;45:90–94.

Hodis HN, Mack WJ. Curr Opin Lipidol 1995;6:209–214.

Hodis HN et al. Circulation 1994;90:42–49.

Hodis HN et al. Circulation 1997;95:2022–2026.

Hokanson JE, Austin MA. J Cardiovasc Risk 1996;3:213–219.

Holvoet P et al. J Clin Invest 1995;95:2611–2619.

Hong MK et al. Curr Prob Cardiol 1997;22:1–36.

Hopkins PN et al. Curr Opin Lipidol 1996;7:241–253.

Hoppichler F et al. Atherosclerosis 1996;126:333–338.

Horie H et al. Circulation 1997;96:166–173.

Hornig B et al. Circulation 1996;93:210–214.

Hosenpud JD et al. J Heart Lung Transplant 1997;16:691–712.

Hotamisligil GS et al. Science 1996;271:665–668.

Howard G et al. Circulation 1996;93:1809–1817.

Howard GC, Pizzo SV. Lab Invest 1993;69:373–386.

Hulley S et al. JAMA 1998;280:605–613.

Hunt SC et al. Arteriosclerosis 1989;9:335–344.

Hurst JW. Circulation 1994;90:2163–2165.

Hwang C-S et al. Annu Rev Cell Dev Biol 1997;13:231–259.

The International Committee for the Evaluation of Hypertriglyceridemia as a Vascular Risk Factor. Am J Cardiol 1991;68(suppl):1A–42A.

Isner JM et al. Lancet 1996;348:370–374.

Iso H et al. Am J Epidemiol 1996;144:1151–1154.

Jacobs DR Jr et al. Am J Epidemiol 1990;131:32–47.

Jarrett RJ. Diabetologia 1994;37:945–947.

Joint National Committee on Detection, Evaluation, and Treatment of High Blood Pressure. Arch Intern Med 1993;153:154–183.

Jones DA et al. In: Granger DN, Schmid-Schönbein GW, eds. Physiology and pathophysiology of leukocyte adhesion. New York: Oxford University Press, 1995:148–168.

Jukema JW et al. Circulation 1995;91:2528–2540.

Kagan AR, Uemura K. Bull World Health Organ 1976;53:489–499.

Kane JP et al. JAMA 1990;264:3007–3012.

Kannel WB. Am J Cardiol 1995;76:69C–77C.

Kannel WB et al. Am Heart J 1990;120:672–676.

Kaplan JR et al. Arterioscler Thromb 1993;13:254–263.

Kaplan NM. Arch Intern Med 1989;149:1514–1520.

Karpe F, Hamsten A. Curr Opin Lipidol 1995;6:123–129.

Karpe F et al. Atherosclerosis 1994;106:83–97.

Katznelson S, Kobashigawa JA. Kidney Int Suppl 1995;52:S112–S115.

Kaul S et al. Cir Res 1993;72:737–743.

Kawai C. Circulation 1994;90:1033–1043.

Keesler GA et al. Arterioscler Thromb 1994;14:1337–1345.

Kemna MS et al. Am Heart J 1994;128:68–72.

Kinlay S et al. Curr Opin Lipidol 1996;7:389–397.

Kirchmair R et al. Baillieres Clin Endocrinol Metab 1995;9:705–719.

Kissebah AH. Diabetes Res Clin Pract 1996;30(suppl):S25–S30.

Kleindienst R et al. Isr J Med Sci 1995;31:596–599.

Kobashigawa JA, Kasiske BL. Transplantation 1997;63:331–338.

Kobashigawa JA et al. N Engl J Med 1995;333:621–627.

Kockx MM et al. Atherosclerosis 1996;120:115–124.

Koo LC. Int J Cancer 1997;suppl 10:22–29.

Kopelman PG, Albon L. Br Med Bull 1997;53:322–340.

Kornowski R et al. Am J Cardiol 1997a;79:1601–1605.

Kornowski R et al. J Am Coll Cardiol 1997b;29(suppl A):365A.

Kortelainen ML. Int J Obesity 1996;20:245–252.

Kortelainen ML, Sarkioja T. Arterioscler Thromb Vasc Biol 1997;17:574–579.

Kramsch DM et al. N Engl J Med 1981;305:1483–1489.

Krasinski K et al. Circulation 1997;95:1768–1772.

Krauss RM. Curr Opin Lipidol 1994;5:339–349.

Krauss RM et al. Lancet 1987;2:62–66.

Kritz H et al. Wien Klin Wochenschr 1996;108:87–97.

Kroon AA et al. Circulation 1996;93:1826–1835.

Kruth HS. Curr Opin Lipidol 1997;8:246–252.

Ku G et al. J Biol Chem 1992;267:14183–14188.

Kuhn FE et al. Am J Cardiol 1991;68:1425–1430.

Kume N et al. J Clin Invest 1992;90:1138–1144.

Kushwaha RS. Curr Opin Lipidol 1992;3:167–172.

Kwiterovich PO Jr et al. Clin Chem 1991;37:317–326.

Laakso M. Am J Epidemiol 1993;137:959–965.

Laakso M. Curr Opin Lipidol 1996;7:217–226.

Lakier JB. Am J Med 1992;93(suppl 1A):8S–12S.

Lamarche B et al. Circulation 1997;95:69–75.

Larkin FA et al. J Am Diet Assoc 1990;90:230–237.

Lawn RM et al. Nature 1992;360:670–672.

Lee YJ et al. Jpn Heart J 1996;37:327–332.

Lefkovits J, Topol EJ. Prog Cardiovasc Dis 1997;40:141–158.

Lehr H-A, Messmer K. In: Granger DN, Schmid-Schönbein GW, eds. Physiology and pathophysiology of leukocyte adhesion. New York: Oxford University Press, 1995:434–446.

Lerner DJ, Kannel WB. Am Heart J 1986;111:383–390.

Leung WH et al. Lancet 1993;341:1496–1500.

Levine GN et al. Circulation 1996;93:1107–1113.

Levy RI et al. Circulation 1984;69:325–337.

Ley K. Cardiovasc Res 1996;32:733–742.

Ley K et al. In: Granger DN, Schmid-Schönbein GW, eds. Physiology and pathophysiology of leukocyte adhesion. New York: Oxford University Press, 1995:217–240.

Libby P. Am J Cardiol 1994;73:508–510.

Libby P. Circulation 1995;91:2844–2850.

Libby P. Lancet 1996;348:s4–s7.

Libby P, Hansson GK. Lab Invest 1991;64:5–15.

Libby P, Tanaka H. Clin Transplant 1994;8:313–318.

Libby P, Tanaka H. Prog Cardiovasc Dis 1997;40:97–106.

Libby P et al. J Heart Lung Transplant 1992;11:S5–S6.

Libby P et al. Ann N Y Acad Sci 1997;11:134–142.

Lip GY, Beevers DG. Lancet 1997;350:378–379.

Liuzzo G et al. N Engl J Med 1994;331:417–424.

Lobo RA. Ann N Y Acad Sci 1990;592:286–294.

Loree HM et al. Arterioscler Thromb 1994;14:230–234.

Loscalzo J. Arteriosclerosis 1990;10:672–679.

Luscher TF. Blood Pressure Suppl 1994;1:18–22.

Luscher TF et al. Hypertension 1987;9: III-193–III-197.

Lyons TJ et al. Mod Med 1993;61(suppl 2):4–8.

MAAS Investigators. Lancet 1994;344:633–638.

Maca T et al. Atherosclerosis 1996;127:27–34.

Mack WJ et al. Stroke 1993;24:1779–1783.

Mack WJ et al. Arterioscler Thromb Vasc Biol 1996;16:697–704.

MacMahon S et al. Lancet 1990;335:765–774.

MacMahon S et al. Circulation 1998;97:1784–1790.

Maher VM et al. JAMA 1995;274:1771–1774.

Maher VMG, Brown BG. Curr Opin Lipidol 1995;6:229–235.

Mahley RW, Innerarity TL. Biochim Biophys Acta 1983;737:197–202.

Majno G, Joris I. Am J Pathol 1995;146:3–15.

Malmros H. Acta Med Scand 1950;246:137–150.

Mangin EL Jr et al. Circ Res 1993;72:161–166.

Mann GV et al. Am J Epidemiol 1972;95:26–37.

Mann JM, Davies MJ. Circulation 1996;94:928–931.

Manninen V et al. Circulation 1992;85:37–45.

Matrisian LM. Bioessays 1992;14:455–463.

Matsuzawa Y. Diabetes Metab Rev 1997;13:3–13.

Matsuzawa Y et al. Ann N Y Acad Sci 1995;748:399–406.

Matsuzawa Y et al. In: Otamura, ed. Progress in obesity research. London: J. Libbey, 1990:309–312.

Mattila KJ. Eur Heart J 1993;14(suppl K):51–53.

Mattila KJ et al. Clin Infect Dis 1995;20:588–592.

McBride PE. Med Clin North Am 1992;76:333–353.

McGill HC. Am Heart J 1988;115:250–257.

McGill JB et al. Diabetes 1994;43:104–109.

McKenzie WB et al. Aust N Z J Med 1985;15(suppl):566–567.

McKeone BJ et al. J Clin Invest 1993;91:1926–1933.

McLean JW et al. Nature 1987;330:132–137.

McPherson DD et al. J Am Coll Cardiol 1991;17:79–86.

Megnien JL et al. Br J Clin Pharmacol 1996;42:187–193.

Melnick JL et al. Eur Heart J 1993;14 (suppl K):39–42.

Mercuri M et al. Am J Med 1996;101:627–634.

Metzler B, Xu Q. Int Arch Allery Immunol 1997;114:10–14.

Miesenböck G et al. J Clin Invest 1993;91:484–490.

Milei J et al. Cardiologia 1996;41:535–542.

Miller GJ et al. Atherosclerosis 1991a;86:163–171.

Miller VT et al. Obstet Gynecol 1991b;77:235–240.

Minick CR et al. Am J Pathol 1979;96:673–706.

Mintz GS et al. J Am Coll Cardiol 1995;25:1479–1485.

Mintz GS et al. Circulation 1997;95:1791–1798.

Mitropoulos KA et al. Atherosclerosis 1989;76:203–208.

Mittleman MA et al. N Engl J Med 1993;329:1679–1683.

Miyazaki A et al. Biochim Biophys Acta 1992;1126:73–80.

Moffatt RJ et al. Metab Clin Exp 1995;44:1536–1539.

Moreno PR et al. Circulation 1994;90:775–778.

Morisaki N et al. Atherosclerosis 1997;131:43–48.

Moskowitz WB et al. Circulation 1990;81:586–592.

Muller JE et al. Circulation 1989;79:733–743.

Muller JE et al. J Am Coll Cardiol 1994;23:809–813.

Müller-Wieland D et al. Curr Opin Lipidol 1997;8:348–353.

Munro JM et al. Hum Pathol 1987;18:375–380.

Munro JM. Eur Heart J 1993;14(suppl K):72–77.

Muramatsu J et al. Atherosclerosis 1997;130:179–182.

Murry CE et al. Am J Pathol 1997;151:697–705.

Nabulsi AA et al. N Engl J Med 1993;328:1069–1075.

Nakamura T et al. Atherosclerosis 1994;107:239–246.

Naruszewicze M et al. Chem Phys Lipids 1994;67:167–174.

Nathan L, Chaudhuri G. Annu Rev Pharmacol Toxicol 1997;37:477–515.

National Institutes of Health. NIH publication no. 98-4080 (November 1997). Bethesda, MD: National Institutes of Health, 1997.

Nelken NA et al. J Clin Invest 1991;88:1121–1127.

Neufeld EJ et al. Circulation 1997;96:1403–1407.

Neutel JM et al. Am Heart J 1992;124:435–440.

Newman WP III et al. N Engl J Med 1987;314:138–144.

Newman WP III et al. Mod Pathol 1988;1:109–113.

Nichols AV et al. Methods Enzymol 1986;128:417–431.

Niemala S et al. Heart 1996;75:573–575.

Nieminen MS et al. Eur Heart J 1993;14 (suppl K):12–16.

Nigon E et al. J Lipid Res 1991;32:1741–1753.

Nissen SE et al. Circulation 1991;84:1087–1099.

Noll G et al. Int J Microcirc Clin Exp 1997;17:273–279.

Nordestgaard BG. Curr Opin Lipidol 1996;7:269–273.

Nordestgaard BG et al. Arterioscler Thromb 1992;12:6–18.

Nordestgaard BG et al. Arterioscler Thromb Vasc Biol 1995;15:534–542.

Ohara Y et al. J Clin Invest 1993;91:2546–2551.

O'Brien KD et al. J Clin Invest 1993;92:945–951.

O'Brien KD et al. Circulation 1996;93:672–682.

O'Driscoll G et al. Circulation 1997;95:1126–1131.

Ohara Y et al. J Clin Invest 1993;91:2546–2551.

Ohman EM et al. Coron Artery Dis 1993;4:957–964.

O'Keefe JH Jr et al. Am J Cardiol 1996;77:649–652.

O'Leary DH et al. Stroke 1992;23:1752–1760.

Ooi TC et al. Arterioscler Thromb 1992;12:1184–1190.

Oram JF et al. J Clin Invest 1983;72:1611–1621.

Ornish D et al. Lancet 1990;336:129–133.

O'Rourke M. Hypertension 1995;26:2–9.

Packard CJ. Ther Exp 1994;85:1–6.

Padgett RC et al. Circ Res 1992;70:423–429.

Paganini-Hill A. Prog Cardiovasc Dis 1995;38:223–242.

Palinski W et al. Arteriosclerosis 1990;10:325–335.

Palinski W et al. Proc Natl Acad Sci U S A 1995;92:821–825.

Pan XM et al. Am J Physiol 1997;272:G158–G163.

Panza JA et al. Circulation 1993a;87:1468–1474.

Panza JA et al. J Am Coll Cardiol 1993b;21:1145–1151.

Papadaki M, Eskin SG. Biotechnol Prog 1997;13:209–221.

Parhami F, Demer LL. Curr Opin Lipidol 1997;8:312–314.

Parhami F et al. J Clin Invest 1993;92:471–478.

Parhami P et al. Arterioscler Thromb Vasc Biol 1997;17:680–687.

Park KS et al. Metabolism 1991;40:600–603.

Pasi KJ et al. Thromb Res 1990;59:581–591.

Pasterkamp G et al. Circulation 1995;91:1444–1449.

Patel P et al. BMJ 1995;311:711–714.

Pathobiological Determinants of Atherosclerosis in Youth (PDAY) Research Group. JAMA 1990;264:3018–3024.

Pathobiological Determinants of Atherosclerosis in Youth (PDAY) Research Group. Arterioscler Thromb 1993;13:1291–1298.

Patsch JR et al. Arterioscler Thromb 1992;12:1336–1345.

Patsch W, Gotto AM Jr. Adv Pharmacol 1995;32:375–427.

Peeples LH et al. Metab Clin Exp 1989;38:1029–1036.

Peiris AN et al. Ann Intern Med 1989;110:867–872.

Pels K et al. Jpn Circ J 1997;61:893–904.

PEPI Writing Group. JAMA 1995;273:199–208.

Pesonen E et al. Eur Heart J 1993;14 (suppl K):7–11.

Phillips NR et al. Circulation 1993;88:2762–2770.

Pieters MN et al. Biochim Biophys Acta 1994;1225:125–134.

Pitt B et al. J Am Coll Cardiol 1995;1133–1139.

Pittilo RM et al. Br J Haematol 1984;58:627–632.

Plotnick GD et al. JAMA 1997;278:1682–1686.

Ponte E et al. Minerva Med 1997;88:143–149.

Porkka KVK, Ehnholm C. Curr Opin Lipidol 1996;7:162–166.

The Post Coronary Artery Bypass Graft Trial Investigators. N Engl J Med 1997;336:153–162.

Preston AM. Prog Food Nutr Sci 1991;15:183–217.

Pucci AM et al. J Heart Transplant 1990;9:339–345.

Quinn MT et al. Proc Natl Acad Sci U S A 1987;84:2995–2998.

Quinn MT et al. Proc Natl Acad Sci U S A 1988;85:2805–2809.

Raines E et al. In: Fuster V et al., eds. Atherosclerosis and coronary artery disease. New York: Lippincott–Raven, 1996:539–568.

Rajman I et al. Q J Med 1994;87:709–720.

Rakugi H et al. Am Heart J 1996;132:213–221.

Ramirez LC et al. Ann Intern Med 1992;117:42–47.

Rapp JH et al. Arterioscler Thromb 1994;14:1767–1774.

Reaven GM. Diabetes 1988;37:1595–1607.

Reaven GM. Annu Rev Med 1993;44:121–131.

Reaven GM. Physiol Rev 1995;75:473–486.

Reaven PD et al. Arterioscler Thromb 1992;12:318–324.

Reddy KG et al. J Am Coll Cardiol 1994;23:833–843.

Reed DM et al. Arteriosclerosis 1989;9:560–564.

Regnstrom J et al. Lancet 1992;339:1183–1144.

Reilly M et al. Circulation 1996;94:19–25.

Rentrop KP et al. Am J Cardiol 1988;61:677–684.

Ridker PM. Circulation 1998;97:1671–1674.

Rigotti NA, Pasternak RC. Cardiol Clin 1996;14:51–68.

Rivas F et al. Circ Res 1976;38:439–447.

Robertson WB, Strong JP. Lab Invest 1968;18:538–551.

Roheim PS, Asztalos BF. Clin Chem 1995;41:147–152.

Rokitansky CF. A manual of pathological anatomy. Philadelphia: Blanchard and Lea, 1855.

Roma P, Catapano AL. Atherosclerosis 1996;127:147–154.

Rosenfeld ME et al. Am J Pathol 1992;140:291–300.

Ross R. Nature 1993;362:801–809.

Ross R. In: Alexander et al., eds. Hurst's the heart arteries and veins, ed. 9, vol. 1. New York: McGraw-Hill, 1998:1139–1159.

Ross R, Glomset JA. Science 1973;180:1332–1339.

Ross R, Glomset JA. N Engl J Med 1976;295:420–425.

Rossouw JE. Am J Cardiol 1995;76:86C–92C.

Sacks FM et al. Lancet 1994;344:1182–1186.

Sacks MN et al. Lancet 1994;343:269–270.

Sakai M et al. Arterioscler Thromb Vasc Biol 1996;16:600–605.

Salonen JT, Salonen R. Arterioscler Thromb Vasc Biol 1991;11:1245–1249.

Salonen JT et al. Lancet 1992;339:883–887.

Salonen R et al. Am J Cardiol 1995a;76:34C–39C.

Salonen R et al. Circulation 1995b;92:1758–1764.

Sammalkorpi K et al. Metab Clin Exp 1988;37:859–865.

Schairer C et al. Epidemiology 1997;8:59–65.

Schaper W. In: Schaper W, Schaper J, eds. Collateral circulation. Norwell, MA: Kluwer Academic Publishers, 1993:41–64.

Schmid-Schönbein GW et al. Atherosclerosis 1997;131(suppl):S23–S25.

Schneider DJ, Sobel BE. Clin Cardiol 1997;20:433–440.

Schuler G et al. Circulation 1992;86:1–11.

Schumacher R et al. Circulation 1998;97:645–650.

Schwartz CJ et al. Am J Cardiol 1993;71:9B–14B.

Schwartz CJ et al. Clin Cardiol 1991;14 (suppl I):I1–I16.

Schwartz SM. J Clin Invest 1997;100(suppl):S87–S89.

Schwartz et al. Atherosclerosis 1995;118(suppl):S125–S140.

Sehayek E, Eisenberg S. Arteriosclerosis 1990;10:1088–1096.

Seiler C et al. Circulation 1993;88 (part 1):2139–2148.

Seiler C et al. J Am Coll Cardiol 1995;26:1615–1622.

Selwyn AP et al. Circulation 1997;95:5–7.

Setsuda M et al. Clin Ther 1993;15:374–382.

Shah PK. Cardiol Clin 1996;14:17–29.

Shah PK. Am J Cardiol 1997;79(suppl 12B):17–23.

Sharrett AR et al. Arterioscler Thromb 1994;14:1098–1104.

Shi C et al. Proc Natl Acad Sci U S A 1996;93:4051–4056.

Shimizu Y et al. [Japanese] Kokyu to Junkan 1991;39:687–690.

Shiode N et al. Am Heart J 1996;131:1051–1057.

Shircore A et al. Circulation 1995;92:2411–2418.

Simpson HC et al. Lancet 1983;1:786–790.

Sing CF et al. In: Woodford FP et al., eds. Atherosclerosis X. Amsterdam: Elsevier, 1995:638–644.

Sirtori CR, Franceschini G. N Engl J Med 1997;337:1918.

Slyper AH. JAMA 1994;272:305–308.

Small DM. Arteriosclerosis 1988;8:103–129.

Small DM et al. J Clin Invest 1984;73:1590–1605.

Sniderman AD et al. Arterioscler Thromb Vasc Biol 1998;18:147–151.

Solberg LA, Strong JP. Arteriosclerosis 1983;3:187–198.

Solerte SB et al. Int J Obes Relat Metab Disord 1997;21:417–423.

Soma MR et al. Arch Intern Med 1993;153:1462–8.

Southworth MR, Mauro VF. Ann Pharmacother 1997;31:489–491.

Sowers JR et al. Am J Hypertens 1993;6:260s–270s.

Sparrow CP et al. J Biol Chem 1989;264:2599–2604.

Spodick DH et al. Am J Cardiol 1984;53:481–482.

Srikanthan VS, Dunn FG. Med Clin North Am 1997;81:1147–1163.

St. Clair RW. Curr Opin Lipidol 1997;8:281–286.

Staab ME et al. Circulation 1995;92(suppl I):I-93.

Stamler J et al. Arch Intern Med 1993a;153:598–615.

Stamler J et al. Diabetes Care 1993b;16:434–444.

Stampfer MJ, Colditz GA. Prev Med 1991;20:47–63.

Stampfer MJ et al. JAMA 1996;276:882–888.

Stary HC et al. Circulation 1992;85:391–405.

Stary HC et al. Arterioscler Thromb 1994;14:840–856.

Stary HC et al. Circulation 1995;92:1355–1374. Copublished in Arterioscler Thromb Vasc Biol 1995;15:1512–1531.

Stein JH, Rosensen RS. Arch Intern Med 1997;157:1170–1176.

Stein O, Stein Y. Curr Opin Lipidol 1995;6:269–274.

Steinberg D. Atherosclerosis 1997a;131(suppl):S5–S7.

Steinberg D. Lewis A. Circulation 1997b;95:1062–1071.

Steinberg D, Witztum JL. JAMA 1990;264:3047–3052.

Steinbrecher UP et al. Proc Natl Acad Sci U S A 1984;81:3883–3887.

Steiner G et al. Circulation 1987;75:124–130.

Stemme S et al. Lab Invest 1991;65:654–660.

Stout RW. Diabetes Care 1990;13:631–654.

Stout RW. Diabetes 1996;45(suppl 3):S45–S46.

Stroes ESG et al. Lancet 1995;336:467–471.

Strong JP. Arch Pathol Lab Med 1992;116:1268–1275.

Subar AF et al. Am J Public Health 1990;80:1323–1329.

Subbiah MT. Proc Soc Exp Biol Med 1998;217:23–29.

Suissa S et al. Contraception 1997;56:141–146.

Sung JJY, Sanderson JE. Heart 1996;76:305–307.

Suurküla M et al. Arterioscler Thromb Vasc Biol 1996;16:462–470.

Tabata H et al. Cardiovasc Res 1997;35:470–479.

Taeymans Y et al. Circulation 1992;85:78–85.

Tamai O et al. Circulation 1997;95:76–82.

Tardif J-C et al. N Engl J Med 1997;337:365–372.

Taskinen MR et al. Arterioscler Thromb Vasc Biol 1996;16:1215–1221.

Teirstein PS et al. N Engl J Med 1997;336:1697–1703.

Teng B et al. J Clin Invest 1986;77:6663–6672.

Terry RB et al. J Clin Endocrinol Metab 1989;68:191–199.

Tesfamariam B et al. J Clin Invest 1991;87:1643–1648.

Thompson GR et al. Lancet 1995;345:811–816.

Tillotson JL et al. Am J Clin Nutr 1997;65(1 suppl):228S–257S.

Topol EJ. Prog Cardiovasc Dis 1997;40:95–96.

Topol EJ, Ellis SG. Circulation 1991;83:1084–1086.

Toussaint J-F et al. Circulation 1996;94:932–938.

Treasure CB et al. N Engl J Med 1995;332:481–487.

Tresch DD, Aronow WS. Clin Geriatr Med 1996;12:23–32.

Tsurumi Y et al. Circulation 1996;94:3281–3290.

Ueno H et al. Arterioscler Thromb Vasc Biol 1997;17:2453–2460.

Uretsky BF et al. Circulation 1987;76:827–834.

Vague P et al. Metabolism 1986;35:250–253.

Valantine HA, Schroeder JS. Circulation 1997;96:1370–1373.

Valentine RJ et al. J Vasc Surg 1994;19:668–674.

Vallabhajosula S, Fuster F. J Nucl Med 1997;38:1788–1796.

Vallance P et al. Lancet 1997;349:1391–1392.

Valtonen V et al. Eur Heart J 1993;14 (suppl K):20–23.

Van Belle E et al. Circulation 1997;96:2667–2674.

van der Heide JJH et al. N Engl J Med 1993;329:769–773.

van der Wal AC et al. Circulation 1994;89:6–44.

van de Stolpe A, van der Saag PT. J Mol Med 1996;74:13–33.

Vanhoutte PM. J Hypertens Suppl 1996;14:S83–S93.

Vanhoutte PM. Eur Heart J 1997;18(suppl E):E19–E29.

Vanoverschelde JJ et al. Circulation 1993;87:1513–1523.

Vaughan CJ et al. Lancet 1996;348:1079–1082.

Vazquez M et al. Br J Pharmacol 1996;117:1155–1162.

Ventura HO et al. Am Heart J 1995;129:791–798.

Verstraete M, Fuster V. In: Alexander RW et al., eds. Hurst's the heart arteries and veins, ed. 9, vol. 1. New York: McGraw-Hill, 1998:1501–1551.

Violaris AG et al. Circulation 1994;90:2267–2279.

Virchow R. Phlogose und Thrombose im Gefasssystem, Gesammelte Abhandlungen zur Wissenschaftlichen Medicin. Frankfurt-am-Main: Meidinger Sohn and Company, 1856:458.

Vischer U. Eur J Endocrinol 1997;137:343–344.

Visser MR, Vercellotti GM. Eur Heart J 1993;14(suppl K):39–42.

Vita JA et al. Circulation 1990;81:491–497.

Vlassara H. J Lab Clin Med 1994;124:19–30.

Vogel RA. Clin Cardiol 1997;20:426–432.

Vogel RA et al. Am J Cardiol 1996;77:37–40.

Vogel RA et al. Am J Cardiol 1997;79:350–354.

Volterrani M et al. Am J Med 1995;99:119–122.

von Eckardstein A et al. Curr Opin Lipidol 1994;5:404–416.

Vos J et al. Prog Cardiovasc Dis 1993;35:435–454.

Wakatsuki A et al. Obstet Gynecol 1997;90:22–25.

Walldius G et al. Am J Cardiol 1994;74:875–883.

Waller BF. In: Pepine C, ed. Acute myocardial infarction. Philadelphia: F. A. Davis, 1989:29–104.

Waller BF. In: Alexander RW et al., eds. Hurst's the heart arteries and veins, ed. 9, vol. 1. New York: McGraw-Hill, 1998:1197–1240.

Waller BF et al. Clin Cardiol 1992a;15:451–457.

Waller BF et al. Clin Cardiol 1992b;15:535–540.

Walsh BW et al. N Engl J Med 1991;325:1196–1204.

Watanabe K et al. Am Heart J 1996;132:23–29.

Waters D. Cardiol Clin 1996;14:31–50.

Waters D et al. Circulation 1993;87:1067–1075.

Waters D et al. Circulation 1994;89:959–968.

Waters D et al. Circulation 1995;92:2404–2410.

Watson KE, Demer LL. Curr Opin Lipidol 1996;7:101–104.

Watson KE et al. J Clin Invest 1994;93:2106–2113.

Watts GF et al. Lancet 1992;339:563–569.

Weber C et al. Circulation 1996a;93:1488–1492.

Weber MA. Am J Hypertens 1994;7:146S–153S.

Weber P et al. Int J Vitam Nutr Res 1996b;66:19–30.

Weinberger J, Simon AD. Curr Opin Cardiol 1997;12:468–474.

Weintraub WS, Pederson JP. Am J Cardiol 1996;78:1036–1038.

Weis M, von Scheidt W. Circulation 1997;96:2069–2077.

Weissman NJ et al. J Am Coll Cardiol 1997;29(suppl A):124A.

Wenke K et al. Circulation 1997;96:1398–1402.

Wenzel K et al. Hum Genet 1996;97:15–20.

Wenzel K et al. J Mol Med 1997;75:57–61.

West of Scotland Coronary Prevention Study Group. Circulation 1998;97:1440–1445.

White FC et al. In: Schaper W, Schaper J, eds. Collateral circulation. Norwell, MA: Kluwer Academic Publishers, 1993:261–289.

Wick G et al. Int Arch Allergy Immunol 1995a;107:130–131.

Wick G et al. Immunol Today 1995b;16:27–32.

Wight TN. Curr Opin Lipidol 1995;6:326–334.

Wild RA. Obstet Gynecol 1996;87(suppl):27S–35S.

Williams JK et al. Circ Res 1988;62:515–523.

Willich SN et al. Circulation 1989;80:853–858.

Willich SN et al. Circulation 1993;87:1442–1450.

Wilson PW. Clin Chem 1995;41:165–169.

Wilson RF, White CW. In: Willerson JT, Cohn JN, eds. Cardiovascular medicine. New York: Churchill Livingstone, 1995:390–463.

Wissler RW, the PDAY Collaborating Investigators. Atherosclerosis 1994;108(suppl):S3–S20.

Wissler RW, Vesselinovitch D. Am J Cardiol 1990;65:33F–40F.

Witztum JL, Hörkkö S. Ann N Y Acad Sci 1997;811:88–99.

Witztum JL, Palinksi W. In: Hansson GK, Libby P, eds. Immune functions of the vessel wall. London: Harwood Academic Publishers, 1996:159–172.

Wong ND et al. Ann Intern Med 1991;115:687–693.

Woolf N, Davies MJ. In: Fuster V, Verstraete M, eds. Thrombosis in cardiovascular disorders. Philadelphia: W. B. Saunders, 1992.

World Health Organization. Hypertension control: Report of a WHO Expert Committee. WHO Technical Report Series 862. Geneva: World Health Organization, 1996.

Xu Q, Wick G. Mol Med Today 1996;2:372–379.

Xu Q et al. Arterioscler Thromb 1992;12:789–799.

Xu Q et al. J Clin Invest 1993a;91:2693–2702.

Xu Q et al. Lancet 1993b;341:255–259.

Yamaguchi H et al. Chem Phys Lipids 1994;67–68:399–403.

Yamamoto H et al. Am Heart J 1995;130:1168–1173.

Yamamoto M et al. Int J Obes Relat Metab Disord 1997;21:948–951.

Yamashita S et al. Diabetes Care 1996;19:287–291.

Yla-Herttuala S et al. J Clin Invest 1989;84:1086–1095.

Yokoi H et al. J Am Coll Cardiol 1997;30:855–862.

Zeiher AM et al. Circulation 1991;84:1984–1992.

Zeiher AM et al. Circulation 1994;89:2525–2532.

Zhang Y et al. Am J Pathol 1993;143:496–506.

Zhang Y et al. Nature 1994;372:425–432.

Zhu W et al. Arterioscler Thromb Vasc Biol 1996;16:1104–1111.

Zilversmit DB. Circ Res 1973;33:633–638.

Zilversmit DB. Circulation 1979;60:473–485.

Zilversmit DB. Clin Chem 1995;41:153–158.

Zweifach BW. In: Granger DN, Schmid-Schönbein GW, eds. Physiology and pathophysiology of leukocyte adhesion. New York: Oxford University Press, 1995:v–vii.

Risk Control

The sole aim of diagnosis and treatment of hyperlipidemia is the prevention or postponement of . . . atherosclerotic arterial disease.

—Tjerk de Bruin et al. (1996)

I believe the chief cause for premature development of arteriosclerosis in diabetes, save for advancing age, is excessive fat: an excess of fat in the body, obesity; an excess of fat in the diet; and an excess of fat in the blood. With an excess of fat diabetes begins and from an excess of fat diabetics die; formerly of coma, recently of arteriosclerosis.

—E. P. Joslin (1927),
quoted by Paul Durrington

The only kind of information that is entirely convincing [is] that from randomized, controlled, clinical trials with clinical outcomes.

—Basil M. Rifkind and Jacques E. Rossouw (1998)

References for Section III (Chapters 11–14) begin on page 241.

Chapter 11

Observational Epidemiology and Risk Factors

In both the United States and most countries of western Europe, CHD remains the leading cause of death despite dramatic declines in the CHD mortality rate (AHA 1997; Thom 1989), including a decline in the United States of about 2% per year for 30 years (Manson et al. 1996). CHD killed about 500,000 Americans in 1995, accounting for 1 in every 4.8 deaths (AHA 1997).

The declines can be attributed to improved medical care and favorable changes in the presence of major risk factors. In the United States, more than one-half of the 20% decline in age-adjusted CHD mortality rate between 1968 and 1976 was attributed to risk factor reduction, in particular smoking cessation and reductions in plasma cholesterol (Goldman and Cook 1984). In the Framingham cohort, more than one-half of the 51% decrease in CHD mortality rate observed in women between 1950 and 1989 and one-third to one-half of the 44% decrease in men could be attributed to improvements in risk factors in the 1970 cohorts (Sytkowski et al. 1996). In The Netherlands, approximately 44% of the decline in the CHD mortality rate from 1978 to 1985 has been credited to primary prevention efforts, including smoking cessation, reduced plasma cholesterol, and treatment of hypertension, and 46% to treatment in coronary care units, postinfarction treatment, and CABG (Bots and Grobbee 1996).

Because of public health initiatives, smoking rates have dropped about 40% among U.S. adults since 1965 (AHA 1997). Between 1960–1962 and 1988–1991, mean TC among U.S. adults decreased 15 mg/dL, and the proportion of individuals with cholesterol of 240 mg/dL or higher decreased from 25% and 28% of men and women in 1976–1980 (NHANES II) to 19% and 20% in 1988–1991 (phase 1 of NHANES III) (Johnson et al. 1993). Initiation in 1972 of the National High Blood Pressure Education Program made the detection and treatment of hypertension a national priority. In 1971, half of Americans with hypertension were unaware of their condition; 20 years later, that proportion had declined to 16% (Burt et al. 1995). However, a large percentage of Americans have remained sedentary and the prevalence of obesity has increased (see later).

In contrast, Central and Eastern European nations are facing increases in CHD rates (Bonita 1994; Rastenyte et al. 1992). The problem is comparable with that faced in the West more than 30 years ago: With regard to cardiovascular health, Eastern Europe has been described as emerging "from 40 years of Communism 40 years behind the times" (Jamrozick 1995). In many Eastern European countries, prevalence is alarmingly high for smoking, elevated blood cholesterol, hypertension, obesity, and alcohol abuse (Kôrv et al. 1996; Ginter 1995; Forster and Józan 1990).

OBSERVATIONAL EPIDEMIOLOGIC STUDIES

Over the last decades, epidemiologic studies have together written a cohesive story that convincingly links a number of major risk factors (see Table 13.4) with the development of CHD. Clearly, these factors do not account entirely for the disease, since a small minority of patients with atherosclerotic events have no known risk factors. Indeed, 20% of MIs in the Framingham cohort occurred at TC concentrations of less than 200 mg/dL (Kannel 1995; Wong et al. 1991), and some individuals with heterozygous familial hypercholesterolemia survive into their 70s without clinical events.

The Framingham study, initiated in 1948 in Framingham, Massachusetts, has been one of the leading longitudinal cohort studies of risk for CVD in both men and women. It has identified many of the major risk factors and has refined risk assessment (Murabito 1995; Levy and Kannel 1988; Castelli 1984). In the Framingham cohort, risk for reinfarction was increased about nine times in women and three times in men with TC greater than 270 mg/dL compared with individuals with cholesterol lower than 190 mg/dL (Wong et al. 1991).

The Seven Countries Study, conducted from 1958 to 1964 and involving 12,763 middle-aged male subjects, remains one of the most comprehensive cross-cultural studies relating differences in lifestyle factors to differences in rates of CHD. Baseline serum cholesterol, which correlated with saturated fat intake, and blood pressure strongly predicted CHD death rates (Keys 1980). Rates in northern European cities, where a diet high in saturated fat was consumed, were about 2.5 times higher than rates in southern European regions typified by a Mediterranean diet. At 25 years' follow-up, late CHD death rates remain largely explained by differences in serum cholesterol concentration during the early phase of the study (Menotti et al. 1997).

The Ni-Hon-San Study, the best-known migration study, showed that middle-aged Japanese men living in Japan (Nippon), Honolulu, and San Francisco had progressively higher serum cholesterol and CHD death rates as lifestyle became progressively westernized, including a shift toward a diet higher in animal fat (Worth et al. 1975; Benfante 1992) (see also "Changing Risk with Acculturation" in Chapter 20).

RISK FACTOR OVERVIEW

More than 200 risk factors for CVD have been described, and in assessing risk it is critical to distinguish between major risk factors (with both strength of epidemiologic association and biologic plausibility) and risk associations based on preliminary or even trivial data. That distinction is often ignored by the news media and is misunderstood by many patients and even some health professionals. CHD risk factors are also categorized as modifiable (lifestyle factors and modifiable disorders), which are the focus of this manual, or unmodifiable (age, sex, hereditary factors); chronic or acute; and proatherogenic or prothrombotic. As seen in the metabolic syndrome, factors related to lifestyle and genetics may tend to cluster.

A recent Bethesda Conference proposed a risk factor classification based on the strength of evidence that intervention affects CVD outcome (Fuster and Pearson 1996). In category I, risk factors for which interventions have been proved to lower risk, are cigarette smoking, elevated LDL-C, a diet high in fat and cholesterol, hypertension, left ventricular hypertrophy (LVH), and the thrombogenic risk factors elevated fibrinogen (observational epidemiologic evidence; measurement may be useful), aspirin, and warfarin. In category II, risk factors for which interventions are likely to lower risk, are diabetes; physical inactivity; reduced HDL-C; plasma TG/small, dense LDL; and postmenopausal status. In category III, risk factors associated with increased risk that if modified might lower risk, are psychosocial factors, elevated Lp[a], elevated homocysteine, oxidative stress, and no alcohol consumption. Category IV comprises the unmodifiable risk factors of age, male sex, low socioeconomic status, and a family history of premature CVD.

Without accounting for the impact of the other risk factors, it has been estimated that TC of 200 mg/dL or more contributes to 42.7% of deaths from CHD in the United States (Hahn et al. 1990). Contributions of other risk factors to CHD deaths are no regular exercise, 34.6%; obesity, 32.1%; SBP of 140 mm Hg or higher, 28.9%; current or former smoking, 25.1%; and diabetes mellitus, 13.1%.

MULTIPLE RISK FACTORS

A very important concept is that multiple risk factors tend to increase CHD risk synergistically. Yusuf et al. (1998) assessed the presence of five risk factors in 12,932 men and women in the NHANES I (1971–1975) Follow-up Study (follow-up through 1992) (Table 11.1 and Figure 11.1). Having three risk factors tripled the risk for a CHD event and nearly doubled

Table 11.1. RELATIVE RISK FOR CHD, STROKE, AND TOTAL MORTALITY ACCORDING TO NUMBER OF RISK FACTORS

Number of risk factors	Prevalence (%)			Relative risk (95% CI)		
	Male	Female	All	Incident CHD	Incident stroke	Total mortality
0	19.9	28.5	25.0	1.0	1.0	1.0
1	36.2	30.5	32.8	1.6 (1.4–1.9)	1.4 (1.1–1.8)	1.2 (1.1–1.3)
2	30.2	26.1	27.8	2.2 (1.9–2.6)	1.9 (1.5–2.4)	1.4 (1.3–1.5)
3	11.7	12.7	12.3	3.1 (2.6–3.6)	2.3 (1.7–3.0)	1.7 (1.5–1.9)
4–5	2.0	2.2	2.1	5.0 (3.9–6.3)	4.3 (3.0–6.3)	3.1 (2.6–3.7)

Note: Risk factors considered were current smoking, high blood cholesterol ($\geq$240 mg/dL), hypertension (SBP $\geq$140 mm Hg, DBP $\geq$90 mm Hg, or taking antihypertensive medication), diabetes (self-reported), and overweight (BMI $\geq$27.8 kg/m^2 for men, $\geq$27.3 kg/m^2 for women). Analysis was of the NHANES I (1971–1975) Follow-up Study (follow-up through 1992) data set, $N = 12,932$.
Source: Data from Yusuf et al. 1998.

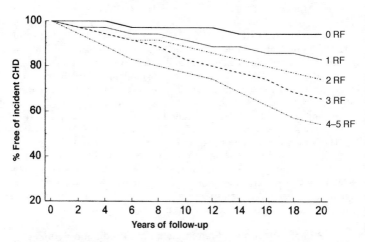

Figure 11.1.   Probability of CHD not developing, according to number of risk factors (RF) (see Table 11.1 for definition of risk factors). (From Yusuf et al. 1998; used with permission.)

the risk for dying of any cause; having four or five risk factors increased the CHD risk fivefold and the risk for death threefold. Such findings emphasize the need for a multifactorial approach to risk factor reduction. Reducing plasma cholesterol or controlling hypertension in a diabetic patient reduces CHD risk just as effectively as controlling hyperglycemia (Grundy et al. 1998). It is important to consider all the major risk factors simultaneously; unfortunately, physicians often fail to collect the necessary data elements in the course of usual medical care (Kottke et al. 1997). American and European risk reduction practice guidelines now emphasize assessment and control of global risk (NCEP 1994; International Task Force 1992; Pyörälä et al. 1994; NIH 1997).

The Münster Heart Study (formerly called the Prospective Cardiovascular Münster, or PROCAM, study) at 6-year follow-up of middle-aged men found that fully one-fourth of CHD events occurred in the 4.3% of men who had plasma TG greater than 200 mg/dL and an LDL-C:HDL-C ratio greater than 5 (Assmann and Schulte 1992). In 8-year follow-up, an LDL-C:HDL-C ratio of 5.0–5.9 was associated with 171 observed events per 1,000 men; this jumped to 278 events per 1,000 with a ratio greater than 7 (Assmann et al. 1998). Interestingly, analysis of the 8-year data showed the correlation between fasting TG and major coronary events to remain after adjustment for LDL-C and HDL-C, even after other risk factors were taken into account. In addition to classic major risk factors, Lp[a] and fibrinogen concentrations were important predictors of risk in the Münster Heart Study. Future efforts of the study will focus on the elaboration of risk algorithms in women.

The Multiple Risk Factor Intervention Trial (MRFIT) screened 350,564 men as possible participants. Only 3% of those screened were considered to be at low risk for CHD because of TC lower than 182 mg/dL; SBP/DBP <120/<80 mm Hg; and absence of diabetes, current smoking, or a history of MI. Twelve years later, when compared with the rest of the subjects, these men had an 89% lower CHD death rate, 53% lower total mortality rate, and an estimated increase in longevity of more than 9 years (Stamler et al. 1993b). The MRFIT data showed that, on average, a male smoker with serum cholesterol and SBP in the highest quintiles is 20 times as likely as a male nonsmoker with cholesterol and SBP in the lowest quintiles to die of CHD during a 12-year period (Neaton and Wentworth 1992).

The Chicago Heart Association Study showed similar benefit according to risk factor levels in women. For middle-aged and older women (N = 8,325), a favorable baseline profile according to serum cholesterol, blood pressure, and smoking status reduced the 15-year CHD risk by 60% and increased longevity by about 5 years (Stamler et al. 1993b).

Primary Prevention Framingham Risk Prediction Score

A variety of CHD risk prediction algorithms have been developed over the years on the basis of the Framingham and other data sets. A recent model (Figures 11.2 and 11.3) for use in primary prevention (only) has been developed using categorical variables based on data on men and women examined in the Framingham Heart Study from 1971 to 1974 and having 12 years of follow-up (Wilson et al. 1998). The subjects were white and ranged in age from 30 to 74 years. Estimates of idealized risk are based on optimal blood pressure, TC of 160–199 mg/dL or LDL-C of 100–129 mg/dL, HDL-C of 45 mg/dL in men or 55 mg/dL in women, no diabetes, and no smoking. The model builds on the lipid and blood pressure categories defined by the second Adult Treatment Panel of the NCEP (NCEP 1994) and the JNC V (Joint National Committee 1993). Not all major risk factors are included because of practical and theoretic considerations.

An AHA statement accompanying the publication of the Framingham risk charts discusses in detail their essential features and appropriate use (Grundy et al. 1998). It is important to note that the presence of a risk factor may not confer high *absolute* risk during the next 10 years but will confer high risk over a lifetime of exposure. Thus, the intent in lowering elevated cholesterol in most young adults, for example, is largely to prevent the development or progression of atherosclerosis rather than to prevent MI in the next decade. Absolute risk for CHD cannot be nearly fully reduced by aggressive therapy initiated after atherosclerosis has become advanced (Grundy et al. 1998), and risk scores may not predict nearly half the future episodes of CHD (Fowkes et al. 1998; Shaper et al. 1986). The risk charts are useful, however, in encouraging clinicians to regard overall risk. They may be used to motivate or reassure patients and may assist in the selection of therapies. The NCEP risk categories are more broadly outlined and refer strongly to clinical judgment.

Metabolic Syndrome

Grundy (1997) has noted that the next step in CHD prevention after current NCEP guidelines (see Chapter 13) may be a focus on control of the metabolic syndrome (Table 11.2), which appears to rival elevated LDL-C in atherogenic potential (see also Chapter 8). In the recent statin trials with clinical endpoints (see Chapter 12), substantial risk reduction was achieved through lowering LDL-C even in the presence of components of the metabolic syndrome.

MAJOR UNMODIFIABLE RISK FACTORS
History of Atherosclerotic Disease

Established CHD or clinical atherosclerotic disease of the aorta, carotid arteries, or arteries to the limbs confers the highest risk for MI or CHD death. Risk is increased five to seven times, and about half of MIs and at least 70% of CHD deaths occur in patients with prior manifestations of atherosclerotic disease (NCEP 1994; Mueller et al. 1995; Pekkanen et al. 1990; Rosengren et al. 1997). Recent studies suggest that one-third of stroke patients have asymptomatic CHD, and cardiac events are the leading cause of death in stroke survivors (Sen and Oppenheimer 1998).

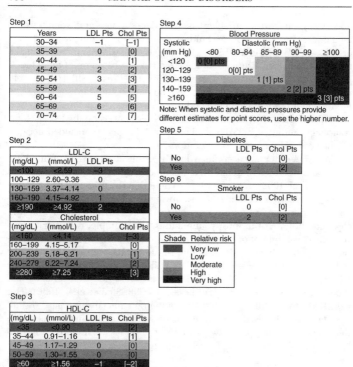

Step 1

Years	LDL Pts	Chol Pts
30–34	−1	[−1]
35–39	0	[0]
40–44	1	[1]
45–49	2	[2]
50–54	3	[3]
55–59	4	[4]
60–64	5	[5]
65–69	6	[6]
70–74	7	[7]

Step 2

LDL-C		
(mg/dL)	(mmol/L)	LDL Pts
<100	<2.59	−3
100–129	2.60–3.36	0
130–159	3.37–4.14	0
160–190	4.15–4.92	1
≥190	≥4.92	2

Cholesterol		
(mg/dL)	(mmol/L)	Chol Pts
<160	<4.14	[−3]
160–199	4.15–5.17	[0]
200–239	5.18–6.21	[1]
240–279	6.22–7.24	[2]
≥280	≥7.25	[3]

Step 3

HDL-C			
(mg/dL)	(mmol/L)	LDL Pts	Chol Pts
<35	<0.90	2	[2]
35–44	0.91–1.16	1	[1]
45–49	1.17–1.29	0	[0]
50–59	1.30–1.55	0	[0]
≥60	≥1.56	−1	[−2]

Step 4

Blood Pressure					
Systolic (mm Hg)	Diastolic (mm Hg)				
	<80	80–84	85–89	90–99	≥100
<120	0 [0] pts				
120–129	0[0] pts				
130–139			1 [1] pts		
140–159				2 [2] pts	
≥160					3 [3] pts

Note: When systolic and diastolic pressures provide different estimates for point scores, use the higher number.

Step 5

Diabetes		
	LDL Pts	Chol Pts
No	0	[0]
Yes	2	[2]

Step 6

Smoker		
	LDL Pts	Chol Pts
No	0	[0]
Yes	2	[2]

Shade	Relative risk
	Very low
	Low
	Moderate
	High
	Very high

Figure 11.2. Score sheet for estimating 10-year risk for CHD for men who do not have known atherosclerotic disease. Use fasting LDL-C when known, rather than TC for step 2. Pts, points. (From Wilson et al. 1998; used with permission. *Note that this simplified risk chart does not replace full clinical evaluation of risk according to NCEP guidelines [Chapter 13] but may be useful in patient counseling or selection of intensity of intervention.*)

Patients with asymptomatic PVD appear to have the same increased risk for CVD events and death as claudicants (Leng et al. 1996). Carotid intima–media thickness as determined by B-mode ultrasound appears to be a useful surrogate endpoint for atherosclerosis in distant beds (Burke et al. 1995) and for clinical coronary events (Hodis et al. 1998).

Family History of Premature Coronary Heart Disease

A family history of premature CHD indicates a high risk independent of traditional and nontraditional risk factors (Eaton et al. 1996; NCEP 1994).

(Sum from steps 1–6)
Step 7

Adding up the points	
Age	_____
LDL-C or TC	_____
HDL-C	_____
Blood pressure	_____
Diabetes	_____
Smoker	_____
Point total	_____

(Determine CHD risk from point total)
Step 8

CHD Risk			
LDL Pts Total	10 Yr CHD Risk	Chol Pts Total	10 Yr CHD Risk
<-3	1%		
-2	2%		
-1	2%	[<-1]	[2%]
0	3%	[0]	[3%]
1	4%	[1]	[3%]
2	4%	[2]	[4%]
3	6%	[3]	[5%]
4	7%	[4]	[7%]
5	9%	[5]	[8%]
6	11%	[6]	[10%]
7	14%	[7]	[13%]
8	18%	[8]	[16%]
9	22%	[9]	[20%]
10	27%	[10]	[25%]
11	33%	[11]	[31%]
12	40%	[12]	[37%]
13	47%	[13]	[45%]
≥14	≥56%	[≥14]	[≥53%]

(Compare with average person your age)
Step 9

Comparative Risk			
Age (years)	Average 10 Yr CHD Risk	Average 10 Yr Hard* CHD Risk	Low** 10 Yr CHD Risk
30–34	1%	1%	2%
35–39	3%	4%	3%
40–44	5%	4%	4%
45–49	7%	8%	4%
50–54	11%	10%	6%
54–59	14%	13%	7%
60–64	16%	20%	9%
64–69	21%	22%	11%
70–74	25%	25%	14%

* Hard CHD events exclude angina pectoris.

**Low risk was calculated for a person the same age, optimal blood pressure, LDL-C 100–129 mg/dL or cholesterol 160–199 mg/dL, HDL-C 45 mg/dL for men or 55 mg/dL for women, nonsmoker, no diabetes.

Risk estimates were derived from the experience of the Framingham Heart Study, a predominantly Caucasian population in Massachusetts, United States.

Figure 11.2.   *Continued.*

Sex and Age

CHD rates in men are similar to those in women 10 years older (Castelli 1984). Absolute risk for CHD increases steeply with age in both sexes, and today most new-onset CHD occurs after age 65 years (Denke and Grundy 1990; Gordon et al. 1977).

MAJOR MODIFIABLE RISK FACTORS

Major dietary contributors to CHD risk are discussed in Chapter 15.

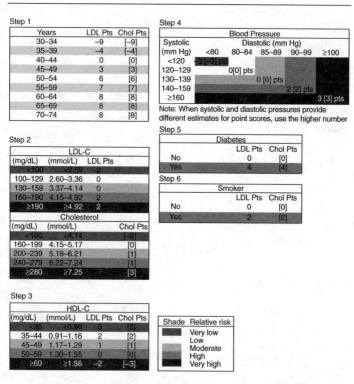

Step 1

Years	LDL Pts	Chol Pts
30–34	–9	[–9]
35–39	–4	[–4]
40–44	0	[0]
45–49	3	[3]
50–54	6	[6]
55–59	7	[7]
60–64	8	[8]
65–69	8	[8]
70–74	8	[8]

Step 4

Blood Pressure					
Systolic	Diastolic (mm Hg)				
(mm Hg)	<80	80–84	85–89	90–99	≥100
<120	–3 [–3] pts				
120–129	0[0] pts				
130–139			0 [0] pts		
140–159				2 [2] pts	
≥160					3 [3] pts

Note: When systolic and diastolic pressures provide different estimates for point scores, use the higher number

Step 5

Diabetes		
	LDL Pts	Chol Pts
No	0	[0]
Yes	4	[4]

Step 6

Smoker		
	LDL Pts	Chol Pts
No	0	[0]
Yes	2	[2]

Step 2

LDL-C			
(mg/dL)	(mmol/L)	LDL Pts	
<100	<2.59	–2	
100–129	2.60–3.36	0	
130–159	3.37–4.14	0	
160–190	4.15–4.92	2	
≥190	≥4.92	2	

Cholesterol		
(mg/dL)	(mmol/L)	Chol Pts
<160	<4.14	[–2]
160–199	4.15–5.17	[0]
200–239	5.18–6.21	[1]
240–279	6.22–7.24	[1]
≥280	≥7.25	[3]

Step 3

HDL-C			
(mg/dL)	(mmol/L)	LDL Pts	Chol Pts
<35	<0.90	5	[5]
35–44	0.91–1.16	2	[2]
45–49	1.17–1.29	1	[1]
50–59	1.30–1.55	0	[0]
≥60	≥1.56	–2	[–3]

Shade	Relative risk
	Very low
	Low
	Moderate
	High
	Very high

Figure 11.3. Score sheet for estimating 10-year risk for CHD for women who do not have known atherosclerotic disease. Use fasting LDL-C value when known rather than TC for step 2. Pts, points. (From Wilson et al. 1998; used with permission. *Note that this simplified risk chart does not replace full clinical evaluation of risk according to NCEP guidelines [Chapter 13] but may be useful in patient counseling or selection of intensity of intervention.*)

Elevated Plasma Cholesterol

The strength of the independent, dose-response relation, the consistency of findings within and among populations, and biologic plausibility all argue for elevated LDL-C as causal in the development of CHD. In addition to the example observational epidemiologic studies cited above and the example interventional trials highlighted in Chapter 12, the meta-analysis by Law et al. (1994) is of particular interest. As seen in Figure 11.4, there is remarkable consistency among large cohort studies in the relation of cholesterol to the incidence of CHD. A risk gradient remains even in rural Chinese communities with mean TC of 115 mg/dL and sometimes nearer 77

(Sum from steps 1-6)
Step 7

Adding up the points	
Age	_____
LDL-C or TC	_____
HDL-C	_____
Blood Pressure	_____
Diabetes	_____
Smoker	_____
Point total	_____

(Determine CHD risk from point total)
Step 8

CHD Risk			
LDL Pts Total	10 Yr CHD Risk	Chol Pts Total	10 Yr CHD Risk
≤−2	1%	[<−2]	[1%]
1	3%	[−1]	[2%]
0	4%	[0]	[2%]
1	4%	[1]	[2%]
2	6%	[2]	[3%]
3	7%	[3]	[3%]
4	9%	[4]	[4%]
5	11%	[5]	[4%]
6	14%	[6]	[5%]
7	18%	[7]	[6%]
8	22%	[8]	[7%]
9	27%	[9]	[8%]
10	33%	[10]	[10%]
11	40%	[11]	[11%]
12	47%	[12]	[13%]
13	≥56%	[13]	[15%]
14	≥56%	[14]	[18%]
15	≥56%	[15]	[20%]
16	≥56%	[16]	[24%]
≥17	≥56%	[≥17]	[≥27%]

(Compare with average person your age)
Step 9

Comparative Risk			
Age (years)	Average 10 Yr CHD Risk	Average 10 Yr Hard* CHD Risk	Low** 10 Yr CHD Risk
30–34	>1%	<1%	<1%
35–39	>1%	<1%	1%
40–44	2%	1%	2%
45–49	5%	2%	3%
50–54	8%	3%	5%
54–59	12%	7%	7%
60–64	12%	8%	8%
64–69	13%	8%	8%
70–74	14%	11%	8%

* Hard CHD events exclude angina pectoris.

**Low risk was calculated for a person the same age, optimal blood pressure, LDL-C 100–129 mg/dL or cholesterol 160–199 mg/dL, HDL-C 45 mg/dL for men or 55 mg/dL for women, nonsmoker, no diabetes.

Risk estimates were derived from the experience of the Framingham Heart Study, a predominantly Caucasian population in Massachusetts, United States.

Figure 11.3. *Continued.*

mg/dL (Chen et al. 1991). The data show that regardless of the overall cholesterol concentration in a population, absolute differences in cholesterol are associated with differences in the incidence of CHD (Betteridge 1996). The true relation between cholesterol concentration and CHD has tended to be underestimated because of regression dilution and surrogate underestimation (Wald and Law 1995). After allowance for these sources of error, analysis of the international studies shows that a 10% difference in cholesterol concentration is associated with a 38% difference in CHD mortality rate. A difference of 23 mg/dL in cholesterol in the cohort studies by this

Table 11.2. THE METABOLIC SYNDROME

Component risk factors
  Atherogenic dyslipidemia
    Borderline–high LDL-C concentration
    Elevated TG
      150–250 mg/dL
      250–500 mg/dl also commonly associated with these clustered lipoprotein abnormalities
    Small LDL particles (LDL phenotype B)
    Low HDL-C
      Categorically, <35 mg/dL
      Also <40 mg/dL in men and <50 mg/dL in women
  Hypertension
  Insulin resistance ± type 2 diabetes mellitus
  Procoagulant state
Contributing causes
  Obesity, especially abdominal obesity
  Physical inactivity
  Cholesterol-raising nutrients
    High intake of saturated fatty acids, *trans* fatty acids, and cholesterol
  Aging
  Genetic factors

Source: Grundy 1997; used with permission.

analysis would be associated with a CHD mortality difference of 54% at age 40, 39% at age 50, 27% at age 60, and 20% at age 70 (Law et al. 1994). Traditionally, CHD risk has been considered to be 2–3% lower for each 1% decrease in TC concentration (Manson et al. 1992).

Reduced High-Density Lipoprotein Cholesterol

The strong inverse relation between HDL-C concentration and CHD risk is well established by observational epidemiologic studies. Each 1-mg/dL increment in HDL-C is associated with a 2% risk decrement in men and 3% risk decrement in women (Gordon et al. 1989). No results from a clinical endpoints trial with the hypothesis of increasing HDL-C concentration have yet been reported. However, in LOCAT, fibrate therapy achieved favorable coronary angiographic changes in men whose chief lipid abnormality was reduced HDL-C (see Chapter 10), and the CHD morbidity and mortality benefits with statin treatment in AFCAPS/TexCAPS occurred in men and women who had reduced HDL-C as an enrollment criterion (see Chapter 12). Also in clinical trials testing LDL-C reduction, including the LRC-CPPT, Helsinki Heart Study, and FATS (see Chapters 10 and 12), treatment-induced increases in HDL-C have been found to be independently associated with a reduction in CHD events and decreased lesion progression (Barter and Rye 1996). The question of whether raising HDL-C will lower CHD risk must be considered in light of the fact that, as reviewed

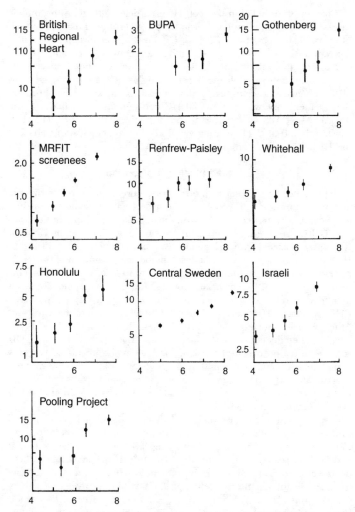

Figure 11.4. Incidence of ischemic heart disease, age adjusted with 95% CIs, according to fifths of the distribution of blood cholesterol in the 10 largest cohort studies. BUPA, British United Provident Association; MRFIT, Multiple Risk Factor Intervention Trial. (From Wald and Law 1995; used with permission.)

in Chapter 8, the relation between HDL particles and atherothrombotic disease is extremely complex. Gordon et al. (1989) found that at least half of the predictive power of HDL-C for CHD is eliminated when non-HDL-C concentration is considered in multivariate analysis. Vega and Grundy (1996) note that this finding may be viewed as welcome news, since statins lower concentrations of all apo B–containing particles in patients with low HDL-C; hence efficacious therapy may already be available for lipoprotein derangements for which a low HDL-C concentration is a marker. The AFCAPS/TexCAPS results appear to be instructive in this regard. The HDL Intervention Trial (HIT) is using gemfibrozil to treat men with CHD and low HDL-C in an effort to prevent new CHD events.

Elevated Plasma Triglyceride

As highlighted in Chapter 8, the relation between hypertriglyceridemia and atherothrombosis is complex. The hypertriglyceridemic state is heterogeneous with respect to underlying metabolic alterations, and the various TGRLs are heterogeneous in atherogenic potential; their metabolism is closely associated with the metabolism and composition of LDL and HDL particles, and they are linked with blood coagulation and fibrinolytic pathways (Hamsten and Karpe 1996). Since the 1980s, a variety of mechanisms whereby TGRLs may be atherogenic and prothrombotic have been identified, and in Europe hypertriglyceridemia is generally accepted as a CHD risk factor (Hamsten and Karpe 1996); it is integral to the European Atherosclerosis Society clinical guidelines (International Task Force 1992). The epidemiologic association of total fasting plasma TG with CHD risk has, thus, been complicated by methodologic difficulties. Whereas earlier analyses tended to find that the predictivity of TG was lost on multivariate analysis, more recent subgroup and meta-analyses as well as indirect data from clinical trials support risk factor status (Austin et al. 1998; Davignon and Cohn 1996).

Austin et al. (1998), on meta-analysis of 17 population-based studies with an average follow-up of 8.4 years in men and 11.4 years in women, found an increase of 88.5 mg/dL in fasting TG to be associated with 32% and 76% increased risks for incident CHD in men and women, which decreased to 14% and 37% after adjustment for HDL-C and other risk factors but remained significant. Miller et al. (1998), in a retrospective cohort study of Johns Hopkins Hospital patients, found that over an 18-year follow-up, independent predictors of CHD events were diabetes mellitus, HDL-C less than 35 mg/dL, and fasting TG greater than 100 mg/dL; they suggested on the basis of their findings that clinical action limits for fasting TG concentration may need to be refined. A number of authors, such as Castelli on the basis of Framingham data (1996), have recommended use of a TG cutpoint of 150 mg/dL. Some workers believe that the conventional epidemiologic approach should be abandoned as regards CHD risk from TG, with a focus instead on metabolic and molecular mechanisms (Hamsten and Karpe 1996).

As discussed in Chapter 8, specific TGRLs and markers of TGRL metabolism have been key correlates of lesion progression in LDL-lowering trials monitored by angiography or B-mode ultrasound (Hodis and Mack 1998). BECAIT results (see Chapter 10) showed improved coronary progression and reduced CHD events with bezafibrate therapy that substantially lowered VLDL-C and plasma TG but did not affect LDL-C concentration. In the Stockholm Ischemic Heart Disease Secondary Prevention Study and the Helsinki Heart Study, fasting TG had a strong relation with effects of therapy on CHD events (see Chapter 12). It is possible that in some of these trials unmonitored LDL particle size may have been favorably affected as well (Havel 1998). Results are needed from large clinical endpoints trials with the hypothesis of lowering TG. The ongoing Bezafibrate Infarction Prevention Trial is treating more than 3,000 patients with angina or recent MI to prevent new CHD events. Some TGRL derangements in patients with TG lower than 200 mg/dL are already being treated (Havel 1998) by LDL-lowering drugs that also lower TG and reduce the cholesterol content of TGRLs disproportionately (Illingworth et al. 1994).

Smoking

What is so unusual is the social and political acceptability of this lethal habit. The tobacco industry is probably responsible for more premature deaths and illness than any other organized commercial enterprise, exceeding the destructive impact of the arms and illicit drugs industries.

—Nicholas J. Wald and Allan K. Hackshaw (1996)

It's good for nothing but to choke a man, and fill him full of smoke and embers. . . . It's little better than ratsbane.

—The water-carrier in Ben Jonson's *Every Man in His Humour* (1598)

Epidemiology of the Risk

A Worldwide Killer. Cigarette smoking is the key public health challenge in developed nations (Peto et al. 1992, 1994; Wald and Hackshaw 1996). In 44 developed countries taken together, tobacco was responsible for 24% of all deaths in males and 7% of all deaths in females in 1990, rising to more than 40% in men in some former socialist economies (Peto et al. 1996). The average loss of life of smokers is 8 years; for those whose deaths are attributable to tobacco, it is about 16 years (Peto et al. 1996). Fifty percent of cigarette smokers die of smoking-related causes (Kottke 1997). Among 1,000 20-year-old Americans who smoke cigarettes regularly, about 6 will die from homicide, 12 will die in a motor vehicle accident, and 250 will die in middle age and 250 in old age from smoking-related disease (Peto et al. 1994). One-third of U.S. deaths in middle age are smoking related (Peto et al. 1994).

Cigarette smoking can kill in at least 24 different ways (Boyle 1997). Among major chronic diseases for which smoking is a risk factor are CVD; cancers, including cancers of the lung and upper aerodigestive system, liver, pancreas, stomach, rectum, renal pelvis, urinary bladder, uterine cervix, and penis, as well as leukemia (Boyle 1997; Hoffmann and Hoffmann 1997; Sherman 1991); and nonmalignant respiratory diseases, for example, emphysema, bronchitis, and pneumonia (ACS 1998; Boyle 1997). Smoking accounts for 90% of cases of lung cancer among U.S. men and for 79% of cases among U.S. women, and it accounts for about 30% of all cancer deaths in the United States (ACS 1995). Chronic obstructive respiratory conditions are the fifth leading cause of death in the United States (Gross 1990), and about 80% of deaths from these conditions can be attributed to smoking (Higgins 1991). Among additional risks are increased risk for cirrhosis of the liver and peptic ulcer disease (Boyle 1997; Sherman 1991). Smokers and their families are more likely to perish in fatal fires (Rigotti and Pasternak 1996). Polycyclic aromatic hydrocarbons and heterocyclic amines are considered the major cancer-causing agents in tobacco smoke; these substances can interfere with cell replication (Skaar et al. 1997).

Women who smoke are more likely to suffer complications of pregnancy, especially in intrauterine growth retardation; miscarriage/spontaneous abortion is more likely (Economides and Braithwaite 1994; Fredricsson and Gilljam 1992; Parazzini et al. 1991; Sherman 1991). Smoking is the leading preventable cause of low birth weight (Rigotti and Pasternak 1996). It is associated with earlier menopause (typically 2 or 3 years) (McBride 1992; Schmeiser-Rieder et al. 1995), decreases women's fecundity (Bolumar et al. 1996), and increases severity of dysmenorrhea (Sundell et al. 1990). (See also the section "Additional Cardiovascular Concerns for Women Who Smoke," later.)

Prevalence. There are about 1 billion smokers in the world today; one-third of them are in China (Wald and Hackshaw 1996), where 61% of men but only 7% of women are smokers. Smoking is a major cause of death in China, and the risks are similar to those in the United States, including an adjusted relative risk for death from CHD of 3.6 in men and 4.7 in women (Lam et al. 1997). In the United States, about 28% of men and 23% of women smoke (nearly the same as rates in the United Kingdom: 28% and 26%), compared with rates of 67% and 25–30% in the Russian Federation, 59% and 15% in Japan, and 40% and 27% in France (WHO 1997). In 1991, only 3% of U.S. physicians but 18% of U.S. registered nurses smoked. In some countries, smoking rates among health care workers are high (e.g., 33% of physicians and 49% of nurses surveyed in Prague in 1994; 48% of male medical students and 14% of female medical students in the Russian Federation in 1993; 48% of general practitioners, 43% of specialists, and 58% of nurses in Tuzla in 1995) (WHO 1997).

From 1970 to 1992, U.S. cigarette consumption decreased 32% (WHO 1997), although that overall decline may be leveling off (AHA 1996). The rate of decline for women was lower than that for men (WHO 1997), although those rates appear now to have equalized (Husten et al. 1996).

Prevalence of smoking among young U.S. women increased in the early 1980s but appears now to be decreasing (Husten et al. 1996). Still, some investigators predict that the United States will soon become the first society in history in which female smokers outnumber male smokers (Perkins et al. 1997).

Smoking and Cardiovascular Disease.   Smoking is the single most important preventable cause of morbidity and mortality from CVD (Lakier 1992). (Mechanisms of cardiovascular damage are discussed in Chapter 8.) In the United States, about one-fifth of deaths from CVD are attributable to smoking (AHA 1997), and CHD accounts for about one-half of those deaths (U.S. Department of Health, Education, and Welfare 1990) (Figure 11.5). Smoking doubles to quadruples the risk for CHD events (Lakier 1992), and the risk is synergistically compounded by hypertension, hypercholesterolemia, glucose intolerance, or diabetes (Lakier 1992). Smoking confers at least a 70% excess rate of death from CHD (Fielding 1985; Lakier 1992). It increases risk for sudden cardiac death 10 times in men and 4.5 times in women (Kannel et al. 1984). Continued smoking after an MI halves life expectancy (Kottke 1997). Smoking is predictive of chronotropic incompetence, and male smokers with chronotropic incompetence are at particularly high risk for death and CHD events (Lauer et al. 1997).

Smoking also increases risk for aortic aneurysm, stroke, TIAs, intermittent claudication/PVD, and arrhythmias (Boyle 1997; Freund et al. 1993; Rigotti and Pasternak 1996). Seventy percent of patients who present with atherosclerosis obliterans (which accounts for about 95% of cases of PVD) are smokers (Hertzer et al. 1979). Thromboangiitis obliterans, the second most common form of PVD, occurs only in smokers; 95% of cases are in male smokers (de Wolfe 1983).

Dose-Response Relation.   The degree of risk of smoking is related to the number of cigarettes smoked and to cumulative consumption (age at beginning and duration) in a strong and consistent dose-response relation (Manson et al. 1992; Rigotti and Pasternak 1996; Tresch and Aronow 1996). Risk for MI and death from CVD is increased even with smoking only one to four cigarettes each day (Rigotti and Pasternak 1996); thus, there is no safe level of tobacco use. Smoking so-called low-yield cigarettes does not reduce smoking-related risk for CVD (Manson et al. 1992; Rigotti and Pasternak 1996; Tresch and Aronow 1996).

Additional Cardiovascular Concerns for Women Who Smoke.   As noted, women who smoke undergo menopause at an earlier age (Schmeiser-Rieder et al. 1995). Estrogen deprivation is a risk factor for CHD in postmenopausal women, whether menopause is natural or surgical (Eaker et al. 1993); thus, smoking hastens the stroke- and CHD-prone years in women. Smoking increases risk for postmenopausal osteoporosis as well (Schmeiser-Rieder et al. 1995).

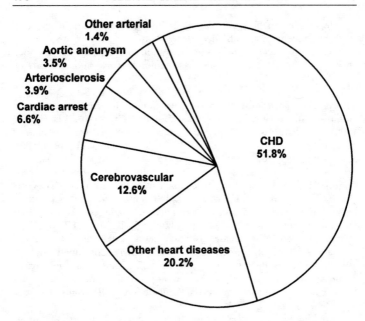

Figure 11.5. CVD deaths attributable to cigarette smoking in the United States, 1988. (Data from U.S. Department of Health, Education, and Welfare 1990.)

Smoking while using oral contraception (OC) is the leading cause of CHD events in U.S. women younger than 50 (Martys 1994) and increases risk for subarachnoid hemorrhage and stroke (Rigotti and Pasternak 1996). Risk for MI is 39 times higher in the heaviest smokers who use OC than in women who neither smoke nor use OC (Manson et al. 1992). Risk calculations include data from studies assessing current OC preparations; in a recent report, the odds ratio for an acute MI was approximately 5 in women who smoked and used OC, rising to greater than 20 with 10 or more cigarettes daily (WHO 1997).

In the Finnmark Study (11,843 men and women 35–52 years of age at entry) at 12-year follow-up, current smoking was a stronger predictor of MI in women than in men (relative risk, 3.3 vs. 1.9), an effect that was more pronounced for subjects younger than 45 (relative risk, 7.1 vs. 2.3). The MI risk for women who smoked heavily was greater than that for men who had never smoked (Njolstad et al. 1996).

Cigar and Pipe Smoking.   Smoking cigars or a pipe also confers significant risk for CHD (Tresch and Aronow 1996). Cigarette smokers who switch to a pipe have a greater risk for all-cause mortality than those who no longer smoke at all (Ben-Shlomo et al. 1994). In the prospective Copen-hagen City Heart Study of 20,000 men and women, the relative risk for a first acute MI increased 2–3% for each gram of tobacco smoked daily, regardless of type of tobacco use (pipe, cigar or cheroot, or plain or fil-tered cigarette) (Nyboe et al. 1991). In a Swedish study of 25,000 men, the amount of tobacco smoked, whether by cigarette, cigar, or pipe, was highly significantly correlated at 16 years with risk for CHD death as well as for a variety of cancers (Carstensen et al. 1987). Cigarette, cigar, and pipe smoking and use of smokeless tobacco are major risk factors for oral cancers; that risk is synergistically increased by excess use of alcohol (ACS 1995).

Smokeless Tobacco.   Observational epidemiologic evidence for a link between smokeless tobacco and risk for CVD is contradictory (Steen 1996). In one recent Swedish study, however, the relative risk for death from CVD was 1.4 (95% CI 1.2–1.6) in snuff users who had never smoked (Bolinder et al. 1994).

Potential roles for nicotine in the development of CVD are briefly reviewed under "Mechanisms," although available data suggest that the prothrombotic effects of cigarette smoke or the effects of carbon monox-ide play a larger role in acute events. Smokeless tobacco not only can lead to nicotine dependence but also can cause cancer and a number of non-cancerous oral conditions; risk for cancer of the cheek and gums is increased almost 50 times in long-term snuff users (ACS 1998).

Environmental Tobacco Smoke.   Environmental tobacco smoke (ETS; also known as passive smoking, second-hand smoke, or side-stream smoke) contains essentially the same toxic agents that are inhaled by smokers (ACS 1995). Living with a smoker increases a nonsmoker's risk for death from CHD by 30% (Glantz and Parmley 1991; Rigotti and Pasternak 1996), and in the United States CHD deaths from passive smoking—which number 35,000–40,000 annually (ACS 1998)—account for 70% of all ETS-attributable deaths (Kritz et al. 1995).

ETS leads to many of the same effects as active smoking, such as induc-tion of platelet abnormalities (Rigotti and Pasternak 1996). Some, such as vasoconstriction, are even more pronounced (Rigotti and Pasternak 1996); it appears that nonsmokers have not "adapted" to smoke's toxic agents (Witschi et al. 1997). ETS has been shown to induce atherosclero-sis in animals (Rigotti and Pasternak 1996); in rats, exposure increased the acute accumulation of LDL in perfused arteries (Roberts et al. 1996).

Classified as a human carcinogen, ETS has a causal association with lung cancer (Rigotti and Pasternak 1996; Witschi et al. 1997). It also increases risk for chronic respiratory symptoms, bronchitis, and pneumo-nia in adults (ACS 1998; Law and Hackshaw 1996; Witschi et al. 1997). The best-documented risks are to the children of parents who smoke; for example, risk is increased for sudden infant death syndrome, chronic oti-tis media, and asthma. Exposure to ETS during pregnancy is associated with small but significant reductions in birth weight (Law and Hackshaw 1996; Rigotti and Pasternak 1996; Witschi et al. 1997).

Coronary Heart Disease Benefits of Smoking Cessation

Reversal of adverse CHD effects occurs rapidly after smoking cessation. Half of the excess risk for nonfatal MI disappears in the first year, and the CHD risk of exsmokers may be nearly that of people who have never smoked within just 2 or 3 years (Manson et al. 1992; Rigotti and Pasternak 1996), regardless of intensity or duration of smoking (Manson et al. 1992). Smoking cessation after an MI reduces death rates 10% to more than 50% (Samet 1992). CHD risk reduction is similar in the elderly (Manson et al. 1992). Thus, it is never too late to stop smoking.

Smoking cessation is also important to prevent other CVDs, such as stroke and PVD (Beilin 1994; Robinson and Leon 1994). The relative risk for cancer death attributable to smoking declines substantially, the extent of risk reduction depending on age at cessation, duration of the habit, and length of abstinence (Skaar et al. 1997). Although cancer risk reduction generally takes longer than CHD risk reduction with smoking cessation, risk for all-cause death in the next 15 years is halved for people who quit smoking before age 50 (ACS 1998).

After cessation, HDL-C rises, on average 6–8 mg/dL (0.2 mmol/L) (Rigotti and Pasternak 1996). Improvements in HDL-C occur quickly, within as little as 30 days (Allen et al. 1994; Feher et al. 1990; Moffatt 1988; Nilsson et al. 1996). Slight decreases in LDL-C have been seen in some studies (Allen et al. 1994; Terres et al. 1994). Cessation decreases fibrinogen and factor VII plasma concentrations, although these improvements may take many years (Samet 1992). Stopping smoking may help inactivate acute atherosclerotic lesions (Weintraub 1990).

Hypertension

Many prospective studies have related increasing SBP and DBP with risk for stroke, MI, congestive heart failure, and renal insufficiency. Average arterial blood pressure and prevalence of hypertension both tend to rise with age, and about one in four adult Americans is hypertensive (Whelton et al. 1996; AHA 1997). Although stroke is often viewed as the chief complication of hypertension, coronary events related to blood pressure are about five times more common in the general population (Sleight 1996). In the MRFIT screenees at 12 years' follow-up (see also Chapter 8), both absolute and relative risk for CHD death increased with progressively higher SBP or DBP, independent of age, race, plasma cholesterol, cigarette smoking status, or income (Stamler et al. 1993a). It is important to note that about two-thirds of hypertension-related CHD deaths in MRFIT occurred in individuals with only mild hypertension, and the relative risk for CHD death also increased with each succeeding SBP level in the normotensive range. The relation between CHD risk and blood pressure is similar for men and women, and both sexes should be treated for hypertension. Whether "white coat hypertension" (blood pressure raised only in the presence of a physician or another health professional) indicates an increased risk for CVD is not yet known (Pyörälä et al. 1994). Because SBP and DBP stand in continuous relation to cardiovascular risk, the classification of blood pressure is somewhat arbitrary (NIH 1997). In the United States, clinical action limits for blood pressure are established by the JNC (see Chapter 16); classification of hypertension by the World Health Organization (WHO 1996) is in general accord with the JNC VI definitions.

Not only the level of blood pressure but also its 24-hour pattern may be critical to risk for CVD (Kaplan 1995). Verdecchia et al. (1994) in a prospective study spanning 7.5 years found that CVD mortality was three times higher in subjects with hypertension who did not have a 10% or greater nocturnal fall in blood pressure (nondippers) from average daytime ambulatory pressure compared with those who did (dippers).

On average, according to meta-analysis (Hebert et al. 1993), antihypertensive drug therapy with lifestyle intervention significantly reduces the relative risk for CHD and for fatal CHD, each by 16% (2–3% for each reduction of 1 mm Hg in DBP, reductions averaging 5–6 mm Hg). Comparable risk reductions are achieved by treating patients with isolated systolic hypertension (Whelton et al. 1996). In comparison, total stroke and stroke mortality rates are reduced 38% and 40% (Hebert et al. 1993). However, the numbers of coronary and stroke deaths prevented are about the same because of the higher prevalence of CHD. There are clear-cut benefits in CVD risk from a decrease of even 5 or 6 mm Hg in DBP (Collins et al. 1990). Unpublished findings from the Hypertension Optimal Treatment trial presented at the International Society of Hypertension meeting in Amsterdam in June 1998 indicate that more aggressive lowering of blood pressure can achieve greater CHD risk reduction. The trial's reduction of DBP from 105 to 83 mm Hg lowered MI risk by 37%. Further reduction was neither beneficial nor harmful. The 5-year trial is the largest ever conducted in the treatment of hypertension, enrolling 19,000 patients in 26 countries, including the United States. Targets in the three treatment groups were DBP less than or equal to 90 mm Hg, less than or equal to 85 mm Hg, and less than or equal to 80 mm Hg (Julius 1996). Recent analyses of prospective data have not shown the J-shaped relation between DBP and CHD incidence described by earlier analyses of smaller data sets (Whelton et al. 1996).

A key to understanding the relation between hypertension and CHD, as discussed in Chapter 8, is the recognition that hypertension rarely occurs as an isolated problem; in general, it is part of a clustering of risk factors or a syndrome also defined by insulin resistance, dyslipidemia, coagulation abnormalities, and other factors, in many cases associated with abdominal obesity, LVH, or both (Weber 1994). Therefore, risk reduction intervention should focus on multiple risk factors for CVD.

Left Ventricular Hypertrophy

LVH is an important but often overlooked risk factor for CVD, as has recently been well reviewed by Lavie et al. (1996). Its consequences include ischemia, arrhythmias, and ventricular dysfunction. It is associated with markedly increased risk for CHD morbidity, CHD mortality, and all-cause mortality; the risk for CHD exceeds that of the accompanying hypertension (Srikanthan and Dunn 1997). In the Framingham Heart Study, each increase of 50 g/m in echocardiographically determined LV mass for height increased the risk for new CHD events by 150% (Levy et al. 1989). An earlier Framingham report showed ECG-detected LVH to be associated with nearly a 10-fold increase in risk for sudden death (Kannel 1983). Framingham data also showed that the presence of LVH on ECG confers an even higher relative risk for congestive heart failure than for CHD (Kannel 1993), although coronary events are more prevalent in the elderly (Lavie et al. 1996).

Risk factors for LVH include age, weight, arterial pressure, sodium intake, and race (hypertension being more common and more severe in blacks); catecholamines, the renin-angiotensin system, and various growth factors also play a role in the pathophysiology of LVH. Because obesity and hypertension tend to increase with age, LVH is a particular problem in the elderly: as many as 50% may have the condition. Echocardiography is considerably more sensitive and specific for LVH than is ECG, and ECG is more sensitive and specific than chest radiography or physical examination. Measures associated with the prevention and reduction of LVH include weight reduction, sodium restriction, and pharmacotherapy (e.g., ACE inhibitors, calcium antagonists, alpha-blockers).

Diabetes Mellitus

The marked increase in CHD risk (two to four times) from type 2 diabetes mellitus is discussed in Chapter 8. Because of the high risk, the absolute benefit of risk factor reduction in diabetic patients is likely to be greater than like intervention in nondiabetic patients. Yet evidence suggests that most diabetic patients do not receive adequate risk factor intervention, which is out of keeping with practice guidelines (Savage 1998).

Haffner et al. (1998), in 7-year follow-up of 2,432 subjects who were part of a well-characterized Finnish population-based cohort, found that adjusted risk for CHD death was not significantly different between diabetic subjects without a previous MI and nondiabetic subjects with a history of MI. Given their results, the clinical evidence of benefit in diabetic subjects in the 4S and CARE trials (see Chapter 12), and the high mortality (including prehospital mortality) after MI in diabetic patients (Abbott et al. 1988; Herliz et al. 1992; Miettinen et al. 1998), the authors suggest that all patients with type 2 diabetes should receive risk intervention as aggressive as that given patients with established atherosclerotic disease. A study by the same group in U.S. subjects showed, according to preliminary results, similar carotid artery intimal wall thickness in diabetic subjects without CHD and nondiabetic subjects with CHD (D'Agostino et al. 1998).

Obesity

As a leading cause of preventable death in the United States, obesity currently follows only smoking, which it will likely surpass in this role in the 21st century (Grundy 1998). About 280,000 deaths in the United States can be attributed each year to "overnutrition" (McGinnis and Foege 1993). Overweight/obesity affects 97 million American adults (55% of the adult population) (NIH 1998). The NHANES III data show an upward trend in the prevalence of overweight and obesity: from 13% of the total U.S. population in 1960 to 23% in 1994, with most of the increase occurring in the 1990s (NIH 1998). There is a disproportionate increase in severe overweight (Kuczmarski et al. 1994). Although U.S. national surveys show that the percentage of calories consumed as fat is decreasing (from about 40–42% in the 1960s to about 34% in the early 1990s), more calories overall are being consumed (Eckel and Krauss 1998). Overweight and obesity are particularly great problems in some U.S. minority groups (see Chapter 20) and in those with lower incomes and less education (NIH 1998).

The definitions of overweight and obesity remain controversial, and a variety of measures have been used to estimate fatness. In its 1998 adult clinical guidelines (see Chapter 16), the NIH has selected BMI criteria with disease risk estimation modified by waist circumference and other risk factors. Waist circumference is used as an estimate of body fat distribution. The upper body, centralized, or abdominal fat pattern ("apple" shape), as contrasted with fat in the thighs and buttocks ("pear" shape), has been correlated with increased risk factors for CVD (Stevens 1995). Although intra-abdominal fat accounts for less than 20% of total body fat, it is a major determinant of postprandial and fasting lipid availability and contributes not only to dyslipidemia but also to beta cell dysfunction and to hepatic and peripheral insulin resistance (Carey 1998) (see also Chapters 3 and 8). Whether simple anthropometric measures such as waist circumference, waist:hip ratio, or sagittal diameter can reliably estimate visceral fat and related CVD risk factors, or which measure or measures might be best, is a matter of scrutiny and debate (Stevens 1995; Pouliot et al. 1994; Rissanen et al. 1997). Height does not appear to have an important influence on anthropometric measures of intra-abdominal fat (Han et al. 1997). For a given waist circumference, Han et al. (1997) found intra-abdominal fat area as determined by magnetic resonance imaging or computed tomography to be higher in older subjects. Assessments by direct methods such as magnetic resonance imaging, spectroscopy, and computed tomography provide much more detailed information about visceral fat but are expensive, and radiation risk with some techniques precludes use in children (Eckel 1997).

Etiology

The development of obesity is incompletely understood but involves social, behavioral, cultural, physiologic, metabolic, and genetic factors (NIH 1998). Lifestyle may play a dominant role (Eckel and Krauss 1998; Grundy 1998). Parental and offspring BMIs are correlated, including between biologic parents and adult adoptees (but not between adoptive parents and adult adoptees); furthermore, similarity of BMI is about twice as great in monozygotic as in dizygotic twins (Sørenson 1995). The complex etiology makes the search for obesity genes challenging; several genome scanning projects with obesity phenotypes as a primary focus are under way (Comuzzie and Allison 1998).

It is being recognized more and more that obesity results in great measure from an environment that promotes excessive food intake and discourages physical activity (through advances in technology and transportation), and that the environment needs to be cured as much as individuals (Hill and Peters 1998; Goodrick et al. 1996). Physiologic mechanisms are strong in the defense against weight loss but weak against weight gain when there is an abundant food supply (Hill and Peters 1998). Nevertheless, altering the environment should not be viewed as insurmountable given the societal gains that have been made in the United States against smoking and a high-fat diet (Hill and Peters 1998). Preventing the development of obesity in young adulthood and middle age should be high on the list of public health priorities, and even if weight control efforts fail in the first generation, they may succeed in later generations (Grundy 1998).

Risks

Obese individuals are at increased risk for multiple health problems (Table 11.3), including CVD and disorders that contribute to the risk for CVD. The obese may also suffer from social stigmatization and discrimination (NIH 1998).

The risks for CHD morbidity and CHD mortality (Table 11.4) are considerably increased in both obese men and women, most studies showing a linear relation (Daly et al. 1996). Until recently, the relation between obesity and CHD risk was viewed as indirect, mediated through covariates such as hypertension, dyslipidemia, and impaired glucose tolerance or type 2 diabetes (Eckel 1997). However, long-term longitudinal studies indicate that obesity independently predicts coronary atherosclerotic disease (Manson et al. 1995; Garrison and Castelli 1985), and growing evidence supports a role for obesity, in particular visceral obesity, in the pathophysiology of atherosclerosis (see Chapter 8). The AHA has now deemed obesity a major risk factor for CHD (Eckel and Krauss 1998): it is no longer viewed that obesity is simply "along for the ride" (Garrison et al.

Table 11.3. MORBIDITY IN OBESITY

Category	Disorder	Category	Disorder
CVD	Hypertension	Breast	Breast cancer
	CHD		Male gynecomastia
	Cerebrovascular disease	Uterine	Endometrial cancer
		Cervical	Cervical cancer
	Varicose veins	Urologic	Prostate cancer
	Deep venous thrombosis		Stress incontinence
	Hypertension	Dermatologic	Sweat rashes
Respiratory	Breathlessness		Fungal infections
	Sleep apnea		Lymphedema
	Hypoventilation syndrome		Cellulitis
Gastrointestinal	Hiatal hernia		Acanthosis nigricans
	Gallstones, cholelithiasis	Orthopedic	Osteoarthritis
			Gout
	Fatty liver, cirrhosis	Endocrine	Growth hormone reduced
	Hemorrhoids		IGF-1 reduced
	Hernia		Reduced prolactin response
	Colorectal cancer		
Metabolic	Dyslipidemia		Hyperdynamic ACTH response to CRH
	Insulin resistance		
	Type 2 diabetes mellitus		Increased urinary free cortisol
	Polycystic ovary syndrome		Altered sex hormones
	Hyperandro-genization	Pregnancy	Obstetric complications
	Menstrual irregularities		Cesarean operation
Neurologic	Nerve entrapment		Large babies
Renal	Proteinuria		Neural tube defects

ACTH, adrenocorticotropic hormone; CRH, corticotropin-releasing hormone; IGF-1, insulin-like growth factor 1.
Source: Jung 1997; used with permission.

1996). Longer periods of follow-up and more complete data have contributed to this shift in understanding (Garrison et al. 1996).

A U- or J-shaped relation has been described between body weight and total mortality rate (Lew and Garfinkel 1979), the excess mortality in the lean subjects probably related to smoking and to diseases such as cancer and digestive diseases (Stern 1995). When smokers and those who died early in follow-up were excluded from analysis, mortality rates have been lowest among the leanest subjects (Manson et al. 1995; Lee et al. 1993). Overweight may pose the greatest health hazard when it is gained in early adulthood and

Table 11.4. MORTALITY RISK IN OBESITY

Disease	Male	Female
Diabetes mellitus	5.19	7.90
Digestive diseases	3.99	7.90
CHD	1.85	2.07
Cerebrovascular disease	2.27	1.52
Cancer: all sites	1.33	1.55
Cancer: colorectal	1.73	
Cancer: prostate	1.29	
Cancer: gallbladder/biliary		3.58
Cancer: endometrial		5.42
Cancer: cervix		2.39
Cancer: ovary		1.63

Note: Risk is for those weighing ≥140% above ideal weight compared with those weighing 90–100% of ideal.
Source: Jung 1997; used with permission. Data from Lew and Garfinkel 1979 (American Cancer Society study).

maintained or increased in middle age (Shaper 1996). In the large population assessed in the American Cancer Society Prevention Study, Stevens et al. (1998) found that relative risk at 12 years' follow-up for all-cause death according to BMI was significantly higher among younger than older adults (ages 30–44 years vs. 65–74 years). The average American, according to data from the 1970s, gains about 10 kg (22 lb) between ages 20 and 50 years (NIH 1979), and muscle mass typically decreases with aging (Visser et al. 1995). Food intake may increase after age 20 years, even though physical activity tends to decline (Grundy 1998).

Benefits of Weight Loss

There is strong evidence from lifestyle intervention trials that weight reduction in overweight/obese subjects reduces plasma TG and increases HDL-C (it also generally produces some decrease in TC and LDL-C), decreases blood pressure (in both hypertensive and nonhypertensive subjects), and decreases fasting blood glucose in subjects without diabetes and in some patients with type 2 diabetes (NIH 1998) (Table 11.5). Meta-analysis of 70 studies on the effects of weight loss on plasma lipid concentrations showed a decrease of 1.9 mg/dL in TC, 0.8 mg/dL in LDL-C, and 1.3 mg/dL in TG and an increase in HDL-C of 0.27 mg/dL during active weight loss and 0.35 mg/dL on weight stabilization for each 1 kg of weight loss (Dattilo and Kris-Etherton 1992). Weight loss also decreases symptoms of angina and lowers total mortality rate (see Table 11.5). The evidence that weight loss per se decreases CHD risk is much less certain than for reduction of risk factors such as LDL-C (Shaper 1996; Daly et al. 1996). Small reductions in weight and sodium restriction can dramatically improve ventricular function and oxygenation in patients with con-

Table 11.5. BENEFITS OF A 10-kg (22-lb) LOSS OF EXCESS WEIGHT

Category	Benefits
Mortality rate	↓ 20–25% total mortality
	↓ 30–40% diabetes-related mortality
	↓ 40–50% obesity-related cancer mortality
Blood pressure	↓ 10 mm Hg SBP
	↓ 20 mm Hg DBP
Angina pectoris	↓ 91% symptoms
	↑ 33% exercise tolerance
Plasma lipids	↓ 30% plasma TG
	↑ 8% HDL-C
	↓ 10% TC
	↓ 15% LDL-C
Diabetes mellitus	↓ 50% risk for developing diabetes
	↓ 30–50% fasting blood glucose
	↓ 15% glycated hemoglobin (HbA1c)

Source: Jung 1997; used with permission.

gestive heart failure, and weight reduction is also associated with shortening of the QT interval (Eckel 1997).

There is suggestive evidence that reduction in abdominal fat decreases blood pressure, improves dyslipidemia, and improves glucose tolerance in subjects who have impaired glucose tolerance; none of these effects, however, was shown to be independent of weight loss (NIH 1998).

Physical Inactivity

In the United States, more than 60% of adults are not regularly active, and 25% are not active at all (U.S. Surgeon General 1996). One-fourth of American youths report no vigorous physical activity. The benefits of increased physical activity are numerous (Table 11.6).

Extensive data document the benefits of physical activity in both primary and secondary prevention of CVD, as summarized in the U.S. Surgeon General's report (1996) and AHA position statements (Fletcher et al. 1995, 1996) and as seen in population studies (Lee et al. 1995; Morris et al. 1990; Blair et al. 1989, 1995; O'Connor et al. 1989). Physical inactivity is an independent predictor of CHD and is directly related to CVD mortality rate (Lee et al. 1995; Morris et al. 1990; Blair et al. 1989). Manifestations of CHD are reduced in people whose jobs are physically demanding or who regularly participate in moderate to strenuous recreational activities (Powell et al. 1987; Morris et al. 1990), and survival rates are increased after MI when behavior is modified to include regular exercise (O'Connor et al. 1989; Oldridge et al. 1988). Most CVD mortality benefits of physical activity can be attained through moderately intense activity (Lee et al. 1995; Blair et al. 1995; Pate et al. 1995; Fletcher et al. 1996).

Table 11.6. SELECTED BENEFITS OF REGULAR EXERCISE

Reduces risk for premature death
Reduces risk for death from CHD
Reduces risk for type 2 diabetes mellitus
Reduces risk for hypertension
Helps reduce blood pressure in hypertensive individuals
Reduces risk for colon cancer
Reduces feelings of depression and anxiety
Helps control weight
Helps build and maintain healthy bones, muscles, and joints
Helps older adults become stronger and better able to move about without falling
Promotes psychologic well-being

Source: U.S. Surgeon General 1996.

Exercise training increases maximum ventilatory oxygen uptake and decreases myocardial oxygen demands, and beneficial changes occur in hemodynamic, hormonal, metabolic, neurologic, and respiratory function (Fletcher et al. 1996). Exercise can help control diabetes and obesity and adds an independent blood pressure–lowering effect in certain hypertensive groups (Fletcher et al. 1996). Below a critical level of physical activity, chances for being overweight become substantial (Ferro-Luzzi and Martino 1996). Exercise training also favorably alters carbohydrate metabolism, adipose tissue distribution, and insulin sensitivity (Mayer-Davis et al. 1998) and decreases fibrinogen concentrations (Fletcher et al. 1996). Although, importantly, unaccustomed vigorous exercise appears to be able to trigger acute coronary ischemic events (see Chapter 6), endurance training reduces risk for thrombosis (Kramsch et al. 1981).

Exercise induces a number of positive changes in lipoprotein metabolism in both diabetic and nondiabetic individuals (Berg et al. 1997; Winslow et al. 1996). It increases HDL-C, in particular "cardioprotective" HDL_2, and reduces, sometimes markedly, plasma TG. Effects on LDL-C are less consistent, although exercise often moderately lowers LDL-C (Wood 1994), and it shifts LDL from small, dense particles to larger particles. In addition, it decreases the extent of postprandial lipemia (Foger and Patsch 1995), and endurance training increases LPL activity (Stefanick and Wood 1994). There appears to be little effect on Lp[a] (Mackinnon et al. 1997). Regular exercise in overweight individuals enhances the beneficial effect of a low-fat diet on lipid concentrations (Wood et al. 1991). Furthermore, exercise protects against the adverse effects of dyslipidemia on the vascular wall (Winslow et al. 1996) and may improve endothelial function (Hornig et al. 1996).

Aerobic exercise is also associated with improvements in indexes of psychologic functioning, including reduced depression, improved self-confidence and self-esteem, and attenuation of cardiovascular and neurohumoral responses to mental stress (Fletcher et al. 1996).

Several studies have found cardiorespiratory fitness gains from physical activity in several short sessions (e.g., 10 minutes each) to be similar to gains achieved with one longer session (e.g., 30 minutes) given the same total amount and intensity of activity. Although further proof of benefit is needed, it is reasonable to expect benefit from short sessions and compliance may be enhanced (U.S. Surgeon General 1996).

Compared with aerobic training, resistance training alone only modestly affects risk factors for CVD (Fletcher et al. 1996), although carbohydrate metabolism is improved through the development of muscle mass and effects on basal metabolism (Kohrt and Holloszy 1995; Evans 1995). Resistance training helps maintain strength, muscle mass, bone mineral density, and functional capacity and assists in the prevention or rehabilitation of musculoskeletal problems (Fletcher et al. 1996).

Additional information on physical activity and disease risk can be obtained by contacting the CDC (National Center for Chronic Disease Prevention and Health Promotion, Division of Nutrition and Physical Activity, MS K-46, 4770 Buford Highway NE, Atlanta, GA 30341-3724; 1-888-232-4674; http://www.cdc.gov) or The President's Council on Physical Fitness and Sports (Box SG, Suite 250, 701 Pennsylvania Avenue NW, Washington, DC 20004).

SOME POTENTIAL RISK FACTORS

- **Small, dense LDL:** See Chapter 8.
- **Lp[a]:** See Chapter 8. Plasma concentrations of Lp[a] are largely genetically determined. Some but not all prospective studies have described Lp[a] concentration as an independent predictor of CHD risk (Stein and Rosenson 1997; Djurovic and Berg 1997; Seed 1996). Nicotinic acid, pharmacologic doses of sex hormones and anabolic steroids, and LDL apheresis may lower Lp[a] to a degree sufficient to allow evaluation of clinical response (Angelin 1997). An Lp[a] concentration lower than 30 mg/dL is considered desirable.
- **Fibrinogen:** Plasma fibrinogen concentration, a measure of thrombotic potential, is associated with the severity and extent of CHD, PVD, and cerebrovascular atherosclerosis. It is an independent predictor of MI in both men and women and is strongly linked to cigarette smoking. Whether it is a cause or consequence of CVD has not been established, and there are no available drugs that selectively lower fibrinogen. Further standardization of measurement is needed (Heinrich and Assmann 1995).
- **Factor VII:** Factor VII has a positive correlation with the death rate from CVD. Its concentrations are linked with fat intake, plasma cholesterol, and plasma TG (Juhan-Vage 1996).
- **PAI-1:** Many longitudinal cohort studies have linked PAI-1 and tPA antigen with CVD risk, in particular MI. PAI-1 concentrations are closely associated with insulin resistance. Impaired fibrinolytic function, mainly due to elevated PAI-1, is a common finding in patients with thrombotic disease. Regulation of plasma PAI-1 concentration is not well understood. Multiple

interactions with disturbance of both carbohydrate and lipoprotein metabolism are evident (Wiman 1995; Juhan-Vage 1996).

- **C-reactive protein:** Systemic inflammation, for which serum C-reactive protein (CRP) is a marker, may be important in the pathogenesis of atherothrombosis. Smoking has been reported to increase concentrations of CRP. Both smoking and CHD may induce an inflammatory condition, but the increase of serum concentrations of inflammatory markers is complex (de Maat et al. 1996; Ridker et al. 1997). In case-control studies, CRP has been a predictor of CVD events, including MI (Ridker et al. 1997; Tracy et al. 1997).

- **Cellular adhesion molecules:** Cellular adhesion molecules have consistently been found in areas of atherosclerosis development and may be useful as indicators of subclinical disease (Ballantyne and Abe 1997). In a case-control analysis of Physicians' Health Study 9-year data, concentration of soluble ICAM-1 in plasma was positively associated with risk for first MI (Ridker et al. 1998). In the Atherosclerosis Risk in Communities study, circulating concentrations of both ICAM-1 and E-selectin were associated with CHD and carotid artery disease (Hwang et al. 1997). In the future, such molecular markers may prove useful in the identification of patients at high risk for cardiovascular events or in the selection of therapy, and antiadhesion therapies might provide a novel preventive intervention.

- **Infectious agents** (see Chapter 9): A large body of evidence implicates a number of microbial agents in atherogenesis. Pathologic changes of atherosclerosis and a range of infections show considerable overlap. A proved role, whether direct or indirect, would have far-reaching implications for prevention and treatment. Such a role is currently uncertain (Cook and Lip 1996; Ellis 1997).

- **Microalbuminuria:** Microalbuminuria is the presence of albumin above normal but below the detectable range by conventional urine dipstick methodology (Bakris 1996). It appears to be a powerful predictor of risk for atherosclerosis in its own right in diabetes mellitus. Data suggest that it is not a predictor in nondiabetic subjects. Data support the notion of early, aggressive intervention to attenuate the rise of microalbuminuria with blood glucose control. ACE inhibitors also attenuate this rise. It has been recommended that microalbuminuria be assessed annually in all diabetic patients (Bakris 1996). Among other novel risk factors proposed in diabetes are insulin resistance, elevated concentrations of proinsulin-line molecules, and PAI-1. Conventional risk factors do not account for all the increased atherosclerotic risk resulting from diabetes (Yudkin 1997).

- **Hyperinsulinemia and insulin resistance:** See Chapter 8.

- **Homocysteine:** See Chapter 15. Research is needed to establish that lowering plasma concentrations of homocysteine, an intermediate compound formed during metabolism of methionine, will reduce atherosclerotic morbidity and mortality.

- **Oxidative stress:** See "Antioxidant Vitamin Supplements" in Chapter 15.

- **Low socioeconomic status:** The increased risk for CVD among people of low socioeconomic status may relate to a higher prevalence of risk factors or less access to care (Kaplan and Keil 1993).
- **Stress, anger, and psychosocial risk factors:** Results of available studies of stress, anger, and psychosocial risk factors in CHD risk are inconsistent (Allan and Scheidt 1996; O'Connor et al. 1995).

Suggested Reading

Multiple Risk Factors

Assmann G, Cullen P, Schulte H. The Münster Heart Study (PROCAM): results of follow-up at 8 years. Eur Heart J 1998;19(suppl A):A2–A11.

Castelli WP. Lipids, risk factors and ischaemic heart disease. Atherosclerosis 1996;124:S1–S9.

Genest J Jr, Cohn JS. Clustering of cardiovascular risk factors: targeting high-risk individuals. Am J Cardiol 1995;76(suppl):8A–20A.

Greenland P, Grundy S, Pasternack RC, Lenfant C. Problems on the pathway from risk assessment to risk reduction (editorial). Circulation 1998;97:1761–1762.

Grundy SM, Balady GJ, Criqui MH, et al. Primary prevention of coronary heart disease: guidance from Framingham. A statement for healthcare professionals from the AHA Task Force on Risk Reduction. Circulation 1998;97:1876–1887.

Kaplan NM. The challenge of managing multiple cardiovascular risk factors. Am J Hypertens 1997;10:167S–169S.

Stamler J, Dyer AR, Shekelle RB, et al. Relationship of baseline major risk factors to coronary and all-cause mortality, and to longevity: findings from long-term follow-up of Chicago cohorts. Cardiology 1993;82:191–222.

Wilson PWF, D'Agostino RB, Levy D, et al. Prediction of coronary heart disease using risk factor categories. Circulation 1998;97:1837–1847.

Yusuf HR, Giles WH, Croft JB, et al. Impact of multiple risk factor profiles on determining CVD risk. Prev Med 1998;27:1–9.

Elevated Plasma Cholesterol

Betteridge DJ. Cholesterol lowering and secondary prevention of CHD—the evidence of benefit is unequivocal. In: Betteridge DJ, ed. Lipids: current perspectives. St. Louis: Mosby, 1996:261–271.

Law MR, Wald NJ, Thompson SG. Serum cholesterol reduction and health: by how much and how quickly is the risk of ischaemic heart disease lowered? BMJ 1994;308:367–372.

Wald NJ, Law MR. Serum cholesterol and ischaemic heart disease. Atherosclerosis 1995;118(suppl):S1–S5.

Reduced High-Density Lipoprotein Cholesterol

Assmann G, Schulte H, von Eckardstein A, Huang Y. High-density lipoprotein cholesterol as a predictor of coronary heart disease risk. The PROCAM experience and pathophysiological implications for reverse cholesterol transport. Atherosclerosis 1996;124(suppl):S11–S20.

Barter PJ, Rye K-A. High density lipoproteins and coronary heart disease (review). Atherosclerosis 1996;121:1–12.

Vega GL, Grundy SM. Hypoalphalipoproteinemia (low high density lipoprotein) as a risk factor for coronary heart disease (review). Curr Opin Lipidol 1996;7:209–216.

Elevated Plasma Triglyceride

Austin MA, Hokanson JE, Edwards KL. Hypertriglyceridemia as a cardiovascular risk factor. Am J Cardiol 1998;81(4A):7B–12B.

Criqui MH. Triglycerides and cardiovascular disease: a focus on clinical trials (review). Eur Heart J 1998;19(suppl A):A36–A39.

Davignon J, Cohn JS. Triglycerides: a risk factor for coronary heart disease (review). Atherosclerosis 1996;124(suppl):S57–S64.

Hamsten A, Karpe F. Triglycerides and coronary heart disease—has epidemiology given us the right answer? In: Betteridge DJ, ed. Lipids: current perspectives. St. Louis: Mosby, 1996:43–68.

Kesäniemi YA. Serum triglycerides and clinical benefit in lipid-lowering trials (review). Am J Cardiol 1998;81(4A):70B–73B.

Smoking

Lakier JB. Smoking and cardiovascular disease. Am J Med 1992;93(suppl 1A):8S–12S.

Peto R, Lopez AD, Boreham J, et al. Mortality from tobacco in developed countries: indirect estimation from national vital statistics. Lancet 1992;339:1268–1278.

Peto R, Lopez AD, Boreham J, et al. Mortality from smoking in developed countries, 1950–2000: indirect estimates from national vital statistics. Oxford: Oxford University Press, 1994.

Rigotti NA, Pasternak RC. Cigarette smoking and coronary heart disease: risks and management. Cardiol Clin 1996;14:51–68.

Skaar KL, Tsoh JY, McClure JB, et al. Smoking cessation 1: an overview of research. Behav Med 1997;23:5–13.

Tresch DD, Aronow WS. Smoking and coronary artery disease. Clin Geriatr Med 1996;12:23–32.

Wald NJ, Hackshaw AK. Cigarette smoking: an epidemiological overview. Br Med Bull 1996;52:3–11.

Hypertension

Lavie CJ, Milani RV, Messerli FH. Prevention and reduction of left ventricular hypertrophy in the elderly (review). Clin Geriatr Med 1996;12:57–68.

Sleight P. Primary prevention of coronary heart disease in hypertension (review). J Hypertens 1996;14(suppl 2):S35–S39.

Srikanthan VS, Dunn FG. Hypertension and coronary artery disease (review). Med Clin North Am 1997;81:1147–1163.

Whelton PK, He J, Appel LJ. Treatment and prevention of hypertension. In: Manson JE, Ridker PM, Gaziano JM, Hennekens CH, eds. Prevention of myocardial infarction. New York: Oxford University Press, 1996:154–171.

Diabetes Mellitus

Haffner SM, Lehto S, Rönnemaa T, et al. Mortality from coronary heart disease in subjects with type 2 diabetes and in nondiabetic subjects with and without prior myocardial infarction. N Engl J Med 1998;339:229–234.

Savage PJ. Treatment of diabetes mellitus to reduce its chronic cardiovascular complications. Curr Opin Cardiol 1998;13:131–138.

Obesity

Carey DGP. Abdominal obesity (review). Curr Opin Lipidol 1998;9:35–40.

Daly PA, Solomon CG, Manson JE. Risk modification in the obese patient. In: Manson JE, Ridker PM, Gaziano JM, Hennekens CH, eds. Prevention of myocardial infarction. New York: Oxford University Press, 1996:203–240.

Eckel RH for the Nutrition Committee. Obesity in heart disease: a statement for healthcare professionals from the Nutrition Committee, American Heart Association. AHA medical/scientific statement. Circulation 1997;96: 3248–3250.

Grundy SM. Multifactorial causation of obesity: implications for prevention (review). Am J Clin Nutr 1998;67(suppl):563S–572S.

Regulation of body weight. Science 1998;280(5368):1363–1390. May 29, 1998, special issue.

Physical Inactivity

Berg A, Halle M, Franz I, Keul J. Physical activity and lipoprotein metabolism: epidemiological evidence and clinical trials (review). Eur J Med Res 1997;2:259–264.

Consensus Development Panel on Physical Activity and Cardiovascular Health. Physical activity and cardiovascular health. JAMA 1996;276:241–246.

Ferro-Luzzi A, Martino L. Obesity and physical activity. Ciba Found Symp 1996;201:207–227.

Fletcher GF, Balady G, Blair SN, et al. Statement on exercise. Benefits and recommendations for physical activity programs for all Americans. A statement for health professionals by the Committee on Exercise and Cardiac Rehabilitation of the Council on Clinical Cardiology, American Heart Association. Circulation 1996;94:857–862.

Paffenbarger RS Jr, Lee I-M. Exercise and fitness. In: Manson JE, Ridker PM, Gaziano JM, Hennekens CH. Prevention of myocardial infarction. New York: Oxford University Press, 1996:172–193.

U.S. Surgeon General. Physical activity and health. Washington, DC: U.S. Department of Health and Human Services, 1996.

Chapter 12

Major Lipid-Lowering Trials Assessing Clinical Events

A number of large clinical trials have examined the hypothesis that reducing TC or LDL-C concentration would reduce rates of morbidity and mortality from CHD in patients both with and without established atherosclerotic disease. The introduction of the potent and safe HMG-CoA reductase inhibitor class of agents has enabled reduction of all-cause mortality rate in addition to the already well-demonstrated reductions in CHD risk. The statins yield LDL-C lowering of a dimension not previously achievable with medication and have been catapulted by the clinical trial results (Tables 12.1–12.3) to the forefront of primary and secondary prevention. Some key trials are briefly reviewed here. None of the trials had raising HDL-C or lowering plasma TG as a hypothesis, although results have shed some light on these questions.

PRIMARY PREVENTION DRUG TRIALS

Early clinical trial attempts to demonstrate reductions in first CHD events by cholesterol lowering were successful despite the modest efficacy of available drugs, although they were troubled by uncertainties about non-CVD morbidity and mortality. These concerns led to debate about the safety of cholesterol lowering (Jacobs et al. 1992; Lewis et al. 1993; Muldoon et al. 1990), although the NCEP (1994) and many other experts (International Task Force 1992; Stamler et al. 1993c) consistently held that CHD benefit from lipid-lowering therapy, including drug therapy, overshadowed any non-CVD risk. Nevertheless, most clinicians did not embrace lipid-regulating drug therapy for primary prevention except in patients with severe genetic dyslipidemia. Now, however, with the availability of the statins, the question of whether cholesterol lowering is beneficial has been very clearly resolved.

Table 12.1. EFFECT OF HMG-CoA REDUCTASE INHIBITOR THERAPY ON CHD: CLINICAL EVENT TRIALS

Trial, agent	Baseline LDL-C (mg/dL)	Decrease in LDL-C (%)	LDL-C achieved (mg/dL)	Events at 5 years	Statin event rate	Placebo event rate	RRR	ARR[a]
Primary prevention								
WOSCOPS,[b] pravastatin	192	26[c]	159	Nonfatal MI or CHD death	174/3,302 5.3%	248/3,293 7.5%	31%	2.2%
AFCAPS/ TexCAPS, lovastatin	150	25[d]	115[d]	Nonfatal or fatal MI, unstable angina, or sudden cardiac death as first event	116/3,304 3.5%	183/3,301 5.5%	37%	2.0%
Secondary prevention								
4S,[e] simvastatin	188	35	122	All-cause death (primary endpoint)	182/2,221 8.2%	256/2,223 11.5%	30%	3.3%
				Nonfatal MI, coronary death, or resuscitated cardiac arrest	431/2,221 19.4%	622/2,223 27.9%	34%	8.5%
CARE,[e] pravastatin	139	32[f]	98	Nonfatal MI or CHD death	212/2,081 10.2%	274/2,078 13.2%	24%	3.0%
LIPID[b] *preliminary,* pravastatin	150	25[g]	112	Nonfatal MI or CHD death	554/4,512 12.3%	706/4,502 15.7%	23%	3.4%

ARR, absolute risk reduction; RRR, relative risk reduction.
[a]ARR was calculated as the placebo event rate minus the statin event rate.
[b]By number of events.
[c]In patients actually treated; LDL-C reduction was 17% in all patients randomized to pravastatin.
[d]At 1 year.
[e]By number of patients.
[f]Reduction from baseline value; 28% reduction compared with placebo.
[g]Percentage average difference between pravastatin and placebo.
Source: Modified from Jacobson et al. in press; used with permission.

Table 12.2. KEY POINTS OF HMG-CoA REDUCTASE INHIBITOR CLINICAL EVENT TRIALS

Trial	Year published	Sex, age (years)	Statin, daily dose (mg)	Enrollment lipids (mg/dL)	Key clinical effect(s)	Benefit Women	Benefit Elderly
Primary prevention							
WOSCOPS*	1995	M, 45–64	Pravastatin, 40	LDL-C ≥155	Coronary events ↓31% No excess non-CVD death Total mortality ↓22%	NA	NA
AFCAPS/ TexCAPS*	1998	M, 45–73 F, 55–73	Lovastatin, 20–40	TC 180–264 LDL-C 130–190 HDL-C ≤45 for men, ≤47 for women	Coronary events ↓37%, including unstable angina No excess non-CVD death	✓	✓
Secondary prevention							
4S	1994	M/F, 35–70	Simvastatin, 20–40	TC 212–309	Total mortality ↓30% Coronary events ↓34%	✓	✓
CARE	1996	M/F, 21–75	Pravastatin, 40	TC <240 LDL-C 115–174	Coronary events ↓24% No excess non-CVD death	✓	✓
LIPID	1996	M/F, 31–75	Pravastatin, 40	TC 155–270	*Preliminary data:* *Coronary death ↓~24%* *Coronary events ↓ ~23%* *Total mortality ↓ ~23%*	✓	✓

*In WOSCOPS, 77% of patients would have been eligible for a drug by 1993 NCEP adult guidelines. In AFCAPS/TexCAPS, 17% would have been drug eligible.

Table 12.3. ESTIMATED NUMBERS OF CLINICAL EVENTS PREVENTED WITH HMG-CoA REDUCTASE INHIBITOR TREATMENT OF 1,000 UNSELECTED PATIENTS

Trial	Patient profile*	Years Rx	Coronary revasc.	MI	Unstable angina	CHD/CVD death
Primary prevention						
WOSCOPS	M, middle aged, ↑ LDL-C	5	8	20 NF	—	7 CVD
AFCAPS/ TexCAPS	M/F, average cholesterol	5	17	12	7	—
Secondary prevention						
4S	M/F, ↑ LDL-C	6	60	70 NF		40 CHD
CARE	M/F, TC <240 mg/dL	5	62	26 NF		11 CHD

Note: Not all reports estimated effects for all events shown; absence of data does not indicate absence of effect. WOSCOPS also estimated prevention of two all-cause deaths, and CARE estimated prevention of 13 strokes or TIAs.
NF, nonfatal.
*Meeting study enrollment criteria (see text).

Nonstatin Trials

Meta-analysis of early primary prevention trials found a 10% reduction in cholesterol to yield 25%, 12%, and 22% reductions in rates of nonfatal, fatal, and all MIs (Rossouw et al. 1990) and a nonsignificant 8% reduction in all-cause mortality rate (Gould et al. 1995).

World Health Organization Clofibrate Trial

The double-blind World Health Organization (WHO) clofibrate trial, begun in 1965 and conducted in Edinburgh, Budapest, and Prague, enrolled 15,745 men aged 30–59 years who did not have manifest CHD. Half of those in the top one-third of the TC distribution among 30,000 participants screened received 1.6 g clofibrate daily (median baseline TC 247 mg/dL); the other half received an olive oil capsule as a placebo. Average time on trial was 5.3 years, although treatment at all centers did not end until 1976. Results were published in 1978 (WHO Principal Investigators 1978). In the clofibrate group, TC was lowered 9% from the baseline value and the coronary event rate was significantly reduced 20%, largely reflecting a 25% decrease in nonfatal MI. However, there was a 47% excess of mortality during treatment in the clofibrate group, a difference not significant when corrected for age at death (WHO Principal Investigators 1980, 1984). Excess mortality was reduced to 5% in 8 years of follow-up after the end of treatment (WHO Principal Investigators 1984). The excess was not accounted for by any particular disease and was not linked causally to clofibrate. The WHO mortality findings remain a subject of debate.

Lipid Research Clinics Coronary Primary Prevention Trial

The Lipid Research Clinics Coronary Primary Prevention Trial (LRC-CPPT) was conducted from 1973 to 1983 at 12 centers in the United States. Results were published in 1984 (Lipid Research Clinics Program 1984a, 1984b) with an average time on trial of 7.4 years. They are considered the first major proof of the lipid-lowering hypothesis and confirmed the 2:1 ratio between CHD risk reduction and cholesterol lowering predicted by observational epidemiologic studies. The double-blind LRC-CPPT randomly assigned 3,806 asymptomatic hypercholesterolemic men aged 35–59 years to diet and cholestyramine or diet and placebo. The men had type II hyperlipidemia, with TC of at least 265 mg/dL; the mean baseline LDL-C was 204 mg/dL. Sequestrant therapy reduced mean TC and LDL-C 8% and 13% more than placebo, and the rate of CHD death or nonfatal MI was a significant 19% lower in the drug group. Cholestyramine's cholesterol-lowering efficacy was limited by the drug's poor tolerability: 68% of patients in the drug group reported gastrointestinal symptoms, and the average daily dose taken was only about 14 g, even though 24 g was prescribed. An unexpected finding was a 1.6-mg/dL increase in HDL-C, which independently accounted for a 2% reduction in CHD risk. Total mortality rate, which the trial was not powered to assess, was reduced by only 7%. There was a nonsignificant increase in non-CVD deaths. The only noteworthy difference was 11 deaths from accidents and violence in the drug group, compared with 4 deaths in the placebo group, a difference that has never been convincingly related to use of the nonabsorbable resin.

Helsinki Heart Study

Screening for the Helsinki Heart Study was performed in 1981–1982, and the results of the double-blind, randomized, 5-year trial were published in 1987 (Frick et al.). The trial enrolled 4,081 asymptomatic men aged 40–55 years who had non-HDL-C of at least 200 mg/dL, assigning them to either gemfibrozil, 600 mg twice daily plus diet, or placebo plus diet. Mean baseline LDL-C was 188 mg/dL. Lipid changes in the gemfibrozil group versus placebo were TC –10%, LDL-C –11%, serum TG –35%, and HDL-C +11%, and the drug therapy significantly reduced CHD incidence (cardiac death plus MI) by 34%. There was no difference in the all-cause mortality rate (which the trial was not designed to assess), and nonsignificantly more deaths occurred in the drug group from accidents and violence (10 vs. 4) and intracranial hemorrhage (5 vs. 1). The deaths could not be attributed to therapy. Taking the LRC-CPPT and Helsinki Heart Study active treatment groups together, the two homicides were victims, five of the eight suicides were trial dropouts, and among the 10 subjects who died in an accident, two were trial dropouts, three had high blood alcohol at autopsy, and another three had a history of psychiatric treatment or symptoms (Wysowski and Gross 1990).

Post hoc analyses of the Helsinki data have proved extremely interesting. Greatest CHD benefit has been narrowed to patients with type IIb hyperlipidemia (elevated LDL-C and TG) (Manninen et al. 1988), more specifically to patients with an LDL-C:HDL-C ratio greater than 5 and TG greater than 200 mg/dL (71% risk reduction) (Manninen et al. 1992), and most specifically to overweight patients, who often had multiple risk factors (78% risk reduction in those with a BMI >26 kg/m^2, TG ≥200 mg/dL, and HDL-C <42 mg/dL) (Tenkanen et al. 1995).

Statin Trials

West of Scotland Coronary Prevention Study

The results of the West of Scotland Coronary Prevention Study (WOSCOPS) (Shepherd et al. 1995) set the stage for a fundamental change in the way clinicians view lipid-lowering pharmacotherapy in primary prevention. In hypercholesterolemic men who were fundamentally healthy—none had a history of MI and only small percentages had a history of angina pectoris according to the Rose questionnaire (5%) or intermittent claudication (3%)—statin therapy achieved substantial reductions in LDL-C, CHD events, and, most important, all-cause mortality rate.

WOSCOPS, which was double-blind, randomized, and placebo controlled, tested pravastatin, 40 mg/day with background diet, in 6,595 hypercholesterolemic men aged 45–64 years. Enrollment required LDL-C of at least 155 mg/dL during two screening visits, with at least one value of at least 174 mg/dL and one value no greater than 232 mg/dL, and fasting TG no higher than 530 mg/dL. Mean baseline LDL-C was 192 mg/dL. The men's cholesterol values were in the highest quartile of the range found in the British population. The LDL-C reduction of 26% from baseline value doubled the efficacy seen in earlier primary prevention drug studies. Treatment also lowered TG by 12% and increased HDL by 5%. Pravastatin treatment yielded a significant 31% reduction in definite coronary events (CHD death or nonfatal MI) at 4.9 years compared with placebo (P <.001). The need for CABG or PTCA was reduced 37% (P = .009). There was no excess of non-CVD deaths in the drug group, and total mortality rate was reduced 22%, a reduction just missing statistical significance (P = .51). Clinical benefit was evident in those subjects with and without prior vascular risk, younger and older than 55 years, and with and without multiple risk factors. A divergence between the pravastatin and placebo groups in CHD events began to emerge as early as 6 months after the start of the trial, although the difference was not significant at that point. Pravastatin therapy was well tolerated.

Post hoc analysis of WOSCOPS data found that there was no reduction in risk for CHD without a reduction in LDL-C, but it did not demonstrate additional benefit beyond a reduction of about 24% (West of Scotland Coronary Prevention Study Group 1998). Whether target-based or percentage-based reduction in LDL-C concentration is more beneficial is currently a topic of speculation, but without prospective, hypothesis-driven data on the question there appears to be no reason to change current target-based guidelines (Gotto and Grundy, in press). WOSCOPS was initiated before development of current NCEP guidelines, but 77% of its patients fell within NCEP categories for consideration of drug therapy, given that all had received dietary therapy (West of Scotland Coronary Prevention Study Group 1997). The WOSCOPS results validated the NCEP recommendation to use drug therapy in high-risk patients without known atherosclerotic disease. Extrapolating the WOSCOPS data from Scotland to the United States has indicated that pravastatin therapy is cost-effective for Americans in primary prevention (findings presented by Joel W. Hay, PhD, at the 70th Scientific Sessions of the American Heart Association, Orlando, 9–12 November 1997). Cost per life-year saved compared favorably with antihypertension medications, smoking cessation programs, exercise programs, CABG, PTCA, and other interventions widely used in CHD prevention (Hay et al. 1997).

Air Force/Texas Coronary Atherosclerosis Prevention Study

The recently published (Downs et al. 1998) Air Force/Texas Coronary Atherosclerosis Prevention Study (AFCAPS/TexCAPS) was the first major primary prevention trial of lipid lowering to include men at least 65 years of age and women, and the first to demonstrate risk reduction in generally healthy men and women with only average LDL-C and below-average HDL-C concentrations.

AFCAPS/TexCAPS, which randomly assigned patients to 20–40 mg/day lovastatin or placebo, both with background diet, was a very pure test of primary prevention. The 6,605 subjects, 997 of them women and 1,416 of them aged 65–73 years, had no history, signs, or symptoms of definite MI, angina, cerebrovascular accident, TIA, or claudication. Mean baseline total and LDL-C concentrations were only 221 and 150 mg/dL, values equal to the 51st and 60th percentiles of the third National Health and Nutrition Examination Survey (NHANES III: 1988–1994) reference population (National Health Center for Health Statistics 1996). Respective enrollment criteria were 180–264 and 130–190 mg/dL, and TG was required to be no more than 400 mg/dL. In addition, patients had decreased HDL-C at baseline: a mean of 36 mg/dL in men and 40 mg/dL in women, equal to the 16th and 25th NHANES III percentiles. The HDL-C enrollment criterion was no more than 45 mg/dL for men and no more than 47 mg/dL for women. Among other enrollment criteria were age 45–73 years in men and age 55–73 years and postmenopausal status in women (among whom about 30% were taking hormone replacement therapy). In contrast to the WOSCOPS, only 17% of the AFCAPS/TexCAPS patients would have been eligible for drug therapy according to current NCEP guidelines.

Lipid changes with lovastatin compared with placebo were LDL-C –25% (to 115 mg/dL), HDL-C +6%, and TG –15%. At 5.2 years' follow-up, active treatment significantly reduced rates of first acute major coronary event (unstable angina, MI, and sudden cardiac death) by 37% ($P < .001$), fatal or nonfatal MI by 40% ($P = .002$), unstable angina by 32% ($P = .02$), and coronary revascularization by 33% ($P = .001$). In each category, a difference between the randomized groups occurred within the first year and continued throughout the trial. There was no difference in non-CVD or total mortality rate between drug and placebo groups. Although the number of events was small, CHD incidence was reduced 46% among women in the drug treatment group compared with women in the placebo group. Treatment benefit on first major CHD event applied equally to patients above and below the median age by sex (57 years in men and 62 years in women). Benefit was also seen in other predefined subgroups such as hypertensive individuals and smokers. Equal clinical benefit occurred in all baseline LDL-C tertiles, with no evidence of a threshold effect. Benefit was greatest in the lowest baseline HDL-C tertile. Lovastatin therapy was well tolerated.

SECONDARY PREVENTION DRUG TRIALS

Nonstatin Trials

Meta-analysis of early secondary prevention trials found a 10% reduction in cholesterol to yield 19%, 12%, and 15% reductions in rates of nonfatal, fatal, and all MIs (Rossouw et al. 1990).

Coronary Drug Project

In the Coronary Drug Project, several interventions were compared with placebo in 8,341 American men who had had at least one MI. Intervention groups received low- or high-dosage estrogen (2.5 or 5 mg/day), dextrothyroxine (6 mg/day), clofibrate (1.8 g/day), or nicotinic acid (3 g/day). The estrogen and dextrothyroxine trials were discontinued because of either increased mortality or side effects. Mean time on trial for the remaining three treatments—clofibrate, nicotinic acid, and placebo—was 6.2 years. No benefit was seen with clofibrate; in addition, the frequency of gallstones was significantly higher in that group. At the end of the active intervention period, the group receiving nicotinic acid showed a 10% reduction in cholesterol from the baseline value and a decrease in nonfatal MI rate (Coronary Drug Project Research Group 1975). Because investigators were focusing on mortality alone, they did not attribute much significance at the time to the reduction in nonfatal MI rate compared with placebo (8.9% vs. 12.2% at 5 years). In mortality follow-up 15 years after the trial began, or 9 years after the interventions ended, the reduction of 11% in all-cause mortality in the nicotinic acid group was highly significant (Canner et al. 1986). The investigators postulated that the reduction in MIs during the intervention period ultimately affected the all-cause mortality rate.

Stockholm Ischemic Heart Disease Secondary Prevention Study

The nonblinded Stockholm Ischemic Heart Disease Secondary Prevention Study randomized 555 men and women with a history of MI to combination therapy with clofibrate (2 g/day) and nicotinic acid (3 g/day) or to a control group. Before randomization, all patients were instructed to reduce their intake of saturated fat, cholesterol, and simple sugars, smokers were counseled to quit smoking, and overweight patients were advised on calorie restriction; also, other medical problems such as hypertension were treated. After 5 years, significant changes in the drug treatment group compared with controls included reductions in TC (13%), TG (19%), CHD mortality rate (36%), and total mortality rate (26%) (Carlson and Rosenhamer 1988). Retrospective subset analysis showed the decrease in CHD mortality to be directly related to the decrease in TG. The reduction in the CHD death rate was 60% in drug recipients whose TG decreased 30% or more, and significant benefit occurred only in patients whose baseline TG was greater than 130 mg/dL (Carlson and Rosenhamer 1988).

Statin Trials

Scandinavian Simvastatin Survival Study

Publication of the Scandinavian Simvastatin Survival Study (4S) in 1994 (Scandinavian Simvastatin Survival Study Group 1994) erased any doubts about the value of cholesterol-lowering therapy in secondary prevention. This multicenter trial examined whether simvastatin therapy would reduce the primary endpoint of total mortality rate. The secondary endpoint was major coronary events, comprising coronary death, nonfatal acute MI, resuscitated cardiac arrest, and definite silent MI. A total of 4,444 men and women aged 35–70 years who had a history of angina pectoris and/or MI were randomized to simvastatin 20 mg/day or placebo, both with background diet. The TC enrollment criterion was 212–309 mg/dL; the mean TC and LDL-C at baseline were 261 and 188 mg/dL. Serum TG was required to be no more than 220 mg/dL. The cholesterol-lowering goal was TC of 115–200 mg/dL, and to that end simvastatin could be titrated up to 40 mg/day (as was done in 37% of patients) or down to 10 mg/day (as was done in two patients).

The trial lasted an average of 5.4 years. Simvastatin therapy reduced LDL-C by 35%, increased HDL-C by 8%, and decreased TG by 10%. The total mortality rate fell by a highly significant 30% ($P = .0003$). Drug therapy also reduced major coronary events by a highly significant 34%, coronary revascularization procedures by 37%, and coronary mortality rate by 42%. Simvastatin therapy caused no serious side effects, nor was non-CVD mortality rate increased. The women receiving simvastatin showed coronary benefit similar to that achieved in the men (35%, $P = .01$). Risk reductions were similar for those older or younger than 60 years, and benefit was not mitigated at all in hypertensive patients, cigarette smokers, or diabetic patients. Benefit was seen across all quartiles of TC, LDL-C, and HDL-C (Scandinavian Simvastatin Survival Study Group 1995), and post hoc analysis suggested that in the main the magnitude of change in LDL-C determined the benefit of simvastatin therapy in individual patients (Pedersen et al. 1998). Benefit began after about 1 year of therapy and increased steadily thereafter.

Post hoc subgroup analysis showed relative risk reductions of 43% for total mortality, 55% for major CHD events, and 37% for any atherosclerotic event in the 202 diabetic subjects of 4S (Pyörälä et al. 1997). The absolute benefit may have been greater in these patients because of their greater absolute risk for an event. Analyses of 4S data showed simvastatin therapy in secondary prevention to be quite cost-effective (Johannesson et al. 1997; Pedersen et al. 1996).

Cholesterol and Recurrent Events Trial

In the Cholesterol and Recurrent Events (CARE) trial (Sacks et al. 1996), TC averaged only 209 mg/dL and LDL-C averaged only 139 mg/dL at baseline, values close to mean concentrations for U.S. adults (206 and 128 mg/dL) (Johnson et al. 1993). Many CARE subjects had undergone coronary revascularization. A total of 4,200 men and postmenopausal women (total age range, 21–75 years) receiving dietary instruction were randomized to either placebo or pravastatin, 40 mg/day. Enrollment required TC of less than 240 mg/dL, LDL-C of 115–174 mg/dL, and TG of less than 350 mg/dL. Lipid changes during follow-up with pravastatin compared with placebo were TC −20%, LDL-C −28%, HDL-C +5%, and TG −14%. At 5 years, pravastatin therapy produced a 24% lower rate of acute MI or coronary death ($P = .003$), the primary endpoint, with a clear difference having occurred since follow-up at 2 years. It decreased the need for CABG or PTCA by 27% ($P <.001$) and decreased the stroke rate by 31% (see later). The non-CVD mortality rate was not increased with pravastatin therapy. Women had even better outcomes than men: a 46% reduction compared with a 20% reduction in major coronary events (both $P = .001$). Coronary benefit was not substantially altered by patient age at baseline, the presence of hypertension or diabetes, smoking status, or LV ejection fraction. Post hoc analysis of CARE data showed no further benefit of LDL-C lowering beyond approximately 125 mg/dL (Sacks et al. 1998), a finding not confirmed by trials such as LCAS (see Chapter 10).

Long-term Intervention with Pravastatin in Ischemic Disease: Preliminary Results

With 9,014 patients enrolled, the Long-term Intervention with Pravastatin in Ischemic Disease (LIPID) trial, conducted in Australia and New Zealand, is the largest trial of an HMG-CoA reductase inhibitor. Results as of this writing are awaiting publication but were presented by prinicpal investigator Andrew Tonkin, MD, at the Scientific Sessions of the AHA (70th sessions, Orlando, November 9–12, 1997) and the American College of Cardiology

(47th session, Atlanta, March 29–April 1, 1998). LIPID was designed, in 1989, to be applicable to as many patients as possible and encompassed enrollment TC of 155–270 mg/dL (The LIPID Study Group 1995). In addition, fasting TG could not exceed 445 mg/dL. Men and women aged 31–75 years were stratified according to qualifying diagnosis of either prior MI (accounting for about two-thirds of patients) or unstable angina pectoris. Treatment with background diet was 40 mg/day pravastatin or placebo.

The mean baseline lipid values of 290, 150, 37, and 161 mg/dL for TC, LDL-C, HDL-C, and TG in LIPID are highly concordant with values in AFCAPS/TexCAPS. The LIPID trial embraces most patients with CHD in a way that the 4S and CARE studies did not; 42% of LIPID patients had TC of no more than 212 mg/dL, and so would have been ineligible for the 4S trial, and about one-third of patients had TC too high for enrollment in the CARE study. Patients were quite representative of the type of patients seen in clinical practice: For example, 82% were taking aspirin, 47% were taking a beta-blocker, and about 40% had undergone previous revascularization (The Lipid Study Group 1995).

With follow-up of approximately 6 years, and only one patient lost to follow-up, preliminary data showed that TC was reduced about 20% and there were significant or highly significant reductions, on the order of 20–25%, in clinical event rates, among them coronary mortality (the primary endpoint), total mortality, and acute MI. There were also significant reductions, according to preliminary data, in all stroke, need for CABG, need for PTCA, and unstable angina. Benefit applied equally to women (17% of the LIPID patients) and to patients 65–69 years of age (24% of patients) or older (15% of patients). Treatment was found to be cost-effective. Thus, the LIPID clinical endpoint results, when published, are expected to confirm the significant reduction in all-cause mortality found in the 4S trial, and to extend that benefit to patients with lower cholesterol.

As noted in Chapter 10, pravastatin treatment in LIPID was shown in a substudy of 522 patients to reduce the development of carotid atherosclerosis across a wide range of pretreatment cholesterol values (MacMahon et al. 1998).

STATIN THERAPY AND STROKE

Each year about 600,000 Americans have a stroke and about 158,000 die of stroke. After CHD and cancer, stroke is the third leading cause of death in the United States, and it is the number one cause of serious disability. More than 70% of those who survive have an impaired ability to work, for an average of 7 years after the event (AHA 1997). Annual expenditures in the United States for stroke have been estimated to be $17–28 billion for direct costs and $13–15 billion for indirect costs (AHA 1997; Dobkin 1995).

Evidence relating plasma cholesterol and stroke has been equivocal; hypertension and smoking are strong modifiable risk factors (Stoy 1997; Postiglione and Napoli 1995; Prospective Studies Collaboration 1995; Tell et al. 1988). However, recent clinical trials have supported significant stroke risk reduction with statin therapy (Table 12.4). Fatal or nonfatal stroke was a specified endpoint in the post-MI CARE trial of pravastatin and significantly reduced the incidence of stroke by 31% with no increase in the risk for hemorrhagic stroke (Sacks et al. 1996). The CARE investigators estimated that treating 1,000 patients with a history of MI and TC less than 240 mg/dL (CARE study criteria) for 5 years would prevent 13 strokes or TIAs in unselected patients. Benefit would be even greater in patients 60 years of age or more and in women, with prevention of 25 and 28 strokes and TIAs. A similar reduction in risk for cerebrovascular events was seen on post hoc analysis of the secondary prevention 4S trial of simvastatin, again with no increased risk for hemorrhagic stroke (Scandinavian Simvastatin Survival Study Group 1994). A nonsignificant benefit was seen in the subset of 4S patients who were diabetic (Pyörälä et al. 1997). In primary prevention, post hoc analysis of WOSCOPS data showed a nonsignificant 11% risk reduction in stroke (Shepherd et al. 1995). In AFCAPS/TexCAPS, the rate of all fatal and nonfatal cardiovascular events was significantly reduced by 25% with lovastatin therapy (Downs et al. 1998). That category included thrombotic cerebrovascular accidents, TIAs, and PVD as well as coronary events. A significant reduction of stroke has also been described in preliminary findings from the LIPID trial of pravastatin (see earlier).

The clinical benefit in stroke reduction has been corroborated by several retrospective meta-analyses of statin trials (Blauw et al. 1997; Crouse et al. 1997; Hebert et al. 1997; Bucher et al. 1998); the 24–31% risk reduction suggests an effect similar to that of aspirin in secondary prevention (Delanty and Vaughan 1997). The pooled odds reduction for nonfatal stroke ranges from 12% to 23% for use of antiplatelet agents in patients with manifested systemic atherosclerosis (Antiplatelet Trialists' Collaboration 1994). Blauw et al. (1997) predicted the prevention of 40 strokes with statin treatment for a considerable length of time in 10,000 patients with CHD. The stroke benefit is supported by imaging studies, such as ACAPS, PLAC II, and KAPS, that have shown improvement in carotid atherosclerosis (see Chapter 10). The intracranial arteries appear relatively resistant to the development of severe atherosclerosis (Postiglione and Napoli 1995). Two of the meta-analyses also examined total mortality rate, finding significant 22% and 20% risk reductions (Hebert et al. 1997; Bucher et al. 1998).

Previous intervention trials using other classes of lipid-lowering drugs showed only equivocal effects on stroke risk (Delanty and Vaughan 1997). Whereas Bucher et al. (1998) on meta-analysis of trials found a risk ratio of 0.76 for fatal and nonfatal stroke for statins (see Table 12.4), the risk ratios with fibrates (5 trials), resins (3 trials), and dietary interventions (10 trials) were all close to 1.0, and null hypothesis estimation showed the effect unlikely to occur by chance. Bucher et al. also found a significant difference ($P = .003$) in CHD mortality reduction between statins and other interventions (31% vs. 10% risk reduction). The explanation for the

Table 12.4. EFFECT OF HMG-CoA REDUCTASE INHIBITOR THERAPY ON RISK FOR STROKE (FATAL AND NONFATAL)

Trial or analysis	Type of analysis	Prevention 1°	Prevention 2°	Total number of subjects	Sex	Number of strokes (incidence, %) Control	Number of strokes (incidence, %) Drug	Relative risk ↓ (%)	Statistical significance
Individual trials[a]									
CARE	Specified endpoint		✓	4,159	M/F	78 (3.8)	54 (2.6)	31	P = .03
4S[b]	Post hoc		✓	4,444	M/F	98 (4.4)	70 (3.2)	30	P = .024
Diabetes subset	Post hoc		✓	202	M/F	—	—	62	P = .071
WOSCOPS	Post hoc	✓		6,595	M	51 (1.5)	46 (1.4)	11	P = .57
LIPID preliminary data	Post hoc		✓	9,014	M/F			≈20	P = .02
Meta-analyses									
Pravastatin regression pooled (Byington et al. 1995)	Post hoc[c]		✓	1,891	M/F	13 (3.9)	5 (5.2)	62	P = .54
Blauw et al. 1997	Retrosp	✓	✓	20,438	M/F	261 (2.6)	181 (1.8)	31	P <.001
Crouse et al. 1997	Retrosp	✓	✓	19,518	M/F	192 (7.3)	134 (5.1)	27[d]	P = .001
Hebert et al. 1997	Retrosp	✓	✓	28,711[e]	M/F	261 (2.2)	193 (1.1)	29	95% CI 14–41%
Bucher et al. 1998	Retrosp	✓	✓	18,125	M/F	—	—	24	95% CI 8–38%

[a]See text for references.

[b]Cerebrovascular disease events.

[c]The Pravastatin Atherosclerosis Intervention Program prospectively pooled results of regression trials, but effect on stroke was not a prior hypothesis.

[d]Risk reduction was 32% in secondary prevention (P = .001) and 15% in primary prevention (P = .48).

[e]The major reason for the larger number is the inclusion of the 8,245 subjects of the Expanded Clinical Evaluation of Lovastatin (EXCEL) study (Bradford et al. 1991).

apparent efficacy of the statins against cerebrovascular disease may lie in an effect (see Chapter 10) of rendering atherosclerotic lesions more stable and less likely to undergo thrombotic disruption (Gotto 1997a; Delanty and Vaughan 1997). Another interpretation, supported by a cohort study associating total cholesterol and stroke (Prospective Studies Collaboration 1995), is that cholesterol level is a causal determinant of stroke (Blauw et al. 1997; Gotto 1997a). In this case, the result may be related to the greater cholesterol-lowering potency of the statins with relative freedom from untoward side effects.

It has been suggested that hemorrhagic stroke may be related to low cholesterol (Law et al. 1994), although it is considered unlikely that the cholesterol concentrations achieved in clinical trials could cause strokes (Gould et al. 1995). Fragmentary evidence of a possible causal relation is viewed as inconclusive (Jacobs et al. 1992). The mechanisms underlying hemorrhagic stroke remain elusive. Indirect evidence from statin trials suggests that reduction in all-cause mortality rate outweighs other risk in populations with a baseline CVD risk of 1–3% (Bucher et al. 1998). Whether cholesterol reduction's outweighing any increased risk for intracranial hemorrhage would apply to individuals or populations in whom the risk for CHD is less than the risk for hemorrhagic stroke (e.g., the Japanese) requires further study (Puddey 1996).

Evidence regarding whether statins reduce the risk for stroke in patients with cerebrovascular disease should become available from the Medical Research Council/British Heart Foundation Heart Protection Study testing simvastatin in patients with a history of TIAs or minor ischemic stroke.

Suggested Reading

Delanty N, Vaughan CJ. Vascular effects of statins in stroke (review). Stroke 1997;28:2315–2320.

Downs JR, Clearfield M, Weis S, et al., for AFCAPS/TexCAPS Research Group. Primary prevention of acute coronary events with lovastatin in men and women with average cholesterol levels. Results of AFCAPS/TexCAPS. JAMA 1998;279:1615–1622.

Gotto AM Jr. Risk factor modification: rationale for management of dyslipidemia (review). Am J Med 1998;104(suppl 2A):6S–8S.

Grundy SM. Statin trials and goals of cholesterol-lowering therapy (editorial). Circulation 1998;97:1436–1439.

Lipid Research Clinics Program. The Lipid Research Clinics Coronary Primary Prevention Trial results. I. Reduction in incidence of coronary heart disease. JAMA 1984;251:351–364.

Lipid Research Clinics Program. The Lipid Research Clinics Coronary Primary Prevention Trial results. II. The relationship of reduction in incidence of coronary heart disease to cholesterol lowering. JAMA 1984;251:365–374.

The LIPID Study Group. Design features and baseline characteristics of the LIPID (Long-term Intervention with Pravastatin in Ischemic Disease) study: a randomized trial in patients with previous acute myocardial infarction and/or unstable angina pectoris. Am J Cardiol 1995;76:474–479.

Manninen V, Tenkanen L, Koskinen P, et al. Joint effects of serum triglyceride and LDL cholesterol and HDL cholesterol concentration on coronary heart disease risk in the Helsinki Heart Study: implications for treatment. Circulation 1992;85:37–45.

Oliver MF. Statins prevent coronary heart disease (commentary). Lancet 1995;346:1378–1379.

Oliver M, Poole-Wilson P, Shepherd J, Tikkanen MJ. Lower patients' cholesterol now: trial evidence shows clear benefits from secondary prevention. BMJ 1995;310:1280–1281.

Sacks FM, Pfeffer MA, Moye LA, et al. The effect of pravastatin on coronary events after myocardial infarction in patients with average cholesterol levels. N Engl J Med 1996;335:1001–1009.

Scandinavian Simvastatin Survival Study Group. Randomised trial of cholesterol lowering in 4444 patients with coronary heart disease: the Scandinavian Simvastatin Survival Study (4S). Lancet 1994;344:1383–1389.

Shepherd J, Cobbe SM, Ford I, et al., for the West of Scotland Coronary Prevention Study Group. Prevention of coronary heart disease with pravastatin in men with hypercholesterolemia. N Engl J Med 1995;333:1301–1307.

Chapter 13

National Cholesterol Education Program Algorithm for Risk Control in Adults

The guidelines of the NCEP second Adult Treatment Panel (ATP II) include a simplified, algorithmic approach to the evaluation and management of dyslipidemia, which is described here. The guidelines have been published both in full (NCEP 1994) and in abbreviated form (Expert Panel 1993). It is critical that physicians familiarize themselves with the ATP II guidelines to enable appropriate risk reduction intervention; a 1992 survey (Tunis et al. 1994) found only 59% of internists to be familiar with ATP I guidelines, which were issued in 1987. It would be incongruous for nonadherent physicians to reproach noncompliant patients.

The lipid focus of the NCEP guidelines is LDL-C because LDL is considered the primary atherogenic lipoprotein, although clinical decision making is informed by HDL-C and TG concentrations. The guidelines stress the idea of overall, or global, risk—the assessment of both lipid and nonlipid risk factors in both number and severity—in case management. In keeping with this focus, the clinical algorithm is stratified according to whether CHD or other atherosclerotic disease is absent (primary prevention) or present (secondary prevention, Table 13.1). Evidence is strong that the presence of multiple risk factors leads to a synergistic elevation of CHD risk (see Chapter 11).

SCREENING

Patients without Known Atherosclerotic Disease

All healthy adults aged 20 or older should have their TC measured at least once every 5 years (minimum approach). HDL-C should be measured at the same time if accurate results are available. Both of these measurements may be made in the patient in a nonfasting state.

Table 13.1. NCEP ADULT GUIDELINES: CLINICAL PRESENCE OF ATHEROSCLEROTIC DISEASE

Vascular bed	Definitions
CHD	• Definite clinical and laboratory evidence of MI • Clinically significant myocardial ischemia • History of coronary artery surgery or angioplasty • Angiogram demonstrating significant coronary atherosclerosis in the presence of clinical symptoms of CHD*
PVD	• Abdominal aortic aneurysm or • Clinical signs and symptoms of ischemia of the extremities Either accompanied by significant atherosclerosis on angiography or abnormalities of segment-to-arm pressure ratios or flow velocities
Carotid athero-sclerosis	• Cerebral symptoms (TIAs or stroke) Accompanied by ultrasound or angiographic demonstration of significant atherosclerosis

Note: All patients with established CHD or clinical atherosclerotic disease of the aorta, arteries of the limbs, or carotid arteries are at high risk for CHD events.
*Not recommended that angiography be performed specifically to classify patients for lipid-lowering therapy.
Source: Data from NCEP 1994.

The physician may prefer as the first assessment in primary prevention the more informative fasting lipoprotein profile, which comprises plasma or serum TC, HDL-C, TG, and LDL-C. The LDL-C value is usually esti-mated by using the Friedewald equation (see Chapter 14). Full lipoprotein analysis is advisable in high-risk asymptomatic patients (Table 13.2). It should be borne in mind that high-risk asymptomatic patients are likely to have significant atherosclerosis; the clinical distinction between primary and secondary prevention is, of course, rather arbitrary.

Patients with Atherosclerotic Disease

All patients with established CHD or clinical atherosclerotic disease of the aorta, arteries of the limbs, or carotid arteries are at high risk for CHD events. The first lipid evaluation in these patients should be full fasting lipoprotein analysis (see Table 13.2).

INITIAL ACTION LIMITS

Verification that dyslipidemia is present requires a fasting lipoprotein analy-sis, and initiation of lipid-lowering therapy requires establishing an eleva-tion of LDL-C by at least two consecutive fasting determinations. Lipid cutpoints or action limits are no more than a guide for risk evaluation and therapy. For example, one simplification used by the NCEP is the definition

NCEP ALGORITHM FOR RISK CONTROL IN ADULTS **209**

Table 13.2. NCEP LIPID SCREENING IN ADULTS

Age[a]	≥20 years
Appropriate screening	Universal, opportunistic
Measure nonfasting TC and HDL-C	• Healthy individuals Proceed to fasting lipoprotein analysis if patient without atherosclerotic disease has high TC, low HDL-C, or borderline-high TC + two or more other risk factors (see Tables 13.3 and 13.4).
Perform full fasting lipoprotein analysis: TC, HDL-C, TG, and LDL-C	• Atherosclerotic disease present or • Diabetes mellitus present[b] • Advisable if patient otherwise at high risk (e.g., hypertension, family history of early CVD, multiple risk factors) • Physician may choose as the initial assessment in healthy individuals

Note: For frequency of follow-up, see Table 13.3.
[a]For NCEP screening recommendations in children and adolescents, see Chapter 19.
[b]The ADA recommends that a full fasting lipoprotein profile be obtained every year in adult patients with diabetes (see Chapter 21).
Source: Data from NCEP 1994.

of a low HDL-C concentration at 35 mg/dL for both sexes. In general, HDL-C concentrations are higher in women than in men; hence the European Atherosclerosis Society sets higher HDL-C cutpoints for women: less than 46 mg/dL for increased risk, less than 39 mg/dL for high risk, and greater than 66 mg/dL for a protective effect, compared with values of less than 39 mg/dL, less than 31 mg/dL, and greater than 58 mg/dL for men (International Task Force 1992). Lipid cutpoints should not be considered set in stone, but they do provide a starting point. Assessment and treatment should be individualized according to overall risk.

Patients without Known Atherosclerotic Disease

As summarized in Table 13.3, initial management of patients without atherosclerotic disease may be based on TC and HDL-C concentrations. Fasting lipoprotein analysis is required if the patient has

• High TC (≥240 mg/dL),
• Low HDL-C (<35 mg/dL), or
• Borderline-high TC (200–239 mg/dL) in the presence of two or more other risk factors.

Additional major risk factors for consideration in the NCEP algorithm are listed in Table 13.4.

   If LDL-C in primary prevention proves to be at an acceptable concentration (<130 mg/dL), lipid re-evaluation may be deferred for up to 5

Table 13.3. NCEP CLINICAL ACTION ACCORDING TO INITIAL CHOLESTEROL VALUES IN ADULTS

Initial assessment	Results and action[a]
Atherosclerotic disease present (secondary prevention)	
Fasting lipoprotein analysis[b]	**LDL-C ≤100:** individualized instruction on Step II Diet and other lifestyle modifications; repeat lipoprotein analysis annually
	LDL-C >100: clinical evaluation; initiate cholesterol-lowering therapy
Atherosclerotic disease absent (primary prevention)	
TC and HDL-C (non-fasting acceptable)	**TC <200**
	HDL-C ≥35: repeat TC and HDL-C determinations within 5 years or with physical examination; provide general educational materials
	HDL-C <35: lipoprotein analysis (see below)
	TC 200–239
	HDL-C ≥35 + <2 other RF: repeat TC and HDL-C determinations in 1–2 years; instruct in diet, physical activity, RF reduction
	HDL-C <35 or ≥2 other RF: lipoprotein analysis (see below)
	TC ≥240: lipoprotein analysis (see below)
After fasting lipoprotein analysis[c]	**LDL-C <130:** Repeat TC and HDL-C determinations within 5 years; provide general educational materials
	LDL-C 130–159
	<2 other RF: provide information on Step I Diet and other lifestyle modifications; re-evaluate annually, including lipoprotein analysis, RF reduction
	≥2 other RF: clinical evaluation; initiate dietary and other lifestyle modifications
	LDL-C ≥160: clinical evaluation; initiate dietary and other lifestyle modifications

RF, risk factor(s).
[a]All lipid values in mg/dL. Other RF for consideration are listed in Table 13.4.
[b]Average of two determinations 1–8 weeks apart (three if variation >30 mg/dL); patient should not be in recovery phase from acute coronary or other medical event.
[c]May also be performed at outset. Assignment to last two categories (high risk) should be based on average of at least two determinations, as in previous footnote.
Source: Data from NCEP 1994.

years. If LDL-C is borderline high (130–159 mg/dL) but risk is otherwise low, risk factor reduction and annual re-evaluation are called for. If LDL-C is high (≥160 mg/dL) or if it is borderline high and two or more other risk factors are present, a full clinical evaluation should be performed (see later) and dietary and other lifestyle modifications initiated (see Chapters 15 and 16).

Table 13.4. OTHER MAJOR RISK FACTORS FOR CHD

Risk factor	Value/Comment
Positive[a]	
Age	Men ≥45 years
	Women ≥55 years, or premature menopause without ERT
Family history of premature CHD	Definite MI or sudden CHD death before age 55 in male first-degree relative, or before age 65 in female first-degree relative
Current cigarette smoking	No level of cigarette smoking is acceptable
Hypertension	Blood pressure ≥140/90 mm Hg or taking antihypertension medication
Low HDL-C	<35 mg/dL
Diabetes mellitus[b]	Taking diabetic agent(s) or meets criteria for diagnosis (see Table 16.17)
Obesity, in particular abdominal obesity[c]	(See Tables 16.7 and 16.8)
Negative (protective)	
High HDL-C	≥60 mg/dL: in adult algorithm, may subtract 1 risk factor other than atherosclerosis or hypercholesterolemia when high HDL-C is present

Note: These are major risk factors for consideration in the NCEP adult algorithm in addition to elevated LDL-C and the presence of CHD or other atherosclerotic disease. High risk for CHD is more often the result of multiple risk factors than of a single risk factor of severe degree.
[a]Physical inactivity should also be a target for intervention.
[b]Authors' note: key points: (1) meticulous control probably decreases macrovascular disease, definitely decreases microvascular sequelae; (2) risk of diabetes approximates that conferred by CHD; (3) diabetes diagnosis cutpoints have been redefined (see Table 16.17).
[c]Obesity was not listed by the NCEP because its risk was considered to be accounted for by other factors (hypertension, hyperlipidemia, low HDL-C, and diabetes mellitus). We have listed it because the AHA has now deemed obesity a major risk factor for CHD.
Source: Data modified from NCEP 1994.

Patients with Atherosclerotic Disease

In adult patients with CHD or other atherosclerotic disease, the initial lipid evaluation, as noted, is a full fasting lipoprotein analysis. LDL-C of no more than 100 mg/dL is considered optimal in these patients. Patients with optimal LDL-C should receive individualized instruction in the Step II Diet and other lifestyle modifications (see Chapters 15 and 16), and the lipoprotein analysis should be repeated annually (see Table 13.3). When LDL-C exceeds 100 mg/dL in secondary prevention, a full clinical evaluation should be performed and lipid-lowering therapy initiated.

Total Cholesterol:High-Density Lipoprotein Cholesterol Ratio

Although the NCEP guidelines do not include lipid ratios in risk stratification, the TC:HDL-C ratio has been shown to be a strong predictor of CHD. The International Lipid Information Bureau considers the TC:HDL-C ratio to be high in primary prevention if it exceeds 5 (<4.5 is desirable). It considers the TC:HDL-C ratio to be high in secondary prevention if it exceeds 4 (<3.5 is desirable) (Gotto et al. 1995). Also, the combination of elevated LDL-C, elevated TG, and low HDL-C appears to confer very high risk.

FREDRICKSON PHENOTYPING

Once hyperlipidemia is confirmed through repeat fasting lipoprotein assessments, it is useful to assign a phenotype according to the Fredrickson classification, which is shown in Table 13.5. This system is based on lipoprotein patterns associated with elevations of cholesterol and/or TG and disregards HDL-C concentration. The Fredrickson phenotype is not an etiologic classification, and establishing the phenotype does not take the place of determining the underlying cause of the dyslipidemia.

It has been estimated that among U.S. patients with hyperlipidemia, less than 1% have type I, 10% have type IIa, 40% have type IIb, less than 1% have type III, 45% have type IV, and 5% have type V hyperlipidemia. In type III hyperlipidemia, cholesterol and TG are typically each elevated to about the same extent.

CLINICAL EVALUATION

A complete clinical evaluation is a key step in evaluating patients with dyslipidemia, since it enables estimation of the level of overall CHD risk and selection of appropriate therapy. The clinical evaluation includes attempting to determine whether the dyslipidemia is a primary disorder or secondary to another condition (see Chapter 14).

Personal and family medical histories need to include any history of dyslipidemia, hypertension, diabetes mellitus, or CVD (see also Chapter 14). Patients with atherosclerotic disease are at highest risk for CHD. Family testing is essential when familial dyslipidemia is suspected.

The **physical examination** should include weight, height, calculated BMI (see Table 16.7), waist:hip ratio (desirable: men <0.9; middle-aged and elderly women <0.8—Grundy et al. 1997b), and blood pressure (see Tables 16.12–16.15). It is also important to look for

• Thyroid abnormalities
• Manifestations of dyslipidemia (e.g., xanthomas, corneal arcus, hepato-splenomegaly)
• Manifestations of atherosclerosis (e.g., vascular bruits, peripheral pulses)

Laboratory tests should include not only full fasting lipoprotein analysis but also routine evaluations such as liver function and thyroid

Table 13.5. FREDRICKSON CLASSIFICATION OF THE HYPERLIPIDEMIAS

Pheno-type	Lipoprotein(s) elevated	Result	Athero-genicity	Associated with genetic disorders	Selected conditions associated with secondary hyperlipidemia
I	Chylomicrons	Very high TG	?	Familial chylomicronemia (familial LPL deficiency, apo C-II deficiency)	Dysglobulinemia, pancreatitis, poorly controlled diabetes mellitus
IIa	LDL	Elevated cholesterol	+++	FH FCH Polygenic hypercholesterolemia Familial defective apo B	Hypothyroidism, acute intermittent porphyria, nephrosis, idiopathic globulinemia, anorexia nervosa
IIb	LDL and VLDL	Elevated cholesterol and TG	+++	FH FCH	Hypothyroidism, acute intermittent porphyria, nephrosis, idiopathic globulinemia, anorexia nervosa
III	IDL	Elevated cholesterol and TG	+++	Familial dysbetalipoproteinemia	Diabetes mellitus, hypothyroidism, dysglobulinemia
IV	VLDL	Elevated TG and normal to slightly elevated cholesterol	+	Familial endogenous hypertriglyceridemia FCH	Glycogen storage disease, hypothyroidism, disseminated lupus erythematosus, diabetes mellitus, nephrotic syndrome, renal failure, ethanol abuse
V	VLDL and chylomicrons	Very high TG and normal to slightly elevated cholesterol	+	Familial mixed hypertriglyceridemia	Poorly controlled diabetes mellitus, glycogen storage disease, hypothyroidism, nephrotic syndrome, dysglobulinemia, pregnancy

tests, CK, fasting blood glucose (see Table 16.17), alkaline phosphatase, urinalysis, and ECG.

Lifestyle components for assessment include smoking habits, type and amount of physical exercise performed, level of life stress, and intake of calories, saturated fat and other types of fat, cholesterol, simple carbohydrates, alcohol, and sodium.

In establishing the risk factor profile, it should be borne in mind that a high risk for CHD is more often the result of multiple risk factors than of a single risk factor of severe degree. As noted in Chapter 11, multiple risk factors tend to increase risk for CHD in a multiplicative rather than an additive manner.

The causes of dyslipidemia are usually multifactorial and polygenic. If dyslipidemia does not respond to treatment of underlying conditions or replacement or reduction of drugs that can cause secondary dyslipidemia (see Chapter 14), it should be treated as a primary disorder. The primary lipid disorders (Chapter 14) most commonly identified in adult clinical practice are FCH, polygenic hypercholesterolemia, FH, and type III hyperlipidemia (Gotto et al. 1995). Searching for a genetic origin through specialized laboratory methods may be useful in family counseling.

LIFESTYLE INTERVENTION

Lifestyle intervention in the NCEP guidelines emphasizes not only a diet low in saturated fat and cholesterol but also weight control, increased physical activity, and cessation of smoking. These modifications are detailed in Chapters 15 and 16; their effects on plasma concentrations of LDL-C, TG, and HDL-C are shown in Table 15.1.

The goal of diet and other lifestyle interventions in the NCEP adult guidelines is to bring LDL-C below the initiation cutpoint, that is as follows:

- <160 mg/dL for patients without known atherosclerotic disease and with fewer than two other CHD risk factors
- <130 mg/dL for patients without known atherosclerosis and with other risk factors
- ≤100 mg/dL for all patients with CHD or other atherosclerotic disease

Monitoring of response to lifestyle intervention is discussed in Chapter 15.

DRUG THERAPY

Drug therapy does not replace lifestyle intervention; it supplements it. Lifestyle modifications often enhance the efficacy of lipid-lowering pharmacotherapy. The goals of drug therapy (Table 13.6) are the same as those for lifestyle intervention, although lower concentrations of LDL-C are desirable for some patients if feasible. Combined drugs may prove necessary in some patients, especially those with severe hyperlipidemia or combined hyperlipidemia. Combination drug therapy is usually considered if 3 months' com-

Table 13.6. NCEP ACTION LIMITS FOR CONSIDERATION OF DRUG THERAPY ACCORDING TO LDL-C CONCENTRATION IN ADULTS

Patient group	Initiation (mg/dL)	Goal (mg/dL)	Notes
No CHD, <2 other risk factors	≥190	<160	• When LDL-C is 190–220 mg/dL and there is *no other risk,* consider delaying drug therapy in both men <35 years old and premenopausal women. • Use clinical judgment as to whether to use drugs after maximum lifestyle intervention when LDL-C is between 160 and 190 mg/dL.
No CHD, 2 or more other risk factors	≥160	<130	• Use clinical judgment as to whether to use drugs after maximum lifestyle intervention when LDL-C is between 130 and 160 mg/dL.
With CHD or other athero-sclerotic disease	≥130	≤100	• Withholding drug therapy in an effort to reach target LDL-C with lifestyle changes is not necessary for LDL-C ≥130 mg/dL. • A 6-week trial of lifestyle therapy is recommended when LDL-C is between 100 and 130 mg/dL.

Note: Additional risk factors to consider are listed in Table 13.4.
Sources: Data from NCEP 1994 and Grundy et al. 1997a.

pliance with pharmacologic monotherapy does not reduce LDL-C to target values. Monitoring is discussed in Chapter 17.

The physician must use individualized clinical judgment in patients who do not meet criteria for drug therapy but who have not attained goals with lifestyle intervention. Clinical judgment is also required to recognize patients in whom lipid-regulating drug therapy is not appropriate, including patients with limited life expectancy. High-risk but otherwise healthy elderly patients are candidates for lipid-lowering drug therapy (see Chapter 19). Target lipid concentrations in the elderly are the same as those in adult practice generally.

All classes of approved lipid-lowering agents are reviewed in detail in Chapter 17; NCEP recommendations for drug selection in adults are shown in Table 17.2. Although estrogens are not classed as lipid-regulating agents, the NCEP notes that ERT may be considered to lower LDL-C moderately and raise HDL-C moderately in some postmenopausal women (see Chapter 18).

Patients without Known Atherosclerotic Disease

In primary prevention, cholesterol-lowering drug therapy should be considered in patients who have remained substantially above their LDL-C goal despite an adequate period of intensive dietary intervention. Candidates for drug therapy include those with LDL-C of 190 mg/dL and those who have two or more other risk factors and LDL-C of 160 mg/dL or higher (see Table 13.6). Patients with less severe LDL-C elevations but with other high risk (e.g., diabetes mellitus or a family history of premature CHD) may also be candidates (Table 13.7) (see Chapter 21 for ADA recommendations in diabetic patients).

Drug therapy should be delayed if possible until later in life in patients with elevated cholesterol who are otherwise at low risk for CHD, particularly men under 35 years of age and premenopausal women. Lipid-regulating drug therapy is often a lifetime commitment that may exact a substantial financial toll, and, as with any drug therapy, adverse effects are possible. It needs to be borne in mind, however, that even though young adults are at less risk than older adults for CHD events in the short term, rates of CHD are higher in people who were hypercholesterolemic in young adulthood than in those who were not. In 27- to 42-year follow-up in the Johns Hopkins Precursors Study (Klag et al. 1993), TC concentration measured early in adulthood in men was strongly predictive of CVD in midlife. Risk for MI was five times as high for the 25% of the men who had the highest cholesterol compared with the 25% who had the lowest cholesterol. A difference of 36 mg/dL in initial cholesterol concentration in the study was significantly associated with an increased risk for death before age 50 years.

Patients with Atherosclerotic Disease

Patients with established CHD or other atherosclerotic disease are candidates for drug therapy when LDL-C remains 130 mg/dL or higher, or 100 mg/dL or higher if the subject's risk profile is sufficiently high (see Table 13.6). Because of the impressive outcomes of the recent large clinical trials using HMG-CoA reductase inhibitors (Chapter 12), a number of clinical experts, including the American College of Cardiology/AHA Task Force on Practice Guidelines (Ryan et al. 1996), have recommended beginning lipid-lowering drug therapy as early as the time of discharge from the hospital when LDL-C is 130 mg/dL or higher. The AHA Task Force on Risk Reduction, chaired by Scott M. Grundy, MD, chairman of the NCEP ATP II, recently concluded that withholding drug therapy in an effort to reach target LDL-C with lifestyle changes is not necessary when LDL-C is 130 mg/dL or higher in patients with CHD, and recommends a 6-week trial of lifestyle therapy when LDL-C is between 100 and 130 mg/dL (Grundy et al. 1997a). The addition of drug therapy before hospital release may be advantageous in terms of compliance, adding to the benefit of greater reductions in LDL-C. It should be remembered that in an infarct patient, lipid determinations need to be made at the time of admission or no later than 24 hours after the event; otherwise, at least a 4-week waiting period should be observed to enable lipoprotein concen-

Table 13.7. RISK STATUS IN PATIENTS WITHOUT KNOWN ATHEROSCLEROTIC DISEASE

High risk		Moderate risk
LDL-C ≥190	↔	LDL-C 190–220 in young adult men (<35 years) and premenopausal women with *no other risk*
or		or
LDL-C between 160 and 190 + ≥2 other CHD risk factors		LDL-C between 160 and 190 + <2 other CHD risk factors
or		or
LDL-C between 130 and 160 + risk of severe degree, e.g., diabetes mellitus* or heavy cigarette smoking	↔	LDL-C between 130 and 160 + ≥2 other CHD risk factors

Note: All LDL-C values are in mg/dL.
*The ADA recommends consideration of drug therapy for LDL-C ≥130 mg/dL in diabetic patients without known atherosclerotic disease (see Table 21.1).
Source: Data from Jones et al. 1998.

trations to stabilize and to ensure accuracy (Ryan et al. 1996) (see also Chapter 14).

NONDRUG THERAPIES FOR SEVERE REFRACTORY HYPERCHOLESTEROLEMIA

LDL apheresis and other nondrug therapies for severe refractory hypercholesterolemia—as seen, for example, in some patients with FH—are discussed in Chapter 17.

MANAGEMENT OF ELEVATED PLASMA TRIGLYCERIDE

There is less agreement among authorities on treatment recommendations for hypertriglyceridemia than for hypercholesterolemia. The link between plasma TG concentration and risk of CHD appears to be complex; however, increased TG often reflects an increase in TGRLs or remnants of TGRLs with atherogenic potential. Plasma TG and HDL-C concentrations may be more important risk predictors in diabetes mellitus, and there is evidence that TG, HDL-C, and diabetes mellitus each are more important risk factors in women than men.

Because the association between fasting plasma TG (VLDL) and risk for CHD is probably not stepwise, as is the case for LDL-C, simple algorithms may be inadequate for managing hypertriglyceridemia. Patients with borderline-high or high TG (Table 13.8) may have accompanying dyslipidemias that increase risk for CHD. When hypertriglyceridemia is an expression of FCH or familial type III hyperlipidemia (dysbetalipopro-

Table 13.8. NCEP RECOMMENDATIONS FOR MANAGEMENT OF HYPERTRIGLYCERIDEMIA (HTG) IN ADULTS

Value (mg/dL)	Category	Primary management	Consideration of drug therapy
<200	Acceptable		
200–400	Borderline high	• Control underlying conditions (see Table 14.1) • Control body weight • Institute diet[a] • Institute regular exercise • Restrict alcohol in selected patients • Stop smoking, for cardiovascular health	• Established atherosclerotic disease • Family history of premature CHD • Concomitant TC ≥240 mg/dL and HDL-C <35 mg/dL • Genetic form of dyslipidemia associated with increased CHD risk (e.g., FCH, familial type III hyperlipidemia) • In some cases, multiple risk factors
400–1,000	High	• As above, with emphasis on controlling causes of secondary HTG • Values labile: can easily become very high	• Definitely use if history of acute pancreatitis • ADA advises strong consideration in diabetes mellitus[b] • See also above
≥1,000	Very high	• Immediate, vigorous TG lowering efforts required because of risk for acute pancreatitis • Drugs are effective to lower VLDL (see Table 17.1), but no available drug is effective in lowering chylomicron concentrations • Treat causes of secondary HTG, including discontinuation of drugs that raise TG (see Table 14.1) • Very low fat diet; avoid alcohol[c]	

Note: Goal is to reduce TG to <200 mg/dL. Some authorities consider TG >150 mg/dL elevated, in particular in diabetes mellitus.

[a]Increasing the ratio of monounsaturated to saturated fatty acids and increasing the proportion of carbohydrate calories obtained from complex carbohydrates are important aspects of the lipid-lowering diet in patients with HTG.

[b]The ADA refers physicians to clinical judgment for values 200–400 mg/dL in diabetes (see Chapter 21).

[c]In type I hyperlipidemia, use diet with <10% of total energy intake as fat and with low intake of simple carbohydrates, alcohol avoidance, and weight control. Substitution of medium-chain for long-chain fatty acids may be helpful in type I.

Source: Data from NCEP 1994.

teinemia), or when aggravating conditions such as diabetes mellitus or renal disease are present, treatment is clearly advisable. Also to be considered are the effects of hypertriglyceridemia on other lipoproteins, such as low HDL-C and reduced LDL size, that may warrant more aggressive treatment (see Chapter 8).

An elevated plasma TG concentration is most often secondary to an underlying disease or condition, such as diabetes mellitus, excess alcohol consumption, high carbohydrate intake, obesity, hypothyroidism, or chronic renal failure, or to the use of certain drugs, such as beta-blockers, diuretics, contraceptive or replacement estrogens, glucocorticoids, or isotretinoin (see Table 14.1). Control of underlying conditions may control the hypertriglyceridemia.

Lifestyle intervention is recommended for all patients with elevated TG. Primary treatment is body weight control; a low-fat, low-cholesterol diet; regular exercise; smoking cessation; and, in selected patients, restriction of alcohol use. Increasing the ratio of monounsaturated to saturated fatty acids and increasing the proportion of carbohydrate calories obtained from complex carbohydrates are important aspects of the lipid-lowering diet in hypertriglyceridemic patients.

Drug therapy is advisable for some patients with elevated TG (see Table 13.8), although, when acute pancreatitis does not threaten, reduction of LDL-C remains the primary goal of lipid-regulating therapy in the NCEP guidelines. Nicotinic acid is the NCEP's drug of choice at this level of TG elevation when diabetes or glucose intolerance is absent; however, nicotinic acid may be poorly tolerated. Fibric acid derivatives are well tolerated and also effectively lower TG and increase HDL-C concentrations; LDL-C may be increased in some patients. Bezafibrate use in BECAIT (see Chapter 10) to lower plasma TG in young MI survivors yielded coronary angiographic and clinical event benefits despite no effect on LDL-C. HMG-CoA reductase inhibitors may also be considered (see Chapter 17). Fish oil supplementation (see Chapter 17) may have a role in the treatment of severe hypertriglyceridemia (in particular the chylomicronemia of type V hyperlipidemia) resistant to other therapies, although it is not recommended as a routine intervention.

TG concentrations of 1,000 mg/dL or higher require vigorous, immediate intervention because of the risk for pancreatitis (see Table 13.8). Very high TG usually cannot be normalized; achievement of TG of less than 500 mg/dL may be considered a success. Familial chylomicronemia (type I hyperlipidemia), which is rare, has not been unambiguously associated with increased risk for CHD (see Table 13.5 and Chapter 14). There are currently no effective drugs to lower chylomicron concentrations. To reduce chylomicrons, use a diet that is low in simple carbohydrates and that contains less than 10% of total energy intake as fat; in practical terms, the patient is taught to count grams of fat in every food, including low-fat foods such as some breads and vegetables. Also, substitution of medium-chain for long-chain fatty acids may be helpful in familial chylomicronemia; medium-chain

Table 13.9. NCEP RECOMMENDATIONS FOR INCREASING LOW HDL-C IN ADULTS

Value (mg/dL)	Category	Primary management	Consideration of drug therapy
<35	Low (high-risk) HDL-C	• Control body weight • Stop smoking • Institute regular exercise • Address concurrent agents that lower HDL-C	• Consider HDL-C value in selection of drug(s) to lower LDL-C • Use not recommended for isolated low HDL-C in low-risk primary prevention

Source: Data from NCEP 1994.

TGs are available as MCT oil from pharmacies. The patient should also avoid alcohol, and weight control is essential.

MANAGEMENT OF LOW HIGH-DENSITY LIPOPROTEIN CHOLESTEROL

Weight control, smoking cessation, and increased physical activity are key to lifestyle management of low HDL-C (Table 13.9), since a low HDL-C concentration often arises from obesity, smoking, and/or a sedentary lifestyle. Among drugs that may give rise to secondary low HDL-C are beta-blockers without intrinsic sympathomimetic activity, isotretinoin, anabolic steroids, progestins, testosterone, and, in some studies, thiazide diuretics.

In primary prevention, isolated low HDL-C is generally not a target of drug therapy; however, elevated LDL-C may be targeted more aggressively when low HDL-C is present, or a treatment that both lowers LDL-C and raises HDL-C may be chosen. In the angiographic LOCAT trial (see Chapter 10), gemfibrozil therapy yielded angiographic coronary benefit in patients with CHD whose predominant lipid abnormality was reduced HDL-C. Nicotinic acid may be the first choice in low HDL-C if diabetes mellitus is not present; the physician may wish to make a greater than usual effort to enable the patient to take nicotinic acid. A fibrate or statin may be an alternative. Bile acid sequestrants have little effect on HDL-C and may increase plasma TG (see Table 17.1).

ADDITIONAL ISSUES

Cost-Effectiveness of Lowering Low-Density Lipoprotein Cholesterol

CHD will cost the United States an estimated $95.6 billion in 1998, comprising $51.1 billion in direct costs and $44.5 billion in lost productivity (AHA 1997). Of these costs, medications will account for $2.9 billion, or only 6% of direct costs and 3% of all costs.

Review of cost-effectiveness analyses of cholesterol lowering supports population-wide educational endeavors and aggressive risk reduction in secondary prevention, but drug therapy in primary prevention tends to be cost-effective only in high-risk groups (NCEP 1994; Goldman et al. 1992; Kupersmith et al. 1995; Martens and Guibert 1995). Targeting by factors such as age, coexisting risk factors, and sex will improve the cost-effectiveness profile in patients who do not have CHD (Kupersmith et al. 1995; Martens and Guibert 1995). As absolute risk increased from 1% to 4% per year in the primary prevention West of Scotland Coronary Prevention Study (WOSCOPS), the number of patients who would need to be treated to prevent one coronary event dropped from 66 to 17 (West of Scotland Coronary Prevention Study Group 1996). The incidence of CHD was greater than 10% across the 5 years of the trial (2% per year) when any one of the following risk factors was present in the middle-aged men in addition to high cholesterol: pre-existing vascular disease (5% of WOSCOPS subjects had angina and 3% had intermittent claudication), minor ECG abnormalities, smoking, HDL-C of less than 42.5 mg/dL, hypertension, or family history of premature CHD. Thus, high-risk men could easily be identified in the population. In the secondary-prevention Scandinavian Simvastatin Survival Study (4S), in which patients had a history of MI or angina, cost-effectiveness was analyzed prospectively, and the investigators found that simvastatin therapy markedly reduced use of hospital services, thereby offsetting most of its cost (Pedersen et al. 1996). Cost-effectiveness analysis of the pooled results of two regression trials using pravastatin showed favorable outcome compared with other widely accepted medical interventions (Ashraf et al. 1996).

Gains in life expectancy with strict control of cholesterol concentrations are similar to those achieved with smoking cessation, control of DBP, or weight control (Tsevat 1992). Given the crucial role of cholesterol lowering in reducing the incidence of CHD, high priority should be given to validating its cost-effectiveness (Gotto 1997b).

Additional Risk Interventions

An AHA consensus panel has provided recommendations for comprehensive CHD risk reduction in secondary prevention (Smith et al. 1995). Risk reduction measures to be considered include use of antiplatelet agents or anticoagulants, ACE inhibitors, beta-blockers, ERT, and blood pressure control (Table 13.10) in addition to smoking cessation, lipid management, increasing physical activity, and weight management. The panel emphasizes that institution of comprehensive risk factor interventions

- Extends overall survival
- Improves quality of life
- Decreases need for interventional procedures such as CABG and PTCA
- Reduces the incidence of MI

Table 13.10. AHA CONSENSUS PANEL RECOMMENDATIONS FOR SECONDARY PREVENTION: RISK REDUCTION STRATEGIES IN ADDITION TO LIPID MANAGEMENT AND LIFESTYLE CHANGES

Risk intervention	Recommendations
Antiplatelet agents/ anticoagulants	• Start aspirin, 80–325 mg/day, if not contraindicated. • Manage warfarin to international normalized ratio = 2.0–3.5 for post-MI patients not able to take aspirin.
ACE inhibitors post-MI	• Start early post-MI in stable high-risk patients (anterior MI, previous MI, Killip class II [S_3 gallop, rales, radiographic congestive heart failure]). Continue indefinitely for all with LV dysfunction (ejection fraction ≤40%) or symptoms of failure. • Use as needed to manage blood pressure or symptoms in all other patients.
Beta-blockers	• Start in high-risk post-MI patients (arrhythmia, LV dysfunction, inducible ischemia) at 5–28 days. • Continue 6 months minimum. Observe usual contraindications. • Use as needed to manage angina, rhythm, or blood pressure in all other patients.
Replacement estrogen	• Consider ERT in all postmenopausal women. Individualize recommendation consistent with other health risks.
Blood pressure control Goal: ≤140/90 mm Hg	• See Chapter 16.

Note: Endorsed by the Board of Trustees of the American College of Cardiology.
Source: Data from Smith et al. 1995.

Future Directions in Antiatherosclerosis Therapy

Possible future strategies against atherosclerosis include further refining of guidelines for the management of dyslipidemia, improving current pharmacologic strategies, developing new pharmacologic strategies (Table 13.11), and using gene-based therapies (Gotto 1996). Although there is reason to be optimistic that future preventive and therapeutic measures will greatly reduce death and disability from CHD, much basic science and clinical research is required to realize that goal. Clinicians should continue to pursue vigorously risk factor reduction according to established guidelines.

American College of Physicians Cholesterol Recommendations

Review by three commissioned authors (Garber et al. 1996) led to the publication by the American College of Physicians (ACP) (1996) of cholesterol control recommendations that were substantially different from the NCEP ATP II guidelines prepared over 18 months by 25 authorities in a

Table 13.11. POTENTIAL MOLECULAR THERAPIES FOR VASCULAR DISEASE

Pathologic event	Therapeutic target
Plaque rupture	Metalloproteinase inhibitors, leukocyte adhesion blockers
Thrombosis	Glycoprotein IIb/IIIa receptor blockers, tissue factor inhibitors, antithrombins
Endothelial dysfunction	Nitric oxide donors, antioxidants
Endothelial injury	Vascular endothelial growth factor, fibroblast growth factor
Dysregulated cell growth	Cell cycle inhibitors
Dysregulated apoptosis	Integrin antagonists
Matrix modification	Metalloproteinase inhibitors, plasmin antagonists

Source: Braunwald 1997; used with permission. Data modified from Gibbons and Dzau 1996.

range of disciplines (LaRosa 1996; Cleeman and Grundy 1997). Although the ACP recommendations are in accord with the NCEP about the high risk conferred by hypercholesterolemia in patients with vascular disease, they maintain that it is not necessary to measure cholesterol in young men (aged 20–35) or premenopausal women (aged 20–45), or in older people (aged >65). In essence, the conclusion is that if the cholesterol value is known, physicians will overprescribe lipid-lowering drugs.

The ACP recommendations cannot be endorsed. Their policy ignores our knowledge that atherosclerosis begins in adolescence and early adulthood (see Chapter 5). Cholesterol-lowering therapy prescribed late in life cannot nullify years of atherosclerosis buildup (Cleeman and Grundy 1997; Stamler et al. 1993c), and the earlier a change is made in plasma cholesterol, the greater the long-term effect on risk for CHD (Law et al. 1994). Cholesterol measurement is an inexpensive, reliable test whose results can save lives, in particular through motivating changes in lifestyle. It must be remembered, too, that approximately one-fourth of first CHD events manifest as sudden death and approximately two-thirds of MI survivors do not make a complete recovery (AHA 1997). FH will be missed in at least one-half of young adults (about 79,000 Americans missed) if family history is relied on to determine who will be screened for elevated cholesterol (Cleeman and Grundy 1997). Although 61% of adults 25–34 years of age have had their cholesterol measured, only 0.2% are taking lipid-lowering drugs; respective proportions for those aged 35–44 are 76% and 1% (NHLBI 1995). The high absolute risk of the elderly for CHD and the benefits of risk reduction in this age group are discussed in Chapter 19.

The NCEP ATP II guidelines have been endorsed by more than 40 medical and health organizations, including the AHA, the American College of Cardiology, the American Medical Association, the American

Academy of Family Physicians, and the American College of Preventive Medicine, and they remain the gold standard.

Suggested Reading

Braunwald E. Shattuck Lecture. Cardiovascular medicine at the turn of the millennium: triumphs, concerns, and opportunities. N Engl J Med 1997; 337:1360–1369.

Expert Panel on Detection, Evaluation, and Treatment of High Blood Cholesterol in Adults. Summary of the second report of the National Cholesterol Education Program (NCEP) Expert Panel on Detection, Evaluation, and Treatment of High Blood Cholesterol in Adults (Adult Treatment Panel II). JAMA 1993;269:3015–3023.

Grundy SM, Balady GJ, Criqui MH, et al. When to start cholesterol-lowering therapy in patients with coronary heart disease: a statement for healthcare professionals from the American Heart Association Task Force on Risk Reduction. AHA medical/scientific statement. Circulation 1997;95: 1683–1685.

Grundy SM, Balady GJ, Criqui MH, et al. Guide to primary prevention of cardiovascular diseases. A statement for healthcare professionals from the Task Force on Risk Reduction. AHA medical/scientific statement. Circulation 1997;95:2329–2331.

Jones PH, Grundy SM, Gotto AM Jr. Assessment and management of lipid abnormalities. In: Alexander RW, Schlant RC, Fuster V, eds. Hurst's the heart, arteries and veins. New York: McGraw-Hill, 1998:1553–1581.

National Cholesterol Education Program. Second report of the Expert Panel on Detection, Evaluation, and Treatment of High Blood Cholesterol in Adults (Adult Treatment Panel II). Circulation 1994;89:1329–1445. (Note: Softbound copies of the NCEP Second Report of the Expert Panel on Detection, Evaluation, and Treatment of High Blood Cholesterol in Adults [NIH publication no. 93-3095] may be obtained by writing the NHLBI Information Center, P.O. Box 30105, Bethesda, MD 20824-0105 [telephone 301-251-1222, fax 301-251-1223]. One copy is gratis.)

Ryan TJ, Anderson JL, Antman EM, et al. ACC/AHA guidelines for the management of patients with acute myocardial infarction: a report of the American College of Cardiology/American Heart Association Task Force on Practice Guidelines (Committee on Management of Acute Myocardial Infarction). J Am Coll Cardiol 1996;28:1328–1428.

Smith SC Jr, Blair SN, Criqui MH, et al., the Secondary Prevention Panel. Preventing heart attack and death in patients with coronary disease. Consensus panel statement. AHA medical/scientific statement. Published simultaneously in Circulation 1995;92:2–4 and J Am Coll Cardiol 1995;26: 292–294.

Chapter 14

Considerations in the Clinical Evaluation of Dyslipidemia

As described in the previous chapter, management of dyslipidemia in CHD risk entails much more than the starting point of determination of lipid values. The full clinical evaluation includes a personal history, family history, evaluation of lifestyle components, physical examination, other laboratory tests, and establishment of the risk factor profile. An effort must be made to determine any causes of secondary dyslipidemia and any familial lipid disorder. Management in the great majority of patients does not require specialist biochemistry.

SELECTED CAUSES OF SECONDARY DYSLIPIDEMIA

Common causes of secondary dyslipidemia need to be excluded before a diagnosis of a primary dyslipidemia can be considered. The underlying disorder, such as type 2 diabetes mellitus, may be an important diagnosis in its own right, and the lipid derangement may play a role in the disorder's development and sequelae.

Common causes of secondary plasma cholesterol elevation include a diet rich in saturated fatty acids, hypothyroidism, nephrotic syndrome, and chronic liver disease. Hypercholesterolemia can also result from the use of some drugs, such as oral contraceptives. Plasma TG elevation may be related to a diet rich in carbohydrates, excessive alcohol consumption, obesity, pregnancy, diabetes mellitus, hypothyroidism, chronic renal failure, or pancreatitis, among other conditions, or to the use of such drugs as beta-blockers, diuretics, isotretinoin, glucocorticoids, or contraceptive or replacement estrogens. These and some other causes of secondary hyperlipidemia are listed in Table 14.1. Diet-induced hyperlipidemia may also be viewed as diet-sensitive primary hyperlipidemia. The development of low HDL-C is often related to elevated plasma TG; cigarette smoking; a sedentary lifestyle; impaired glucose tolerance; or a very high carbohydrate, very low fat diet.

Table 14.1. SELECTED CAUSES OF SECONDARY HYPERLIPIDEMIA

Related to plasma cholesterol elevation	Related to plasma TG elevation
Diet rich in saturated fatty acids	Diet rich in carbohydrates
Hypothyroidism	Excessive alcohol consumption*
Nephrotic syndrome	Obesity
Chronic liver disease (mainly primary biliary cirrhosis)	Pregnancy
Cholestasis	Diabetes mellitus
Dysglobulinemia	Hypothyroidism
Cushing's syndrome	Chronic renal failure
Oral contraceptives	Pancreatitis
Anorexia nervosa	Bulimia
Acute intermittent porphyria	Cushing's syndrome
	Hypopituitarism
	Dysglobulinemia
	Glycogen storage disease
	Lipodystrophy
	Acute intermittent porphyria
	Systemic lupus erythematosus
	Beta-blocker, diuretic use
	Estrogen use (contraceptive or replacement)
	Glucocorticoid use
	Isotretinoin use

*More than 40 g/day ethanol is considered excessive. See Table 16.16 for recommendations of maximum alcohol intake.
Source: Gotto et al. 1995; used with permission.

In children and adolescents (see Chapter 19), some conditions to consider in particular in relation to the development of dyslipidemia are overweight and the use of isotretinoin, anabolic steroids, or oral contraceptives.

SELECTED PRIMARY DYSLIPIDEMIAS

A family history (Table 14.2) will help determine the likelihood of an inherited dyslipidemia. Fredrickson phenotypes for some primary hyperlipidemias are shown in Table 13.5. The primary lipid disorders most often encountered in adult clinical practice are FCH, polygenic hypercholesterolemia, FH, and type III hyperlipidemia (Gotto et al. 1995).

Familial Hypercholesterolemia

FH (Goldstein et al. 1995; Bild and Williams 1993) has been recognized for many years. It is a common autosomal dominant disorder in which LDL clearance from the circulation is impaired. The heterozygous form has a frequency of about 1 in 500, whereas the homozygous form occurs in only 1 in 1 million. In most populations, more than 150 mutations are

Table 14.2. STEP-BY-STEP FAMILY HISTORY

1. Draw a pedigree	Index patient, parents, siblings, children, grandparents, aunts, uncles
2. Check	Are all blood relatives?
3. Ask	Is relative alive or dead?
If relative is alive	How old?
	Any CVD?
	If so, at what age?
	Smoke?
	Other risk factors for CVD?
If relative has died	Age at death?
	Cause of death?
	Other major illness?
	If CVD was present, at what age?
	Risk factors for CVD?
4. Discard	All uncertain information
5. Assume	Family history is uninformative but not negative for CVD if patient knows little about relatives' cardiovascular health
6. Consider in general	Number and sex of relatives at risk
	Current age and age when CVD developed
	Additional risk factors in those positive for disease
	Number of expected cases of CVD given family risk factors
	Number of observed vs. number of expected cases
7. Negative history significant when	Longevity in most members

Note: A family history chart for patients to complete is available in DeBakey ME et al. The new living heart diet. New York: Simon and Schuster, 1996.
Source: Gotto et al. 1995; used with permission. Data from the European Atherosclerosis Society (International Task Force 1992).

responsible for the disease; molecular diagnosis can be made through linkage analysis in families. However, in some inbred populations, a small number of mutations predominate, and screening at the DNA level is feasible. These populations include Ashkenazi Jews of Lithuanian ancestry living in South Africa, Afrikaners in South Africa, Christian Lebanese in Lebanon and Syria, French Canadians in Quebec Province, and the Finns. The prevalence of heterozygous FH is increased in some of these groups: 1 in 67 among the Ashkenazi Jews, 1 in 100 among the Afrikaners, 1 in 170 among the Christian Lebanese, and 1 in 270 among the French Canadians. Brown and Goldstein demonstrated that the relevant genetic defect in FH is in the gene controlling the LDL receptor protein (Goldstein and Brown 1973, 1979, 1985). Mutations in the LDL receptor gene may result in complete loss of activity in cultured fibroblasts, or there may be as much as 25% residual function.

The elevation of LDL-C that results from the impaired catabolism promotes cholesterol deposition in arteries, skin, and tendons. Cholesterol is usually elevated at birth. Generally, TG and HDL-C concentrations are normal in heterozygous FH; HDL-C is frequently decreased in homozygous FH. The Fredrickson phenotype is IIa (IIb is rare). In FH heterozygotes, in whom the number of functional LDL receptors is halved, LDL-C is elevated twofold to threefold, and symptomatic CHD typically develops after age 35 years (on average, at about age 45 in untreated men and age 55 in untreated women). Among people in the United States and western Europe who have an MI before age 60 years, about 5% are FH heterozygotes. In FH homozygotes, in whom functional LDL receptors are absent, LDL-C is elevated six to eight times and death from MI often occurs during the first two decades of life.

Clinical diagnosis may be established by LDL-C above the 90th percentile in two or more first-degree relatives and the presence of tendinous xanthomas within the kindred. Typical clinical manifestations include cholesteryl ester deposits on the Achilles tendons and the extensor tendons of the hands. These deposits may occur elsewhere as well, for example, over the tibial tuberositas and elbows. Xanthomas in the palpebral fissure are also common, where they are called xanthelasmas. In the homozygous form, "buttery" xanthomas may be present over the thighs and buttocks. Another characteristic finding in FH is premature corneal arcus. Widespread, severe early atherosclerosis, including aortic stenosis, is usual in homozygotes. Heterozygous FH can be difficult to diagnose; the differential diagnosis should include familial defective apo B-100 and FCH (see later). Humphries et al. (1997) consider DNA testing appropriate for (1) diagnosis of FH when physical signs or family history is equivocal or absent, and (2) detection of a mutation causing FH in immediate family members (particularly children) when there is a family history of premature CHD. In children, plasma lipid concentrations may not be diagnostic; some may initially present with values within the normal range.

Diet remains a critical component of therapy in heterozygous FH, for correction of coexisting risk factors as well as LDL-C lowering. Some evidence exists that patients with FH may be more sensitive to dietary cholesterol than subjects with less severe cholesterol elevations (Connor and Connor 1993). In animal studies, both dietary cholesterol and saturated fatty acids down-regulate hepatic LDL receptor activity (Spady and Dietschy 1988). Increased monounsaturated fatty acids (olive oil) may be advisable (Packard and Shepherd 1995) because of evidence that they reduce LDL susceptibility to oxidation (Reaven et al. 1991; Sorgato et al. 1992).

Generally, FH heterozygotes also require lipid-lowering pharmacotherapy, and the availability of the HMG-CoA reductase inhibitors has revolutionized this treatment. Hypercholesterolemia in most heterozygotes can now be controlled by statin monotherapy or by statin-resin combination drug therapy (Packard and Shepherd 1995), whereas before statin availability it was generally uncontrolled. Therapy for homozygous FH is difficult because the condition is usually diet and drug resistant, although some benefit from statins has recently been reported (see Chapter 17). Probucol can achieve regression of xanthomas. FH homozygotes are often treated with LDL apheresis, a modality also used in some heterozygotes (see Chapter 17). Liver transplantation, portacaval shunting, and gene therapy remain experimental (see also Chapter 17).

Familial Defective Apolipoprotein B-100

In familial defective apo B-100 (Zulewski et al. 1998; Soria et al. 1989), LDL particles are cleared more slowly from plasma because of a reduced affinity of LDL for the LDL receptor. The most common form results from a single nucleotide mutation that produces a substitution of glutamine for arginine at amino acid position 3,500 in apo B. Inheritance is autosomal dominant. Prevalence is uncertain and varies by ethnicity; it may range from rare to 1 in 600. The plasma lipoprotein concentrations and clinical features may resemble those of heterozygous FH or may be more moderate, and treatment is the same as in heterozygous FH. Definitive diagnosis is by molecular analysis.

Polygenic Hypercholesterolemia

The most common genetic cause of an isolated increase in TC or LDL-C concentration is polygenic hypercholesterolemia (Durrington 1995). The causes of this disorder, which is associated with increased risk for CHD, are poorly defined, but as the name sets forth, more than one gene is implicated. Genetic and dietary or other environmental factors may interact to stimulate LDL production or to decrease its clearance. Individuals with polygenic hypercholesterolemia may be hypersensitive to dietary saturated fats or cholesterol.

The prevalence of polygenic hypercholesterolemia is unknown, but it is thought to be between 1 in 20 and 1 in 100 in the United States. TC concentration is usually lower than in heterozygous FH, and xanthomas are absent or very rare. Only about 7% of first-degree relatives of patients with polygenic hypercholesterolemia have high LDL-C. Treatment of severe cases is essentially identical to treatment of heterozygous FH, although combination-drug therapy may not be required.

Familial Combined Hyperlipidemia

FCH (de Bruin et al. 1996; de Graaf and Stalenhoef 1998; Wijsman et al. 1998; Kwiterovich 1993) is the most common genetic hyperlipidemia in which multiple lipoprotein phenotypes are manifested. It may present with elevated VLDL (type IV hyperlipidemia), elevated LDL (type IIa), or both (type IIb). All three patterns may be seen within a family, and the pattern may change within an individual. The disorder is quite common, with a prevalence of 0.5–1.0% in the general population. It was first described in 1973 by Goldstein and colleagues as the most common dyslipidemic syndrome in families of survivors of premature MI, and it is associated with an increased risk for CHD. The fundamental basis of FCH remains to be elucidated, as does its kinship with hyperapobetalipoproteinemia (hyper–apo B), LDL phenotype B, familial dyslipidemic hypertension, and insulin resistance syndrome (metabolic syndrome X) (see Chapter 8). FCH may be considered more like a syndrome; it might turn out that patients manifest a mixture of disease entities, with a variety of metabolic defects and possible genetic markers (de Graaf and Stalenhoef 1998). The difference between FCH and hyper–apo B (Sniderman et al. 1982, 1985) may be largely definitional; in the latter, the LDL-C concentration is within the "normal" range, even though plasma apo B values are above the 90th percentile for age and sex. Hyper–apo B has been found in 5% of CHD kindreds.

Specific diagnostic criteria have not been firmly established. Generally, we accept a diagnosis if the index patient and a first-degree relative have one of the phenotypes IIa, IIb, or IV and if there is a strong family history of hyperlipidemia and early coronary disease. The occurrence of more than one lipoprotein phenotype within the family, the absence of xanthomas, and the absence of affected children are useful clinical findings. FCH does not often occur before age 20 years; the diagnosis is usually one of adulthood. Patients are often hypertensive and overweight and may be diabetic and have gout. When TC is elevated, it is generally in the range of 250 to 350 mg/dL. Two-thirds of FCH patients with hypertriglyceridemia have a mild to moderate TG elevation. However, TG elevation may be severe; chylomicronemia may occur, especially when the patient is diabetic.

Treatment of FCH follows standard clinical guidelines for hypercholesterolemia, hypertriglyceridemia, or combined hyperlipidemia. A lipid-lowering diet, weight control, and control of diabetes (if present) are important. Patients with hypertriglyceridemia should avoid exogenous estrogen therapy and alcohol. The use of nicotinic acid may aggravate glucose intolerance, and resins may raise plasma TG concentrations. A statin may be selected if the chief hyperlipidemia is hypercholesterolemia, and a fibrate may be selected if hypertriglyceridemia predominates.

Type III Hyperlipidemia

Familial dysbetalipoproteinemia, or type III hyperlipidemia (Mahley and Rall 1995), is a dramatic demonstration of the atherogenic potential of remnant lipoproteins. It is sometimes referred to as broad-beta disease because the VLDL remnants that define the phenotype migrate as a broad band encompassing both the beta and pre-beta regions. The disorder stems from an apo E–linked metabolic defect; transmission usually mimics an autosomal recessive mode. Besides homozygosity for a receptor binding–defective isoform of apo E, additional genes for familial lipoprotein disorders might operate in the pathogenesis (Feussner et al. 1997). More than 90% of patients with dysbetalipoproteinemia have the apo $E_{2/2}$ phenotype. Other variants of apo E that bind defectively to the LDL receptor have been described in type III (Walden and Hegele 1994); rarely, the defect is apo E deficiency. Yet even though the frequency of apo E_2 homozygosity in the general population is about 1 in 100, the disorder occurs in only about 1 in 5,000. Additional metabolic factors (a "second hit") are usually required for full clinical expression; the patients are often obese and have diabetes mellitus, hypertension, hyperuricemia, hypothyroidism, and/or another familial lipid disorder such as FCH.

Typical clinical manifestations of dysbetalipoproteinemia are planar xanthomas on the hands and tuberous xanthomas, typically over the knees and elbows but not attached to tendons. Usually, cholesterol and TG are increased to nearly equal concentrations, with cholesterol between 300 and 600 mg/dL and TG between 400 and 800 mg/dL, although values may be much higher. A VLDL cholesterol:plasma TG ratio greater than 0.3 supports the diagnosis. It is unusual to encounter type III hyperlipidemia before the end of the second decade. The disorder is more common in men; signs may not occur in women until after menopause. Premature atherosclerosis may present as MI, stroke, or PVD. Diagnosis of dysbetalipoproteinemia can often be made on clinical grounds, although ultracentrifugation or apo E isoelectric focusing is valuable.

Dysbetalipoproteinemia is extremely sensitive to dietary therapy, and a reduction in saturated fat intake together with weight reduction as needed frequently corrects the dyslipidemia. Treatment by diet and fibric acid derivatives results in rapid normalization of lipids and shrinkage of xanthomas. Other drugs that may be considered are HMG-CoA reductase inhibitors and, if diabetes or glucose intolerance is absent, nicotinic acid. Concomitant aggravating conditions need to be treated.

Familial Endogenous and Familial Mixed Hypertriglyceridemias

Hypertriglyceridemia is a major aspect of some genetic lipid disorders (Assmann and Brewer 1991), including FCH, dysbetalipoproteinemia, chylomicronemia, familial endogenous hypertriglyceridemia (type IV hyperlipidemia; elevated VLDL), and familial mixed hypertriglyceridemia (type V hyperlipidemia; elevated VLDL and chylomicrons). It should be borne in mind that hypertriglyceridemia can be secondary to such conditions as diabetes mellitus, renal failure, and excess alcohol intake, and to the use of such drugs as estrogens, diuretics, and beta-blockers.

Familial endogenous hypertriglyceridemia may be an autosomal dominant trait; it is fairly common, occurring in about 1 in 300 people. It is believed to be associated with hepatic overproduction of TG and large VLDL particles. TG concentrations generally range from 200 to 500 mg/dL, and HDL-C is decreased. Uncommonly, TG exceeds 1,000 mg/dL in "pure" type IV (chylomicrons absent). Type IV is often associated with a modest chylomicronemia, giving a type V pattern in which the VLDL component remains predominant. CHD is common in some kindreds but not in others with familial endogenous hypertriglyceridemia. Alcohol restriction and weight control are central to controlling familial endogenous hypertriglyceridemia. Patients often have abnormal glucose tolerance and hyperuricemia. When drug treatment is warranted, the agent of choice is a fibrate or, if abnormal glucose tolerance is absent, nicotinic acid.

Type V hyperlipidemia is rare, although it may be diagnosed in the emergency room as a cause of abdominal pain and pancreatitis. TG concentrations generally exceed 1,000 mg/dL. LPL activity is probably decreased in this disorder, and VLDL is overproduced by the liver. The genetics of familial mixed hypertriglyceridemia have not been well worked out. Typical clinical manifestations are hyperuricemia and abnormal glucose tolerance. Estrogen therapy, alcohol consumption, and obesity all exacerbate the disorder.

Controlling the hypertriglyceridemia in type V hyperlipidemia substantially reduces the risk for pancreatitis. Severe fat restriction should be undertaken, alcohol should be forbidden, and every attempt should be made to encourage the patient to reduce his or her weight, exercise regularly, and control diabetes. A fibrate is a good drug choice, because nicotinic acid may worsen glucose intolerance. When type V is treated, there may be a reversion to a type IV or type IIb pattern.

Familial Chylomicronemia

Chylomicrons are not normally present in the plasma of fasting individuals. Failure to clear chylomicrons can represent their impaired lipolysis due to a deficiency of LPL or apo C-II. Either deficiency can be caused by decreased protein synthesis or synthesis of dysfunctional protein. Both the apo C-II and LPL disorders are rare and inherited as autosomal recessive traits. More than 60 mutations of the LPL gene can cause LPL deficiency (Hayden et al. 1991); 3–7% of whites are heterozygous carriers (Reymer et al. 1995; Bijvoet et al. 1996; Jemaa et al. 1995). Heterozygotes show normal or only slightly elevated TG concentrations in the absence of other conditions associated with hypertriglyceridemia; in homozygotes, fasting TG concentrations may exceed 1,000 mg/dL because of the accumulation of chylomicrons in the blood. The diagnosis of familial apo C-II or LPL deficiency can be made based on the presence of decreased postheparin LPL activity. In the assay, apo C-II deficiency and LPL deficiency can be distinguished by the addition of exogenous apo C-II, which restores LPL activity in the former but not the latter. Homozygosity for LDL deficiency is often associated with HDL-C between 5 and 15 mg/dL (Funke 1997).

Familial chylomicronemia (Brunzell 1995; Chait and Brunzell 1991) is usually diagnosed in childhood by recurrent abdominal pain and pancreatitis. Infants typically show intolerance to fatty foods. Lipemia retinalis, eruptive xanthomas on extensor surfaces and the buttocks, hepatosplenomegaly, and, occasionally, splenomegaly may occur. Eruptive xanthomas are raised, superficial yellow papular lesions surrounded by an erythematous base. Lipemia retinalis is recognized by a pale appearance to the optic vessels, in contrast to the normal finding of dark vessels standing out against a pink background. Clinical manifestations of chylomicronemia may also include paresthesias of the hands, peripheral neuropathy, dyspnea, and dementia manifested mainly as memory loss, in particular for recent events. The manifestation of symptoms and signs does not appear to be related to the degree of the hypertriglyceridemia; some patients with TG as high as 30,000 mg/dL have been asymptomatic. Prolonged misdiagnosis may occur (Chait and Brunzell 1991). One case report of a female patient with familial LPL deficiency, in whom plasma TG concentration increased dramatically at puberty, indicates that phenotypic expression of familial chylomicronemia may be modified by hormonal status (Bucher et al. 1997).

Individuals with chylomicronemia syndrome are at an increased risk for pancreatitis because of sludging of blood flow in the pancreatic circulation caused by the increased viscosity of lipemic plasma. Familial chylomicronemia has traditionally not been associated with premature atherosclerosis, although in 1996 Benlian et al. reported such disease in four patients with LPL deficiency. The authors suggested that defective lipolysis may increase the risk for atherosclerosis; aspects of the risk include elevated fasting TG, reduced HDL-C, and severely delayed clearance of postprandial TGRLs, perhaps enhancing oxidation susceptibility and prothrombin activation. Additional reports are needed to confirm the finding of premature atherosclerosis in this disorder.

Treatment of chylomicronemia syndrome should be guided by the goal of maintaining fasting TG concentrations below 500 mg/dL to minimize the risk for pancreatitis; normalization of TG concentrations is usually not achievable. Treatment should include a diet low in simple sugars and fat (<10% of total calories from fat), avoidance of alcohol, and, if necessary, weight reduction. The replacement of dietary long-chain fatty acids with medium-chain fatty acids (available at pharmacies as MCT oil) may also be beneficial because medium-chain fatty acids are absorbed directly into the portal vein instead of being formed into chylomicrons in the intestine. Drug therapy is generally ineffective in chylomicronemia.

Familial Low High-Density Lipoprotein Cholesterol

Familial low HDL-C (familial hypoalphalipoproteinemia) (Assmann et al. 1990, 1995; Funke 1997; Breslow 1995; Klein et al. 1995) is an interim term encompassing a heterogeneous group of rare disorders. The molecular basis has been elucidated for some, but in others the etiology is unclear. Much remains to be understood in the process of HDL formation. Some of the familial low HDL-C disorders have been associated with premature CHD; others have not. Some examples from the diverse group are described here. Patients with these disorders should be referred to a lipid specialist for treatment.

Although there is no doubt of the strong epidemiologic association between reduced HDL-C concentration and increased risk for atherosclerosis, the lack of a relation between CHD and absence of HDL in monogenic disorders in humans or in knockout mice makes it clear that etiologic and modifying factors play important roles (Funke 1997).

Tangier Disease

The prototypical HDL deficiency disorder is Tangier disease (Funke 1997; Mentis 1996; Walter et al. 1996), so named because it was first discovered in patients on Tangier Island in the Chesapeake Bay (United States). In this rare autosomal recessive disorder, the major proteins apo A-I and apo A-II are in short supply and normal HDL is absent. Instead, a small quantity of the abnormal lipoprotein $HDL_{Tangier}$ is found. There is an increased ratio of pro-apo A-I to apo A-I. The severe deficiency of HDL is associated with the deposition of cholesteryl ester in the tissues of the reticuloendothelial system. This produces the orange tonsils that are pathognomonic when accompanied by low plasma cholesterol and normal or elevated TG concentrations. Splenomegaly, neuropathy, and ocular abnormalities may be present. Whereas coronary disease has been reported in patients over 40 years old, overwhelming early atherosclerosis is not a feature of Tangier disease.

Familial Lecithin:Cholesterol Acyltransferase Deficiency

In familial LCAT deficiency (Kuinenhoven et al. 1997; Glomset et al. 1995; Assmann et al. 1991), LCAT activity is virtually absent, resulting in decreased plasma concentrations of cholesteryl ester and lysolecithin and increased plasma concentrations of cholesterol and lecithin. In all the lipoprotein fractions, composition, structure, and concentration are altered. Clinical features include corneal opacities, anemia, and, frequently, proteinuria; renal failure can be life-threatening. Despite decreased HDL-C, CHD risk is usually not increased, but planar and tendon xanthomas and atherosclerosis may result from hypertension and hyperlipidemia secondary to renal failure. The relatively small number of reported cases of LCAT deficiency syndromes, however, allows only speculation about the relation between LCAT function and atherosclerosis (Kuinenhoven et al. 1997).

Fish-eye Disease

Fish-eye disease, or partial LCAT deficiency (Kuinenhoven et al. 1997; Glomset et al. 1995; Assmann et al. 1991), is characterized by age-dependent corneal opacification, but the other clinical features of familial LCAT deficiency are absent. Among lipoprotein changes are HDL deficiency and elevated plasma TG. Premature atherosclerosis has now been described in about one-third of reported cases (6 of 19), although meaningful conclusions about the link cannot be drawn because of the small number of cases (Kuinenhoven et al. 1997). Both fish-eye disease and familial LCAT deficiency appear to be inherited in an autosomal recessive manner.

Apolipoprotein A-I$_{Milano}$

Individuals who have the apo A-I$_{Milano}$ mutant form of apo A-I have severely reduced HDL-C; some have elevated plasma TG as well. The mutation is associated with longevity and has been reported in individuals living into the ninth decade (Franceschini et al. 1980; Roma et al. 1993; Andersson 1997).

Hypobetalipoproteinemia

LDL-C values at the 5th percentile (approximately 90 mg/dL in western populations) or lower define hypobetalipoproteinemia (Schonfeld 1995). The low LDL-C values have been associated with a reduced risk for CHD (Glueck et al. 1997). When hypobetalipoproteinemia is not associated with an underlying disease such as alcoholism, intestinal malabsorption, or hyperthyroidism, it is generally heritable. Heterozygosity for genetic hypobetalipoproteinemia may occur in about 1 in 10,000 persons (Wagner et al. 1991); it rarely leads to symptoms and may increase longevity. In some well-studied kindreds, inheritance is autosomal dominant. In a subset of kindreds, the phenotype has been linked to truncation-producing mutations of the apo B-100 gene. Diverse physiologic mechanisms have been described. Other low-cholesterol syndromes include autosomal recessive hypobetalipoproteinemia, chylomicron retention disease, and abetalipoproteinemia (see next section), all conditions characterized by low concentrations of circulating lipoproteins, dietary fat malabsorption, and failure to thrive in infancy (Schonfeld 1995; Levy 1996).

Abetalipoproteinemia

The rare abetalipoproteinemia (Kane and Havel 1995) is the most severe manifestation of apo B deficiency. It was first described as a syndrome of retinitis pigmentosa, unusually shaped erythrocytes, a syndrome resembling Friedreich's ataxia, and steatorrhea (Bassen and Kornzweig 1950). LDL and VLDL are virtually absent in this disorder, and chylomicrons are not produced after a meal. Plasma cholesterol, typically less than 50 mg/dL, occurs in HDL. Spinocerebellar degeneration is the most devastating effect; there may be response to supplementation with vitamins A and E. Pedigrees described to date are compatible with autosomal recessive inheritance; the condition has been shown to arise from mutations of the microsomal TG transfer protein (Schonfeld 1995).

LABORATORY CONSIDERATIONS

There may be differences in whole blood lipid measurements obtained from a fingerstick versus a venous puncture. For screening (TC, HDL-C, and TG), fingertip blood and dry chemistry techniques may be used; clinical decision making, however, requires follow-up testing with venous blood. It is best to obtain and average two or more cholesterol values as a baseline for several reasons. Cholesterol values normally fluctuate day to day, by perhaps 3% or more. (Seasonal variation also occurs: Cholesterol concentrations increase in spring and decrease in autumn.) Variation is also inherent in the measurement methodology. For example, posture affects cholesterol concentrations significantly. If a patient lies down for 10 or 15 minutes before the blood sample is drawn, the plasma can re-equilibrate, and the measured plasma or serum cholesterol value may be lower than it would be otherwise. Plasma lipid concentrations are about 4% lower than serum lipid concentrations. The CDC has established a series of primary and secondary standardized laboratories throughout the United States. One should inquire as to whether a given laboratory is standardized against the CDC. The Abell-Kendall method for measuring cholesterol is the gold standard used by the CDC for standardization of cholesterol values. See Jacobs et al. (1982) and Chambless et al. (1992) for discussion of lipid retest reliability. Home tests for cholesterol are not reliable because there is no quality control, although they can sometimes identify individuals with very high cholesterol.

After an MI, lipids should be measured within 24 hours (and preferably within 12 hours) of the onset of chest pain; thereafter, LDL-C concentrations usually decrease for up to 12 weeks. Lipid assessment is usually deferred until 4–6 weeks after an MI. Lipid assessment should be deferred for 3 months when there is other major illness or surgery, or for 3 weeks when the patient has had a minor illness. In pregnancy, it is customary to defer routine lipid evaluation until after delivery because of physiologic dyslipidemia (see Chapter 18), although evaluation should be done when there is a history of hypertriglyceridemia because of the risk for acute pancreatitis with very high TG concentrations.

Major lipid values are reported in conventional units (mg/dL) or Système International (SI) units (mmol/L). Conversion values between mg/dL and mmol/L are 0.02586 for cholesterol (including TC, LDL-C, and HDL-C) and 0.01129 for TG (as multipliers from conventional to SI, and as divisors from SI to conventional). (See also Chart 1 on page 401.)

Triglyceride and Chylomicrons

Measurement of TG requires a 9- to 12-hour fast (water and calorie-free liquids permitted) because of the postprandial fluctuation of TG concentration. Visual inspection of the sample should not be neglected. Chylomicronemia can be recognized by refrigerating the plasma or serum for 12 hours; the finding of a creamy supernatant indicates the presence of chylomicrons. A simple rule of thumb is that TG greater than 300 mg/dL confers turbidity to plasma. For practical purposes, chylomicrons can be assumed to be present when fasting TG exceeds 1,000 mg/dL. No reliable and practical sophisticated laboratory tests are available to recognize chylomicronemia, although the occurrence of apo B-48 is specific for chylomicrons and their remnants.

Low-Density Lipoprotein

The two common methods of laboratory determination of LDL-C concentration combine the cholesterol contributions of LDL, IDL, and Lp[a] into a single value. The methods are ultracentrifugation to separate

VLDL at a density of 1.006 g/mL, with precipitation of apo B–containing particles to separate HDL (Lipid Research Clinics Program 1982), and use of the Friedewald formula (Friedewald et al. 1972):

$$\text{LDL-C (mg/dL)} = \text{TC} - \text{HDL-C} - (\text{TG}/5)$$
$$\text{or}$$
$$\text{LDL-C (mmol/L)} = \text{TC} - \text{HDL-C} - (\text{TG}/2.2)$$

The Friedewald formula does not apply if

- TG exceeds 400 mg/dL,
- Fredrickson type III hyperlipidemia is present, or
- Apo $E_{2/2}$ phenotype is present.

In each of these instances, direct determination of the LDL-C value is warranted. A high Lp[a] value diminishes the accuracy of the Friedewald formula; under these circumstances, the calculated LDL-C value should be adjusted to reflect the contribution of Lp[a] cholesterol (Gotto et al. 1995), if known:

$$\text{LDL-C (mg/dL)} = \text{LDL-C (calculated)} - (\text{Lp[a]}/3)$$

Lp[a] below 30 mg/dL is desirable. Typically, about 10–15% of the cholesterol in estimated LDL-C is in IDL (Grundy 1997). Summing IDL-C and LDL-C seems acceptable because IDL may rival LDL in atherogenic potential (Kirchmair et al. 1995; Hodis et al. 1997). Inherent in precipitation methods, the HDL-C value is not precise, particularly against a background of elevated TG, whether representing postprandial lipemia or endogenous hypertriglyceridemia. Direct measurement of LDL can also be accomplished by immunoprecipitation, in which VLDL is precipitated by using anti–apo C, then HDL is precipitated by using anti–apo A-I and anti–apo A-II. The immunoprecipitation method is much faster and less expensive than ultracentrifugation.

   LDL apo B concentration accurately defines LDL particle number, because there is one molecule of apo B-100 per LDL particle. The ratio of cholesterol to apo B protein in LDL varies interindividually (Abate et al. 1993). In small, dense LDL, cholesterol is reduced; thus, in LDL phenotype B, in which small, dense LDL particles predominate, LDL-C concentration may inadequately reflect the number of LDL particles. Although determination of the plasma concentration of small, dense LDL is not routinely done in most clinical laboratories, the value can easily be obtained by nondenaturing gel electrophoresis (Nichols et al. 1986). As a rule of thumb, a preponderance of small, dense LDL in the LDL fraction is likely when fasting TG exceeds 190 mg/dL and normal LDL is likely when fasting TG is below 105 mg/dL (Gotto et al. 1995).

Non–High-Density Lipoprotein Cholesterol

Some investigators have suggested that non-HDL-C—that is, LDL-C + IDL-C + VLDL-C, a measure of all lipoproteins that contain apo B (Grundy

1997)—is a better representation of "atherogenic cholesterol" than is LDL-C (Havel and Rapaport 1995; Abate et al. 1993; Garg and Grundy 1990). The summed cholesterol content of LDL + IDL + VLDL strongly correlates with total apo B concentration (Abate et al. 1993; Vega and Grundy 1990). As discussed in Chapter 8, IDL and some lipoproteins in the VLDL class are probably atherogenic; larger VLDL particles, which are TG rich, are probably less directly atherogenic (Grundy 1997). Moreover, elevated TG induces modifications in other lipoproteins (including reduced HDL-C concentration and conversion of LDL to small LDL) and may produce a procoagulant state (Grundy 1997). At present, routine laboratory measurements cannot distinguish whether hypertriglyceridemia is caused by small or large particles.

Lipoprotein Profiles by Nuclear Magnetic Resonance Spectroscopy

Applications of nuclear magnetic resonance (NMR)-based analyzing techniques are growing in medicine as in other fields. In atherosclerotic disease, NMR is of interest for analysis of the composition, function, and concentration of plasma lipoproteins (Otvos 1997; de Certaines et al. 1996; Engan 1996) as well as for in vivo imaging of human plaque components (see Chapter 7). For measurement of plasma lipoproteins, NMR competes with a variety of methods, including ultracentrifugation, chromatography, electrophoresis, and various immunochemical techniques. Its advantages in this application include short analysis time (with ^{1}H NMR spectroscopy, processing takes at most a few minutes), information-rich spectra that provide data on multiple chemical compounds and lipoprotein species simultaneously, no need for complex processing of samples, and small sample requirements (samples, moreover, remain intact) (Engan 1996). An obvious disadvantage is the large capital cost of the spectrometer and the need for complex software for data analysis (Engan 1996), although high sample throughput can make the methodology cost-effective. However, there may be significant cost savings in time and labor compared with traditional lipoprotein measurement methods, which all require physical separation steps. The techniques most commonly used for subclass fractionation often take several hours to several days to complete, and usually only partial resolution of the subclasses is achieved; accuracy and precision are limited by the sources of analytic error during the separation process (Otvos 1997).

Fourier transform ^{1}H NMR has the potential to replace ultracentrifugal fractionation of lipoproteins if it stands the test of multicenter trials (de Certaines et al. 1996). (For brief reviews of technical problems and alternatives in NMR analysis of lipoproteins, see de Certaines et al. 1996 and Engan 1996.) Using methyl lipid resonances (e.g., fatty acyl and cholesteryl), Otvos and colleagues (Otvos et al. 1991, 1992, 1996; Otvos 1997) have demonstrated that the major lipoprotein classes have NMR spectra distinct enough to be quantifiable by computer-assisted lineshape analysis (de Certaines et al. 1996). Because the method entails a fitting procedure, a priori knowledge of lineshapes for different lipoprotein fractions is required. Preliminary results have shown good agreement between chemically measured and NMR-calculated lipoprotein concentrations (de Certaines et al. 1996); correlation coefficients are typically in the range of 0.91–0.95 for LDL-C and 0.93–0.97 for HDL-C (Otvos 1997).

Development work on the process by Otvos and colleagues is now largely complete. The process uses a dedicated intermediate-field (400-MHz) NMR spectrometer to quantify chylomicrons and 15 subclasses of VLDL, LDL, and HDL. The measurement step, performed automatically on serum or plasma samples (approximately 0.5 mL) takes less than 1 minute, and the deconvolution and calculation steps (performed on the digitized data using specialized analysis software running off-line on a personal computer) require only a few seconds. It is important to note that the subclasses represent groupings of particles of similar but not identical size; there is no implication of metabolic distinctness (Otvos 1997). HDL subclasses are the best resolved spectroscopically, followed by VLDL subclasses. LDL subclasses are the least distinct spectrally, although a clear distinction can be made between individuals with predominantly large or small particles (LDL phenotypes A and B) (presented by James D. Otvos, PhD, to the Interdisciplinary Council on Reducing the Risk for Coronary Heart Disease, 9th meeting, Washington, DC, September 6–7, 1997). The approximate diameters (in nanometers) of the subclasses quantified by NMR, defined by electron microscopy and polyacrylamide gel electrophoresis, are chylomicrons greater than 220, V6 = 150 ± 70, V5 = 70 ± 10, V4 = 50 ± 10, V3 = 38 ± 3, V2 = 33 ± 2, V1 = 29 ± 2, where V signifies VLDL; IDL = 25 ± 2; L3 = 22 ± 0.7, L2 = 20.5 ± 0.7, L1 = 19 ± 0.7, where L signifies LDL (corresponding to large, intermediate, and small LDL); H5 = 11.5 ± 1.5, H4 = 9.4 ± 0.6, H3 = 8.5 ± 0.3, H2 = 8.0 ± 0.2, H1 = 7.5 ± 0.2, where H signifies HDL (corresponding to the 2b, 2a, 3a, 3b, and 3c HDL subclasses). Lp[a], which may be an independent predictor of risk for CHD, cannot be distinguished from LDL (Otvos 1997). Also, the NMR method is insensitive to the exchange of cholesteryl esters for TGs (presented to the Interdisciplinary Council, September 1997). Subclass concentrations are summed to provide values for TC, LDL-C, and HDL-C, total TG, VLDL TG, and LDL particle concentration (analogous to the information supplied by measuring apo B concentration), and average particle diameters are provided for VLDL, LDL, and HDL (Otvos 1997). All these data are provided in the NMR LipoProfile™ printout, which is now commercially available (LipoMed, Inc., Raleigh, NC).

There is hope that measurement of lipoprotein subclasses, such as that provided by NMR analysis, may eventually help improve the recognition of individuals at increased risk for CHD. As discussed in Chapter 8, evidence suggests that small, dense LDL is a risk factor for CHD. Within the HDL family, risk may also vary according to size, density, or composition (Tailleux and Fruchart 1996; Roheim and Asztalos 1995). A recent NMR study (Freedman et al. 1998) supports earlier reports (Wilson et al. 1990; Johansson et al. 1991) that concentrations of subclasses of small HDL are positively associated with the severity of CHD; thus, unlike larger HDL, small HDL particles may not provide protection against disease. The HDL_2:HDL_3 ratio appears to be a reliable indicator of the efficiency of postprandial lipolysis, which evidence suggests to be related to the risk for CHD (Patsch et al. 1983; Kirchmair et al. 1995), but measurement of HDL_2 and HDL_3 cholesterol may offer no advantage over total HDL-C for prediction of CHD (Wilson 1995). It is not yet recommended that clinicians extend measurement of HDL-C to include the determination of HDL subclasses (NCEP 1994; von Eckardstein et al. 1994). In addition, as discussed in Chapter 8, increased concentrations of IDL (VLDL remnants) have been associated with increased risk, and the TGRLs are increasingly recognized for their heterogeneous roles in atherosclerosis. As noted, IDL is operationally part of the LDL fraction as measured by standard methods (see "Low-Density Lipoprotein"). NMR has promising potential for rapid measurement of plasma lipoprotein classes and subclasses. The next few years will show whether risk estimation will be enhanced by such subclass information and whether NMR will be recommended for use in clinical laboratories.

Suggested Reading

Betteridge DJ, ed. Lipids: current perspectives. St. Louis: Mosby, 1996.

Durrington PN. Hyperlipidaemia: diagnosis and management, ed. 2. Oxford: Butterworth–Heinemann, 1995.

Grundy SM. Small LDL, atherogenic dyslipidemia, and the metabolic syndrome (editorial). Circulation 1997;95:1–4.

Humphries SE, Galton D, Nicholls P. Genetic testing for familial hypercholesterolaemia: practical and ethical issues (review). QJM 1997;90:169–181.

Jialal I. A practical approach to the laboratory diagnosis of dyslipidemia (review). Clin Chem 1996;106:128–138.

Mancini M, Steiner G, Betteridge DJ, Pometta D. Acquired (secondary) forms of hypertriglyceridemia (review). Am J Cardiol 1991;68(suppl):18A–21A.

Packard CJ, Shepherd J. Current concepts in the treatment of familial hypercholesterolaemia (review). Curr Opin Lipidol 1995;6:57–61.

Rader DJ. Gene therapy for atherosclerosis (review). Int J Clin Lab Res 1997; 27:35–43.

Rifai N, Warnick GR, Dominiczak MH, eds. Handbook of lipoprotein testing. Washington, DC: AACC Press, 1997. (Available from the American Association for Clinical Chemistry, telephone 202-857-0717.)

Schaefer EJ. Familial lipoprotein disorders and premature coronary artery disease. Med Clin North Am 1994;78:21–39.

Scriver CR, Beaudet AL, Sly WS, Valle D, eds. The metabolic and molecular bases of inherited disease, ed. 7, vol. 2. New York: McGraw-Hill, 1995. (See Part 8: Lipoprotein and lipid metabolism disorders, pp. 1841–2099.)

Zannis VI, Kardassis D, Zanni EE. Genetic mutations affecting human lipoproteins, their receptors, and their enzymes (review). Adv Hum Genet 1993;21:145–319.

REFERENCES

Abate N et al. Atherosclerosis 1993;104:159–171.

Abbott RD et al. JAMA 1988;260:3456–3460. Erratum JAMA 1989;261:1884.

Allan R, Scheidt S. In: Manson JE et al., eds. Prevention of myocardial infarction. New York: Oxford University Press, 1996:274–299.

Allen SS et al. for the Transdermal Nicotine Study Group. Prev Med 1994;23:190–196.

American Cancer Society. Cancer facts and figures—1995. Atlanta: American Cancer Society, 1995.

American Cancer Society. Cancer facts and figures—1998. Atlanta: American Cancer Society, 1998.

American College of Physicians. Ann Intern Med 1996;124:515–517.

American Heart Association. 1997 heart and stroke statistical update. Dallas: American Heart Association, 1996.

American Heart Association. 1998 heart and stroke statistical update. Dallas: American Heart Association, 1997.

Andersson L-O. Curr Opin Lipidol 1997;8:225–228.

Angelin B. Curr Opin Lipidol 1997;8:337–341.

Antiplatelet Trialists' Collaboration. BMJ 1994;308:81–106.

Ashraf T et al. Am J Cardiol 1996;78:409–414.

Assmann G, Brewer HB Jr. Am J Cardiol 1991;68(suppl):13A–16A.

Assmann G, Schulte H. Am J Cardiol 1992;70:733–737.

Assmann G et al. Curr Opin Lipidol 1990;1:110–115.

Assmann G et al. Curr Opin Lipidol 1991;2:110–117.

Assmann G et al. In: Scriver CR et al., eds. The metabolic and molecular bases of inherited disease, ed. 7, vol. 2. New York: McGraw-Hill, 1995:2053–2072.

Assmann G et al. Atherosclerosis 1996;124(suppl):S11–S20.

Assmann G et al. Eur Heart J 1998;19(suppl A):A2–A11.

Austin MA et al. Am J Cardiol 1998;81(4A):7B–12B.

Bakris GL. Curr Opin Nephrol Hypertens 1996;5:219–223.

Ballantyne CM, Aby Y. J Cardiovasc Risk 1997;4:353–356

Barter PJ, Rye K-A. Atherosclerosis 1996;121:1–12.

Bassen FA, Kornzweig AL. Blood 1950;5:381–387.

Beilin LJ. J Hypertens Suppl 1994;12:S71–S81.

Benfante R. Hum Biol 1992;64:791–805.

Benlian P et al. N Engl J Med 1996;335:848–854.

Ben-Shlomo Y et al. Am J Public Health 1994;84:1235–1242.

Berg A et al. Eur J Med Res 1997;2:259–264.

Betteridge DJ. In: Betteridge DJ, ed. Lipids: current perspectives. St. Louis: Mosby, 1996:261–271.

Bijvoet S et al. J Lipid Res 1996;37:640–650.

Bild DE, Williams RR, eds. Am J Cardiol 1993;72(suppl):1D–84D.

Blair SN et al. JAMA 1989;262:2395–2401.

Blair SN et al. JAMA 1995;273:1093–1098.

Blauw GJ et al. Stroke 1997;28:946–950.

Bolinder G et al. Am J Public Health 1994;84:399–404.

Bolumar F et al. Am J Epidemiol 1996;143:578–587.

Bonita R. BMJ 1994;309:684–685.

Botts ML, Grobbee DE. J Cardiovasc Risk 1996;3:271–276.

Boyle P. Lung Cancer 1997;17:1–60.

Bradford RH et al. Arch Intern Med 1991;151:43–49.

Braunwald E. N Engl J Med 1997;337:1360–1369.

Breslow JL. In: Scriver CR et al., eds. The metabolic and molecular bases of inherited disease, ed. 7, vol. 2. New York: McGraw-Hill, 1995:2031–2052.

Brunzell JD. In: Scriver CR et al., eds. The metabolic and molecular bases of inherited disease, ed. 7, vol. 2. New York: McGraw-Hill, 1995:1913–1932.

Bucher H et al. Eur J Pediatr 1997;156:121–125.

Bucher HC et al. Ann Intern Med 1998;128:89–95.

Burke GL et al. Stroke 1995;26:386–391.

Burt V et al. Hypertension 1995;26:60–69.

Byington RP et al. Circulation 1995;92:2419–2425.

Canner PL et al. J Am Coll Cardiol 1986; 8:1245–1255.

Carey DGP. Curr Opin Lipidol 1998;9:35–40.

Carlson LA, Rosenhamer G. Acta Med Scand 1988; 223:405–418.

Carstensen JM et al. J Epidemiol Community Health 1987;41:166–172.

Castelli WP. Am J Med 1984;76(2A):4–12.

Castelli WP. Atherosclerosis 1996;124:S1–S9.

Chait A, Brunzell JD. Adv Intern Med 1991;37:249–273.

Chambless LE et al. Am J Epidemiol 1992;136:1069–1081.

Chen ZM et al. BMJ 1991;303:276–282.

Cleeman JI, Grundy SM. Circulation 1997;95:1646–1650.

Collins R et al. Lancet 1990;335:827–838.

Comuzzie AG, Allison DB. Science 1998;280:1374–1377.

Connor WE, Connor SL. Am J Cardiol 1993;72:43D–53D.

Cook PJ, Lip GY. QJM 1996;89:727–735.

Coronary Drug Project Research Group. JAMA 1975;231:360–381.

Craig WY et al. BMJ 1989;298:784–788.

Criqui MH. Eur Heart J 1998;19(suppl A):A36–A39.

Crouse JR III et al. Arch Intern Med 1997;157:1305–1310.

D'Agostino RB Jr et al. Presented at the American Heart Association 38th Annual Conference on Cardiovascular Disease Epidemiology and Prevention, Santa Fe, NM, March 18–21, 1998.

Daly PA et al. In: Manson JE et al., eds. Prevention of myocardial infarction. New York: Oxford University Press, 1996:203–240.

Dattilo AM, Kris-Etherton M. Am J Clin Nutr 1992;56:320–328.

Davignon J, Cohn JS. Atherosclerosis 1996;124(suppl):S57–S64.

de Bruin TWA et al. In: Betteridge DJ, ed. Lipids: current perspectives. St. Louis: Mosby, 1996:101–114.

de Certaines JD et al. Anticancer Res 1996;16:1451–1460.

de Graaf J, Stalenhoef AFH. Curr Opin Lipidol 1998;9:189–196.

Delanty N, Vaughan CJ. Stroke 1997;28:2315–2320.

de Maat MP et al. Atherosclerosis 1996;121:185–191.

Denke MA, Grundy SM. Ann Intern Med 1990;112:780–792.

de Wolfe VG. Cardiovasc Clin 1983;13:15–35.

Djurovic S, Berg K. Clin Genet 1997;52:281–292.

Dobkin B. Neurology 1995;45(suppl 1):S6–S9.

Downs JR et al. JAMA 1998;279:1615–1622.

Duell PB, Malinow MR. Curr Opin Lipidol 1997;8:28–34.

Durrington PN. Hyperlipidaemia: diagnosis and management, ed. 2. Oxford: Butterworth–Heinemann, 1995.

Eaker ED et al. Circulation 1993;88:1999–2009.

Eaton CB et al. J Am Board Fam Pract 1996;9:312–318.

Eckel RH for the Nutrition Committee. Circulation 1997;96:3248–3250.

Eckel RH, Krauss RM for the AHA Nutrition Committee. Circulation 1998;97:2099–2100.

Economides D, Braithwaite J. J R Soc Health 1994;114:198–201.

Ellis RW. J Med Microbiol 1997;46:535–539.

Engan T. Anticancer Res 1996;16:1461–1472.

Evans WJ. J Gerontol A Biol Sci Med Sci 1995;50:147–150.

Expert Panel on Detection, Evaluation, and Treatment of High Blood Cholesterol in Adults. JAMA 1993;269:3015–3023.

Fagerberg B et al. Am J Hypertens 1998;11:14–22.

Feher MD et al. J R Soc Med 1990;83:146–148.

Ferro-Luzzi A, Martino L. Ciba Found Symp 1996;201:207–227.

Feussner G et al. Genet Epidemiol 1997;14:283–297.

Fielding JE. N Engl J Med 1985;313:491–498, 555–561.

Fletcher GF et al. Circulation 1995;91:580–615.

Fletcher GF et al. Circulation 1996;94:857–862.

Foger B, Patsch JR. J Cardiovasc Risk 1995;2:316–322.

Forster DP, Józan P. Lancet 1990;335:458–460.

Fowkes FGR et al. BMJ 1998;316:1764.

Franceschini G et al. J Clin Invest 1980;66:892–900.

Fredricsson B, Gilljam H. Acta Obstet Gynecol Scand 1992;71:580–592.

Freedman DS et al. Arterioscler Thromb Vasc Biol 1998;18:1046–1053.

Freund KM et al. Ann Epidemiol 1993;3:417–424.

Frick MH et al. N Engl J Med 1987; 317:1237–1245.

Friedewald WT et al. Clin Chem 1972;18:499–502.

Funke H. Curr Opin Lipidol 1997;8:189–196.

Fuster V, Pearson TA. J Am Coll Cardiol 1996;27:957–1047.

Garber AM et al. Ann Intern Med 1996;124:518–531.

Garg A, Grundy SM. Diabetes Care 1990;13:153–169.

Garrison RJ, Castelli WP. Ann Intern Med 1985;103:1006–1009.

Garrison RJ et al. Curr Opin Lipidol 1996;7:199–202.

Gibbons GH, Dzau VJ. Science 1996;272:689–693.

Ginter E. Eur J Epidemiol 1995;11:199–205.

Glantz SA, Parmley WW. Circulation 1991;83:1–12.

Glomset JA et al. In: Scriver CR et al., eds. The metabolic and molecular bases of inherited disease, ed. 7, vol. 2. New York: McGraw-Hill, 1995:1933–1951.

Glueck CJ et al. Metab Clin Exp 1997;46:625–633.

Goldman L, Cook EF. Ann Intern Med 1984;101:825–830.

Goldman L et al. Circulation 1992;85:1960–1968.

Goldstein JL, Brown MS. Proc Natl Acad Sci U S A 1973;70:2804–2808.

Goldstein JL, Brown MS. Annu Rev Genet 1979;13:259–289.

Goldstein JL, Brown MS. J Lipid Res 1985;25:1450–1461.

Goldstein JL et al. J Clin Invest 1973;52:1533–1543, 1544–1568, 1569–1577.

Goldstein JL et al. In: Scriver CR et al., eds. The metabolic and molecular bases of inherited disease, ed. 7, vol. 2. New York: McGraw-Hill, 1995:1981–2030.

Goodrick GK et al. Nutrition 1996;12:672–676.

Gordon DJ et al. Circulation 1989;79:8–15.

Gordon T et al. JAMA 1977;238:497–499.

Gotto AM Jr. Cleve Clin J Med 1996;63:31–41.

Gotto AM Jr. Arch Intern Med 1997a;157:1283–1284.

Gotto AM Jr. Circulation 1997b;96:4424–4430.

Gotto AM Jr, Grundy SM. Lowering LDL cholesterol: questions from recent subset and meta-analyses of clinical trial data. Circulation, in press.

Gotto AM Jr et al. The ILIB lipid handbook for clinical practice: blood lipids and coronary heart disease. Houston: International Lipid Information Bureau, 1995.

Gould AL et al. Circulation 1995;91:2274–2282.

Gross NJ. Chest 1990;97(2 suppl):19S–23S.

Grundy SM. Circulation 1997;95:1–4.

Grundy SM. Am J Clin Nutr 1998;67(suppl):563S–572S.

Grundy SM et al. Circulation 1997a;95:1683–1685.

Grundy SM et al. Circulation 1997b;95:2329–2331.

Grundy SM et al. Circulation 1998;97:1876–1887.

Haffner SM et al. N Engl J Med 1998;339:229–234.

Hahn RA et al. JAMA 1990;264:2654–2659.

Hamsten A, Karpe F. In: Betteridge DJ, ed. Lipids: current perspectives. St. Louis: Mosby, 1996:43–68.

Han TS et al. Int J Obes Relat Metabol Disord 1997;21:587–593.

Havel RJ. J Am Coll Cardiol 1998;31:1258–1259.

Havel RJ, Rapaport E. N Engl J Med 1995;332:1491–1498.

Hay JW et al. Circulation 1997;96(suppl. I):I-184.

Hayden MR et al. Curr Opin Lipidol 1991;2:104–109.

Hebert P et al. Arch Intern Med 1993;153:578–581.

Hebert PR et al. JAMA 1997;278:313–321.

Heinrich J, Assmann G. J Cardiovasc Risk 1995;2:197–205.

Herliz J et al. Cardiology 1992;80:237–245.

Hertzer NR et al. Arch Surg 1979;114:1336–1344.

Higgins M. Ann N Y Acad Sci 1991;624:7–17.

Hill JO, Peters JC. Science 1998;280:1371–1374.

Hodis HN, Mack WJ. Eur Heart J 1998;19 (suppl A):A40–A44.

Hodis HN et al. Circulation 1997;95:2022–2026.

Hodis HN et al. Ann Intern Med 1998;128:262–269.

Hoffmann D, Hoffmann I. J Toxicol Environ Health 1997;50:307–364.

Hornig B et al. Circulation 1996;93:210–214.

Humphries SE et al. Q J Med 1997;90:169–181.

Husten CG et al. J Am Med Womens Assoc 1996;51:11–18.

Hwang SJ et al. Circulation 1997;96:4219–4225.

Illingworth DR et al. Arch Intern Med 1994;154:1586–1595.

International Task Force. Nutr Metab Cardiovasc Dis 1992;2:113–156.

Jacobs D et al. Circulation 1992;86:1046–1060.

Jacobs DR Jr et al. Am J Epidemiol 1982;116:878–885.

Jacobson TA et al. Maximizing the cost-effectiveness of lipid-lowering therapy. Arch Intern Med, in press.

Jamrozik K. Med J Aust 1995;163:643–645.

Jemaa R et al. J Lipid Res 1995;36:2141–2146.

Johannesson M et al. for the Scandinavian Simvastatin Survival Study Group. N Engl J Med 1997;336:332–336.

Johansson J et al. Arterioscler Thromb 1991;11:174–182.

Johnson CL et al. JAMA 1993;269:3002–3008.

Joint National Committee. Arch Intern Med 1993;153:154–183.

Jones PH et al. In: Alexander RW et al., eds. Hurst's the heart, arteries and veins, ed. 9. New York: McGraw-Hill, 1998:1553–1581.

Juhan-Vague I. Atherosclerosis 1996;124(suppl):S49–55.

Julius S. Am J Hypertens 1996;9(suppl):41S–44S.

Jung RT. Br Med Bull 1997;53:307–321.

Kane JP, Havel RJ. In: Scriver CR et al., eds. The metabolic and molecular bases of inherited disease, ed. 7, vol. 2. New York: McGraw-Hill, 1995:1853–1885.

Kannel WB. Am J Med 1983;75(suppl 3A):4–11.

Kannel WB. Cardiol Elderly 1993;1:359–363.

Kannel WB. Am J Cardiol 1995;76(suppl):69C–77C.

Kannel WB et al. J Card Rehabil 1984;4:267–277.

Kaplan GA, Keil JE. Circulation 1993;88:1973–1998.

Kaplan NM. J Hypertens 1995;13(suppl 2):S1–S5.

Kesäniemi YA. Am J Cardiol 1998;81(4A):70B–73B.

Keys A. Seven Countries. Cambridge, MA: Harvard University Press, 1980.

Kirchmair R et al. Baillieres Clin Endocrinol Metab 1995;9:705–719.

Klag MJ et al. N Engl J Med 1993;328:313–8.

Klein HG et al. J Biol Chem 1995;270:9443–9447.

Kohrt WM, Holloszy JO. J Gerontol A Biol Sci Med Sci 1995;50:68–72.

Kôrv J et al. Stroke 1996;27:199–203.

Kottke TE. J Am Coll Cardiol 1997;30:131–2.

Kottke TE et al. Mayo Clin Proc 1997;72:515–523.

Kramsch DM et al. N Engl J Med 1981;305:1483–1489.

Kritz H et al. Arch Intern Med 1995;155:1942–1948.

Kuczmarski RJ et al. JAMA 1994;273:205–211.

Kuinenhoven JA et al. J Lipid Res 1997;38:191–205.

Kupersmith J et al. Prog Cardiovasc Dis 1995;37:243–271.

Kwiterovich PO Jr. Curr Opin Lipidol 1993;4:133–143.

Lakier JB. Am J Med 1992;93(suppl 1A):8S–12S.

Lam TH et al. JAMA 1997;278:1505–1508.

LaRosa JC. Ann Intern Med 1996;124:505–508.

Lauer MS et al. Circulation 1997;96:897–903.

Lavie CJ et al. Clin Geriatr Med 1996;12:57–68.

Law MR, Hackshaw AK. Br Med Bull 1996;52:22–34.

Law MR et al. BMJ 1994;308:367–379.

Lee IM et al. JAMA 1993;270:2823–2828.

Lee IM et al. JAMA 1995;273:1179–1184.

Leng GC et al. Int J Epidemiol 1996;25:1172–1181.

Levy D, Kannel WB. Am Heart J 1988;116:266–272.

Levy D et al. Ann Intern Med 1989;110:101–107.

Levy E. Clin Invest Med 1996;19:317–324.

Lew EA, Garfinkel L. J Chronic Dis 1979;32:563–576.

Lewis B et al., eds. Low blood cholesterol: health implications. London: Current Medical Literature, 1993.

Lipid Research Clinics Program. Manual of laboratory operations: lipid and lipoprotein analysis, ed. 2. DHEW publication no. NIH 75-628. Washington, DC: U.S. Government Printing Office, 1982.

Lipid Research Clinics Program. JAMA 1984a;251:351–364.

Lipid Research Clinics Program. JAMA 1984b;251:365–374.

The LIPID Study Group. Am J Cardiol 1995;76:474–479.

Mackinnon LT et al. Med Sci Sports Exerc 1997;29:1429–1436.

MacMahon S et al. Lancet 1990;335:765–774.

MacMahon S et al. Circulation 1998;97:1784–1790.

Mahley RW, Rall SC Jr. In: Scriver CR et al., eds. The metabolic and molecular bases of inherited disease, ed. 7, vol. 2. New York: McGraw-Hill, 1995:1953–1980.

Manninen V et al. JAMA 1988;260:641–651.

Manninen V et al. Circulation 1992;85:37–45.

Manson JE et al. N Engl J Med 1992;326:1406–1416.

Manson JE et al. N Engl J Med 1995;333:677–685.

Manson JE et al. In: Manson JE et al., eds. Prevention of myocardial infarction. New York: Oxford University Press, 1996:3–31.

Martens LL, Guibert R. Clin Ther 1995;17:572–580.

Martys R. Wien Med Wochenschr 1994;144:556–560.

Mayer-Davis EJ et al. JAMA 1998;279:669–674.

McBride PE. Med Clin North Am 1992;76:333–353.

McGinnis JM, Foege WH. JAMA 1993;270:2207–2212.

Menotti A et al. Eur Heart J 1997;18:566–571.

Mentis SW. Anesth Analg 1996;83:427–429.

Miettinen H et al. Diabetes Care 1998;21:69–75.

Miller M et al. J Am Coll Cardiol 1998;31:1252–1257.

Moffatt RJ. Atherosclerosis. 1988;74:85–89.

Morris JN et al. Br Heart J 1990;63:325–334.

Mueller HS et al. J Am Coll Cardiol 1995;26:900–907.

Muldoon MF et al. BMJ 1990;301:309–314.

Murabito JM. J Am Med Womens Assoc 1995;50:35–39.

National Cholesterol Education Program. Circulation 1994;89:1329–1445.

National Health Center for Health Statistics. Third National Health and Nutrition Examination Survey, 1988–94, US NHANES III Examination Data File [CD-ROM]. DHHS public use data file 76200. Hyattsville, MD: Centers for Disease Control and Prevention, 1996.

National Heart, Lung, and Blood Institute Cholesterol Awareness Surveys, 1995. NHLBI press conference information, Bethesda, MD, December 4, 1995.

National Institutes of Health. The lipid research clinics population studies data book: The Prevalence Study. Publication no. 79-1527. Bethesda, MD: National Institutes of Health, 1979.

National Institutes of Health. The sixth report of the Joint National Committee on Prevention, Detection, Evaluation, and Treatment of High Blood Pressure. NIH publication no. 98-4080 (November 1997). Bethesda, MD: National Institutes of Health, 1997.

National Institutes of Health. Clinical guidelines on the identification, evaluation, and treatment of overweight and obesity in adults. Bethesda, MD: National Institutes of Health, 1998.

Neaton JD, Wentworth D. Arch Intern Med 1992;152:56–64.

Nichols AV et al. Methods Enzymol 1986;128:417–431.

Nilsson P et al. J Intern Med 1996;240:189–194.

Njolstad I et al. Circulation 1996;93:450–456.

Nyboe J et al. Am Heart J 1991;122:438–447.

O'Connor GT et al. Circulation 1989;80:234–244.

O'Connor NJ et al. Circulation 1995;92:1458–1464.

Oldridge NB et al. JAMA 1988;260:945–950.

Otvos JD. In: Rifai N et al., eds. Handbook of lipoprotein testing. Washington, DC: AACC Press, 1997:497–508.

Otvos JD et al. Clin Chem 1991;37:377–386.

Otvos JD et al. Clin Chem 1992;38:1632–1638.

Otvos J et al. J Clin Lig Assay 1996;19:184–189.

Packard CJ, Shepherd J. Curr Opin Lipidol 1995;6:57–61.

Parazzini F et al. Int J Epidemiol 1991;20:157–161.

Pate RR et al. JAMA 1995;273:402–407.

Patsch JR et al. Proc Natl Acad Sci U S A 1983;80:1449–1453.

Pedersen TR et al. for the Scandinavian Simvastatin Survival Study Group. Circulation 1996;93:1796–1802.

Pedersen TR et al. Circulation 1998;97:1453–1460.

Pekkanen J et al. N Engl J Med 1990;322:1700–1707.

Pérez-Stable EJ et al. JAMA 1998;280:152–156.

Perkins KA et al. J Subst Abuse Treat 1997;14:173–182.

Peto R et al. Lancet 1992;339:1268–1278.

Peto R et al. Mortality from smoking in developed countries, 1950–2000: indirect estimates from national vital statistics. Oxford: Oxford University Press, 1994.

Peto R et al. Br Med Bull 1996;52:12–21.

Postiglione A, Napoli C. Curr Opin Lipidol 1995;6:236–242.

Pouliot MC et al. Am J Cardiol 1994;73:460–468.

Powell KE et al. Annu Rev Public Health 1987;8:253–287.

Prospective Studies Collaboration. Lancet 1995;346:1647–1653.

Puddey IB. Atherosclerosis 1996;119:1–6.

Pyörälä K et al. on behalf of the Task Force. Eur Heart J 1994;15:1300–1331.

Pyörälä K et al. Diabetes Care 1997;20:614–620.

Rastenyte D et al. Br Heart J 1992;68:516–523.

Reaven P et al. Am J Clin Nutr 1991;54:701–706.

Reymer PWA et al. Nat Genet 1995;10:28–34.

Ridker PM et al. N Engl J Med 1997;336:973–979.

Ridker PM et al. Lancet 1998;351:88–92.

Rigotti NA, Pasternak RC. Cardiol Clin 1996;14:51–68.

Rissanen P et al. Int J Obes Relat Metab Disord 1997;21:367–371.

Roberts KA et al. Circulation 1996;94:2248–2253.

Robinson JG, Leon AS. Med Clin North Am 1994;78:69–98.

Roehim PS, Asztalos BF. Clin Chem 1995;41:147–152.

Roma P et al. J Clin Invest 1993;91:1445–1452.

Rosengren A et al. Eur Heart J 1997;18:754–761.

Rossouw JE et al. N Engl J Med 1990;323:1112–1119.

Ryan TJ et al. J Am Coll Cardiol 1996;28:1328–1428.

Sacks FM et al. N Engl J Med 1996;335:1001–1009.

Sacks FM et al. Circulation 1998;97:1446–1452.

Samet JM. Med Clin North Am 1992;76:399–414.

Savage PJ. Curr Opin Cardiol 1998;13:131–138.

Scandinavian Simvastatin Survival Study Group. Lancet 1994;344:1383–1389.

Scandinavian Simvastatin Survival Study Group. Lancet 1995;345:1274–1275.

Schmeiser-Rieder A et al. Wien Med Wochenschr 1995;145:73–76.

Schonfeld G. Annu Rev Nutr 1995;15:23–34.

Seed M. In: Betteridge DJ, ed. Lipids: current perspectives. St. Louis: Mosby, 1996:69–88.

Sen S, Oppenheimer SM. Curr Opin Neurol 1998;11:51–56.

Shaper AG. Ciba Found Symp 1996;201:90–107.

Shaper AG et al. BMJ 1986;293:474–479.

Shepherd J et al. N Engl J Med 1995;333:1301–1307.

Sherman CB. Clin Chest Med 1991;12:643–658.

Skaar KL et al. Behav Med 1997;23:5–13.

Sleight P. J Hypertens 1996;14(suppl 2):S35–S39.

Smith SC Jr et al. Circulation 1995;92:2–4 and J Am Coll Cardiol 1995;26:292–294.

Sniderman AD et al. Ann Intern Med 1982;97:833–839.

Sniderman A et al. Am J Cardiol 1985;55:291–295.

Sørenson TIA. Metabolism 1995;44(suppl 3):4–6.

Sorgato F et al. Arterioscler Thromb 1992;12:529–533.

Soria LF et al. Proc Natl Acad Sci U S A 1989;86:587–591.

Spady DK, Dietschy JM. J Clin Invest 1988;81:300–309.

Srikanthan VS, Dunn FG. Med Clin North Am 1997;81:1147–1163.

Stamler J et al. Arch Intern Med 1993a;153:598–615.

Stamler J et al. Cardiology 1993b;82:191–222.

Stamler J et al. Circulation 1993c;88:1954–1960.

Steen T. Tidsskr Nor Laegeforen 1996;116:625–627.

Stefanick ML, Wood PD. In: Bouchard C et al., eds. Physical activity, fitness, and health. Champaign, IL: Human Kinetics, 1994:417–431.

Stein JH, Rosenson RS. Arch Intern Med 1997;157:1170–1176.

Stern M. Metab Clin Exp 1995;44(suppl 3):1–3.

Stevens J. Adv Exp Med Biol 1995;369:21–27.

Stevens J et al. N Engl J Med 1998;338:1–7.

Stoy NS. J R Coll Physicians Lond 1997;31:521–526.

Sundell G et al. Br J Obstet Gynaecol 1990;97:588–594.

Sytkowski PA et al. Am J Epidemiol 1996;143:338–350.

Tailleux A, Fruchart JC. Crit Rev Clin Lab Sci 1996;33:163–201.

Tell GS et al. Stroke 1988;19:423–430.

Tenkanen L et al. Circulation 1995;92:1779–1785.

Terres W et al. Am J Med 1994;97:242–249.

Thom TJ. Int J Epidemiol 1989;18:S20–S28.

Tracy RP et al. Arterioscler Thromb Vasc Biol 1997;17:1121–1127.

Tresch DD, Aronow WS. Clin Geriatr Med 1996;12:23–32.

Tsevat J. Am J Med 1992;93(suppl 1A):43S–47S.

Tunis SR et al. Ann Intern Med 1994;120:956–963.

U.S. Department of Health, Education, and Welfare. The health benefits of smoking cessation: a report of the Surgeon General. DHHS publication no. CDC 90-8416. Washington, DC: U.S. Department of Health and Human Services, 1990.

U.S. Surgeon General. Physical activity and health. Washington, DC: U.S. Department of Health and Human Services, 1996.

Vega GL, Grundy SM. Arteriosclerosis 1990;10:668–671.

Vega GL, Grundy SM. Curr Opin Lipidol 1996;7:209:216.

Verdecchia P et al. Hypertension 1994;24:793–801.

Visser M et al. Am J Clin Nutr 1995;61:772–778.

von Eckardstein A et al. Curr Opin Lipidol 1994;5:404–416.

Wagner RD et al. J Lipid Res 1991;32:1001–1011.

Wald NJ, Hackshaw AK. Br Med Bull 1996;52:3–11.

Wald NJ, Law MR. Atherosclerosis 1995;118(suppl):S1–S5.

Walden CC, Hegele RA. Ann Intern Med 1994;120:1026–1036.

Walter M et al. J Clin Invest 1996;98:2315–2323.

Weber MA. Am J Hypertens 1994;7(suppl):146S–153S.

Weintraub WS. Adv Exp Med Biol 1990;273:27–37.

West of Scotland Coronary Prevention Study Group. Lancet 1996;348:1339–1342.

West of Scotland Coronary Prevention Study Group. Am J Cardiol 1997;79:756–762.

West of Scotland Coronary Prevention Study Group. Circulation 1998;97:1440–1445.

Whelton PK et al. In: Manson JE et al., eds. Prevention of myocardial infarction. New York: Oxford University Press, 1996:154–171.

WHO Collaborative Study of Cardiovascular Disease and Steroid Hormone Contraception. Lancet 1997;349(9060):1202–1209.

WHO Principal Investigators. Br Heart J 1978;40:1069–1118.

WHO Principal Investigators. Lancet 1980;2:379–385.

WHO Principal Investigators. Lancet 1984;2:600–604.

Wijsman EM et al. Arterioscler Thromb Vasc Biol 1998;18:215–226.

Wilson HM et al. Biochem Soc Trans 1990;18:1175–1176.

Wilson PW. Clin Chem 1995;41:165–169.

Wilson PWF et al. Circulation 1998;97:1837–1847.

Wiman B. Thromb Haemost 1995;74:71–76.

Winslow E et al. Am J Med 1996;101(suppl 4A): 25S–33S.

Witschi H et al. Annu Rev Pharmacol Toxicol 1997;37:29–52.

Wong ND et al. Ann Intern Med 1991;115:687–693.

Wood PD. Med Sci Sports Exerc 1994;26:838–843.

Wood PD et al. N Engl J Med 1991;325:461–466.

World Health Organization. Hypertension control: report of a WHO Expert Committee. WHO Technical Report Series 862. Geneva: World Health Organization, 1996.

Worth RM et al. Am J Epidemiol 1975;102:481–490.

Wysowski DK, Gross TP. Arch Intern Med 1990;150:2169–2172.

Yudkin JS. J Diabetes Complications 1997;11:100–103.

Yusuf HR et al. Prev Med 1998;27:1–9.

Zulewski H et al. J Lipid Res 1998;39:380–387.

Therapeutic Interventions

Coronary disease does not really begin with crushing chest pain, pulmonary edema, shock, angina or ventricular fibrillation, but rather with more subtle signs like a poor coronary risk profile.

—William Kannel (1976)

A very substantial portion of the U.S. population is not yet receiving the preventive or therapeutic measures that have been proved to be effective against cardiovascular disease.

—Eugene Braunwald, Shattuck Lecture (1997)

References for Section IV (Chapters 15–17) begin on page 324.

Chapter 15

Dietary Modification

Dietary modification is the cornerstone of prevention and treatment of dyslipidemia. Its purpose is to reduce the risk for CHD by limiting the intake of saturated fat, cholesterol, and excess calories while maintaining a nutritious diet and an appropriate calorie level. According to some authorities, the typical American diet is a major cause of lipoprotein disorders leading to premature CHD in the United States. Lifestyle intervention in the NCEP guidelines (NCEP 1994) also emphasizes weight control, physical activity, and cessation of smoking, modifications that are detailed in Chapter 16. All these modifications have beneficial lipid effects (Table 15.1). In addition, weight reduction and exercise decrease blood pressure and the risk for diabetes mellitus. Physicians should instruct *all* patients about adopting healthy life habits to prevent the development or intensification of risk factors (Grundy et al. 1997b). Lifestyle measures are also the focus of population strategies to prevent CVD. Furthermore, although NCEP/AHA dietary guidelines were developed specifically for the prevention of CVD, they can contribute to prevention of other diseases such as some cancers, renal disease, and osteoporosis (Krauss et al. 1996).

The three most important dietary risk factors for atherosclerotic disease are saturated fat, cholesterol, and excess calories that lead to obesity. Although news media attention has helped increase public awareness of CHD risk factors, many patients may become confused about interventions of proved, major benefit and reports that represent simply trivial or preliminary data.

STEP I AND II DIETS

The NCEP uses a two-step cholesterol-lowering diet, as shown in Table 15.2. The emphasis is reducing intake of saturated fatty acids and cholesterol. *Trans* fatty acids should also be decreased. It is important to understand that the intake levels shown are to represent averages over a few days or a week. The Step I Diet is the dietary pattern recommended for all healthy people aged 2 years and older.

To decrease intake of saturated fat and cholesterol, the diet should include emphasis on consumption of

Table 15.1. MAJOR EFFECTS OF LIFESTYLE MODIFICATIONS ON PLASMA LIPIDS

Intervention	Major lipid benefit[a]		
	↓ LDL-C	↓ TG[b]	↑ HDL-C[c]
Decreased saturated fat	✓	✓	
Decreased dietary cholesterol	✓		
Decreased weight in overweight	✓	✓	✓
Increased physical activity	✓	✓	✓
Cessation of smoking[d]			✓

[a]Coordinate benefits of interventions include decreased blood pressure, increased glucose tolerance, decreased coronary thrombosis, likely inherent protection from CVD from weight control, exercise, and consumption of fruits, vegetables, and grains. Regular moderate exercise is an important component of weight control.
[b]For hypertriglyceridemia, decreased alcohol intake is beneficial in some patients; increased fatty fish consumption may be helpful; also emphasize smoking cessation.
[c]Physical inactivity, obesity, and smoking are major causes of secondary decreased HDL-C.
[d]Another major beneficial effect of smoking cessation is lowering of plasma fibrinogen concentration. Slight decreases of LDL-C were apparent in some studies.
Source: Gotto et al. 1995; used with permission.

- Vegetables and fruits
- Whole-grain breads, cereals, rice, legumes, and pasta
- Nonfat and low-fat dairy products
- Lean meat, skinless poultry, and fish

It appears prudent to replace most saturated and *trans* fatty acids by oils high in monounsaturated fatty acids, such as canola (rapeseed) oil and olive oil (Katan et al. 1997). Grundy (1997) notes that reducing intake of animal fat as well as gradually reducing intake of *trans* fatty acids should decrease levels of cholesterol-raising fatty acids by about one-third, from an average current U.S. intake level of about 12% to 7–8%. For the average American, simply changing selections in the dairy food group could reduce fat calories from 36% to 24% (Hyson and Mueller 1998). Also, evidence is available to indicate that consumption of vegetables, fruits, and grains may supply substances, such as plant sterols, flavonoids, sulfur-containing compounds, antioxidant vitamins, phytoestrogens, and trace minerals, that may protect against CHD (Howard and Kritchevsky 1997). In a cohort study by Key et al. (1996) in the United Kingdom, the all-cause mortality rate was reduced by about half at 17-year follow-up in the 11,000 vegetarians and health-conscious people recruited compared with the general population; daily consumption of fresh fruit significantly reduced death rates from

**Table 15.2. DIETARY THERAPY OF HYPERLIPIDEMIA:
NCEP/AHA STEP I AND II DIETS**

	Recommended intake	
Nutrient[a]	Step I Diet (primary prevention)	Step II Diet (primary or secondary prevention[b])
Total fat[c]	≤30% of total calories	
Saturated fatty acids	8–10% of total calories	<7% of total calories
Polyunsaturated fatty acids	≤10% of total calories	
Monounsaturated fatty acids	≤15% of total calories	
Carbohydrates	≥55% of total calories	
Protein	~15% of total calories	
Cholesterol	<300 mg/day	<200 mg/day
Total calories	Adults: to achieve and maintain desirable weight	
	Children and adolescents: to promote normal growth and development and to reach or maintain desirable weight	

Note: For cardiovascular health, it is also advisable to limit sodium intake to <2,400 mg/day and to limit alcohol intake to moderate levels (see Table 16.16).
[a]Calories from alcohol not included.
[b]The Step II Diet is initial dietary intervention in patients with atherosclerotic disease; it may be initial dietary intervention in primary prevention if the patient has already been complying with a diet equivalent to the Step I Diet.
[c]It is also advisable to limit intake of foods high in *trans* fatty acids.
Source: NCEP 1994.

CHD, cerebrovascular disease, and all causes. Healthy individuals should obtain adequate nutrient intake from foods eaten in balance, variety, and moderation. Vitamin and mineral supplements are not a substitute for a balanced, nutritious diet (Krauss et al. 1996).

If the patient is in compliance with the Step I Diet at the time of evaluation, or if the diet proves insufficient, the patient should proceed to the Step II Diet. The Step II Diet is initial dietary therapy in secondary prevention; too often, the Step I Diet may be prescribed inappropriately for patients with CHD. The Step II Diet more rigorously limits intake of saturated fat (to <7% of calories) and cholesterol (to <200 mg/day) but is otherwise identical to the Step I Diet. The Step II Diet may require a substantial modification of food choices; the advice of a registered dietitian is valuable in maximizing patient compliance and tailoring a diet that avoids less obvious sources of fat. The Step II Diet may be too rigorous for some elderly people; professional guidance is particularly important in this age group to ensure adequate nutrition.

Safety and Efficacy

Dietary modification judiciously used is a risk-free intervention whose efficacy has been demonstrated in clinical trials (for reviews see Denke 1995 and Willett 1990). In patients previously consuming a typical western diet, institution of the Step I Diet generally decreases TC 5–7%, and institution of the Step II Diet decreases TC an additional 3–7% (NCEP 1994). Response to diet, however, is highly variable: Some patients show dramatic lipid improvements, whereas others do not respond at all (Denke 1995). Emerging evidence supports genetic influences in interindividual variability of certain responses to diet, including weight loss and LDL-C reduction with a low-fat, low-cholesterol diet (Dreon and Krauss 1992).

Hypertriglyceridemia

Patients with hypertriglyceridemia may need more detailed dietary guidance, because intake of alcohol, carbohydrates (particularly simple carbohydrates), and saturated fat can all contribute to elevated TG. For these patients, increased emphasis should be placed on increasing the ratio of monounsaturated to saturated fatty acids, and on increasing the proportion of calories obtained from complex carbohydrates without increasing the total proportion of calories derived from all carbohydrates. Central to raising low concentrations of HDL-C are weight loss as necessary, increased physical activity, and cessation of smoking.

Follow-up

In patients with CHD or other atherosclerotic disease in whom LDL-C is 130 mg/dL or higher, withholding lipid-regulating drug therapy in an effort to lower cholesterol with lifestyle measures alone is not necessary; pharmacotherapy and lifestyle therapy may be initiated concurrently. When LDL-C is 100–129 mg/dL in secondary prevention, maximal dietary therapy with other lifestyle interventions may be tried for 6 weeks before consideration, according to clinical judgment, of drug therapy (Grundy et al. 1997a).

In general, in patients without atherosclerotic disease, dietary intervention must be allowed ample time to be effective before drug therapy is used, especially if significant weight loss is anticipated. Plasma cholesterol should be measured and patient compliance assessed 4–6 weeks and 3 months after the diet is initiated. For the purpose of monitoring treatment efficacy, TC is often a suitable surrogate for LDL-C. For most patients, TC concentrations of 240 and 200 mg/dL correspond roughly to LDL-C concentrations of 160 and 130 mg/dL. Initiating or changing therapy or verification of reaching a lipid goal requires fasting lipoprotein analysis. In most cases in primary prevention, at least 6 months of intensive dietary intervention is required to evaluate the program's effectiveness; however, patients with severe elevation of LDL-C (≥220 mg/dL) or otherwise at very high risk because of diabetes mellitus or a strong family history may be con-

sidered for pharmacotherapy in addition to intensive diet after shorter periods of diet alone (NCEP 1994). ADA recommendations regarding when to
consider lipid-regulating drug therapy are outlined in Chapter 21; the recommendations encompass beginning pharmacotherapy at the same time
as lifestyle therapy in diabetic patients who have other risk factors and an
averaged LDL-C value exceeding goal by more than 25 mg/dL.

Maximal lifestyle interventions need to be continued even when drug
therapy is used. Lifestyle modifications enhance drug actions and help
reduce risk for CVD through other mechanisms (Grundy et al. 1997a;
NCEP 1994).

Compliance

Enough studies of compliance to dietary regimens have shown positive results
to lead to the conclusion that meaningful dietary modification is possible
(Brownell and Cohen 1995). Among MRFIT participants, subjective ratings
and food record ratings showed 40–65% to be good or excellent adherers,
with declining compliance over time (Van Horn et al. 1997). Simply providing information is rarely sufficient to change dietary habits (Brownell and
Cohen 1995). Lowering fat and saturated fat intake to meet national guidelines can be daunting to both physician and patient, and success is most often
hindered by the complexity of dietary information and the challenge of translating guidelines into daily life (Hyson and Mueller 1998). A registered dietitian is a valuable resource for developing a practical strategy from the
confusing array of data* (Hyson and Mueller 1998). Tactics for enhancing
compliance with lipid-lowering therapeutic regimens are listed in Table 17.4.

Major Dietary Components in the Step I and Step II Diets

The actions of the diet on lipoprotein metabolism are complex, and they
are modified by an individual's overall nutritional status, primarily as
determined by the proportion of body fat and state of physical fitness.

Saturated Fatty Acids

Saturated fatty acid intake is the strongest dietary determinant of plasma
LDL-C concentration (Keys et al. 1965; Hegsted et al. 1965). Not all saturated
fatty acids, however, have the same effect on plasma cholesterol (NCEP 1994).
The major culprits in raising plasma cholesterol appear to be lauric acid
(12:0), myristic acid (14:0), and palmitic acid (16:0). Stearic acid (18:0)
appears to have no effect on plasma cholesterol. Nevertheless, the greatest
reductions in plasma cholesterol concentrations are seen not with the reduction of any particular saturated fat but with the reduction of total saturated fat
intake. Animal fats provide most of the saturated fat in the American diet,

---

*To identify a registered dietitian who can join or consult with your team, contact the
Consumer Nutrition Hotline at 1-800-366-1655 or the American Dietetic Association at
www.eatright.org (see "Find a Dietitian").

including butterfat (in butter, milk, cream, ice cream, and cheese) and the fat of beef, pork, lamb, and poultry. Plant oils that are high in saturated fat and that should be avoided include palm oil, palm kernel oil, and coconut oil.

The French Paradox. An apparent exception to the relation between consumption of saturated fat and CHD risk is France. Higher rates of coronary morbidity and mortality would be predicted there on the basis of the fat content of the diet, as well as plasma cholesterol, blood pressure, and prevalence of smoking that are not lower than in countries with higher CHD rates. The reason for the apparent discrepancy, or the so-called French paradox, is not known. Explanations proffered have included a protective effect of red wine, antioxidant, or garlic consumption and the method of death reporting (Burr 1995; Constant 1997). A cardioprotective effect of red wine may reside in its flavonoid content; resveratrol has antioxidant properties that are more potent than vitamin E. Grape juice has about half the amount of flavonoids, by volume, of red wine (Constant 1997).

Polyunsaturated Fatty Acids

The two major categories of polyunsaturated fat are omega-6 and omega-3 fatty acids. The major omega-6 fatty acid in the diet is linoleic acid, which when substituted for saturated fatty acids in the diet results in decreases in LDL-C. Vegetable oils rich in linoleic acid include soybean oil, corn oil, and high-linoleic forms of sunflower and safflower seed oils. Increased intake of linoleic acid is not recommended because of lack of epidemiologic data to support safety of higher intake. Moreover, linoleic acid can promote carcinogenesis in some animals and is prone to free radical oxidation in the body (Jones et al. 1998a). The AHA recommends that no more than 10% of total calories be consumed as polyunsaturated fatty acids (Table 15.2); other authorities recommend that consumption not exceed the current average U.S. intake of about 7% of total energy (Grundy 1997).

The major source of omega-3 fatty acids in the U.S. diet is fish; the predominant omega-3 fatty acids are eicosapentaenoic acid (EPA) and docosahexaenoic acid (DHA). These fatty acids increase the fluidity of the membranes of cold-water fish at low temperatures. Interest in omega-3 fatty acids has grown since observations some 20 years ago that Greenland Eskimos had a lower CHD incidence than a comparison population in Denmark. Diets of both populations were high in fat, but in Denmark more saturated fat was consumed and in Greenland more omega-3 fatty acids. Fish oil supplementation is discussed as a drug in Chapter 17.

There are convincing data from cohort studies that men who consume fish once a week have a lower CHD death rate than men who do not eat fish (Kromhout 1998). In addition, some studies have found reduction of cardiac arrest with consumption of fatty fish (Albert et al. 1998; Siscovick et al. 1995; Burr et al. 1989), a finding suggested to be attributable to an antiarrhythmic effect. Therefore, consumption of a serving of fish, in particular cold-water fish, once a week in healthy individuals and twice a week in patients with CHD seems advisable as part of a balanced diet (Kromhout

1998). Fish is a good source of protein and is low in saturated fat (Stone 1996a). Seafood rich in omega-3 fatty acids includes, in descending order of EPA and DHA content, Atlantic herring, Atlantic mackerel, sockeye salmon, blue mussels, whiting, rainbow trout, and albacore tuna.

Monounsaturated Fatty Acids

The major monounsaturated fat found in the diet is oleic acid, which is found in olive oil, canola oil, and high-oleic forms of sunflower and safflower seed oils. Other good sources are avocados and nuts (hazelnuts, pecans, and macadamia nuts). Monounsaturated fatty acids are neutral with respect to lipoproteins, neither raising nor lowering concentrations of LDL-C, HDL-C, or TG (Jones et al. 1998a). High intakes of oleic acid appear to be safe, and monounsaturates are not as susceptible to oxidation as polyunsaturates (Krauss et al. 1996). In general, CHD as well as cancer rates are lower in populations that consume a traditional Mediterranean diet, which is relatively rich in oleic acid through olive oil consumption and rich in intake of fruits and vegetables (Sacks and Willett 1991; Trichopoulou et al. 1994) (see later).

Cholesterol

Dietary cholesterol definitely raises plasma cholesterol concentrations in some individuals. Therefore, intake needs to be kept relatively low (Krauss et al. 1996). What accounts for these differences in response is not clear; two of the major variables are the percentage of dietary cholesterol absorbed in the intestine and the efficiency of converting cholesterol to bile acids in the liver (Gotto 1991). There is some evidence that dietary cholesterol augments the plasma cholesterol–raising effect of saturated fatty acids, and some epidemiologic data suggest that dietary cholesterol may increase CHD risk beyond its cholesterol-raising effect. An interesting example, reported by Kern (1991), of a hyporesponder to dietary cholesterol was an 88-year-old man who had normal plasma cholesterol concentrations despite having eaten, because of a compulsive disorder, 25 eggs a day for at least 15 years. Staprans et al. (1998) recently provided the first evidence in an animal model that oxidized cholesterol in the diet accelerates the development of atherosclerosis. In the human diet, oxidized lipids are common in such foods as meat, deep-fried foods, baked products containing eggs and butter, and foods processed by heat or drying.

The three major sources of dietary cholesterol are egg yolk, animal fat, and meat. The primary targets for reduction in intake should be egg yolk and animal fat; if they are curtailed, the cholesterol remaining in the lean, well-trimmed meat and in low-fat and fat-free dairy products usually will not be excessive (Jones et al. 1998).

Carbohydrates

Carbohydrates in the diet are sugars and starches. In either form, carbohydrates are neutral with respect to LDL-C. Consumed in large amounts, however, carbohydrates, compared with monounsaturated fatty acids, raise plasma TG and reduce HDL-C concentrations (Jones et al. 1998a). Excessive intake of sugar should be avoided. Although sugar intake has not been directly related to CVD risk, diets high in refined carbohydrates are often high in calories and low in complex carbohydrates, fiber, and essential vitamins and minerals. The AHA encourages consumption of complex carbohydrates in the form of vegetables, bread, cereal, grains, and legumes (Krauss et al. 1996).

Excess Calories

Consumption of excess calories leads to obesity, which is frequently accompanied by elevations in both plasma TG and cholesterol and a reduction in HDL-C. The increasing prevalence of obesity in the United States makes excess caloric intake a major cause of dyslipidemia in this country. Many Americans believe that low-fat foods may be eaten ad libitum; however, many very palatable low-fat commercial foods have added sweetening agents such as high-fructose sweeteners, sugar, or corn syrup, as well as other energy-bearing substances (Rolls and Miller 1997).

ADDITIONAL ISSUES

Other Nutrients

Sodium

For cardiovascular health, it is advisable to limit sodium intake to less than 2,400 mg/day (see "Blood Pressure Control" in Chapter 16).

Alcohol

Moderate alcohol consumption has a well-demonstrated cardioprotective effect (Stampfer et al 1993a; Pearson 1994, 1996), about half of the effect attributed to beneficial effects on HDL-C concentration (Criqui 1996). A consistent 20–40% reduction in CHD has been reported among moderate drinkers in disparate populations (Stampfer et al. 1993a). The effect contributes to the J-shaped relation between alcohol and total mortality rate: lowest mortality occurs in those who consume one or two drinks per day, and total mortality rises rapidly with increasing number of drinks as they exceed three per day (Pearson 1996).

Most health care organizations, including the AHA (Krauss et al. 1996), are in agreement that daily ethanol intake, when ethanol is not contraindicated, should not exceed about 30 g, the amount in about two drinks; the JNC VI hypertension guidelines recommend no more than half that amount for women and lighter-weight men (see Table 16.16). More than 40 g/day ethanol would be considered excessive (Gotto et al. 1995). Children, adolescents, and pregnant women should abstain from alcohol. Because of the intrinsic risks of alcohol use, the AHA considers it inadvisable to issue general population guidelines recommending alcohol use. For an individual patient, advisability of consuming alcohol in moderation is best determined in consultation with the primary care physician (Krauss et al. 1996). Elevated fasting TG concentrations normalize with discontinuation of alcohol in some patients, in some instances dramatically and in particular in type V hyperlipidemia (Erkelens and Brunzell 1980; Schlesinger et al. 1979; Simons et al. 1975; Titanji and Paz-Guevara 1992). In hypertriglyceridemia, therefore, use should be restricted, after a trial period, in selected patients (NCEP 1994). Alcohol is frequently consumed with fatty foods and, at least in normolipidemic subjects, the combination of fat and alcohol has a synergistic effect in increasing plasma TG; this effect is more profound with saturated fat than with polyunsaturated fat (Brewster et al. 1966; Wilson et al. 1970; Pownall 1994). Alcohol should not be consumed at all in pancreatitis, porphyria, and some other conditions (Krauss et al. 1996).

Trans Fatty Acids

The production of partially hydrogenated vegetable oils has increased steadily this century because of their low cost, long shelf life, and suitability for commercial frying (Ascherio and Willett 1997). When vegetable oils are partially hydrogenated to make them more solid, *trans* fatty acids are produced. *Trans* fatty acids raise LDL-C concentrations more than the native oils and less than saturated fatty acids (Lichtenstein 1997). They also lower HDL-C and increase the putative risk factor Lp[a] relative to the parent natural fat (Ascherio and Willett 1997). Ascherio and Willett (1997) estimate that each year at least 30,000 premature deaths in the United States are attributable to consumption of *trans* fatty acids. It is advisable to limit intake of foods high in *trans* fatty acids, such as shortening, some margarines, and some baked goods (e.g., some cookies). The goal would best be achieved by the food industry's substituting other types of fat for *trans* fatty acids in food items (Jones et al. 1998a). Oils and margariness low in *trans* fatty acids can be used at home for food preparation.

Soluble Fiber

As part of a low-fat diet, foods rich in soluble fiber (e.g., oats, barley, beans, soy products, guar gum, and pectin found in apples, cranberries, currants, and gooseberries) can help maximize plasma cholesterol lowering (Bell et al. 1990; Whyte et al. 1992; Ripsin et al. 1992). Total daily dietary fiber intake of 25–30 g from foods (not supplements) is recommended by the AHA (Krauss et al. 1996). Daily fiber intake among U.S. adults averages only about 15 g (Van Horn 1997). Insoluble fiber, which is found in the skin, peels, and husks of fruits, vegetables, and whole-grain products, does not appear to affect plasma cholesterol.

Soy Protein

Many studies have demonstrated that substituting soy protein for animal protein lowers cholesterol concentrations (Potter 1996; Messena and Erdman 1995). Meta-analysis of 38 clinical trials found significant reductions of 9.3% in TC and 12.9% in LDL-C; HDL-C increased 2.4% and TG decreased 10.5%, neither of these changes significant (Anderson et al. 1995). Neither the type of soy protein ingested (isolated or texturized) nor the amount used in the trials had an effect on the findings. Studies that used whole soybeans, which contain a large amount of lipid, or other vegetable protein were excluded. The mechanism for soy protein's lipid-regulating effects is not yet established; proposed mechanisms include impairment of cholesterol absorption or bile acid reabsorption (or both), changes in endocrine status, increases in LDL receptor activity, and isoflavone activity (Potter 1996). Lower serum TC has been associated with high intake of soy products in Japanese men and women (Nagata et al. 1998).

Antioxidant Vitamin Supplements

There is considerable interest in the use of supplemental antioxidant vitamins to reduce CHD risk. Inverse associations between dietary intake of antioxidant vitamins and CHD incidence have been described by case-control, descriptive, and prospective cohort studies; randomized clinical trials have shown no benefit with beta-carotene and possible benefit with vitamin E (Diaz et al. 1997). The Health Professionals Follow-up Study (Rimm et al. 1993) and the Nurses' Health Study (Stampfer et al. 1993b) found 36% and 34% reductions in CHD risk with vitamin E supplementation of at least 100 IU/day for at least 1–2 years. In the prospective, randomized, controlled Cambridge Heart Antioxidant Study in patients with angiographic CHD (Stephens et al. 1996), considered a real test of the antioxidant hypothesis, nonfatal MI rate was reduced 77% over 3 years, although total mortality rate was not affected. Vitamin C is of theoretic benefit for rejuvenating vitamin E (Plotnick et al. 1997). Anti-iron therapy has not yet been tested in animals or humans (Olsson and Yuan 1996).

Individuals may wish to consider supplementation with vitamin E, 1,000 mg/day, and vitamin C, 500 mg/day, so long as it is understood that vitamin supplementation does not lessen risks of major risk factors or substitute for a balanced diet. Supplementation with vitamins E and C at these (and higher) dosages is considered safe (Weber et al. 1996, 1997). Meyers et al. (1996) noted that case reports of vitamin E toxicity at dosages of less than 3,200 mg/day have been few, and that vitamin C toxic reactions are rare at dosages of less than 4,000 mg/day. Prudence may dictate avoidance by women of child-bearing potential and by individuals with liver disease or renal dysfunction or who are taking certain medications or undergoing specific laboratory tests (Meyers et al. 1996). The AHA recommends that antioxidant vitamins and other nutrients be derived from foods, not supplements (Krauss et al. 1996).

Vitamins Affecting Homocysteine Concentration

Many recent observational epidemiologic studies have linked elevated plasma homocysteine with increased risk for CHD, PVD, cerebrovascular disease, and thrombosis; some describe the predictivity to be as strong as that of hypercholesterolemia or smoking (Duell and Malinow 1997). Concentrations of homocysteine can be reduced with pharmacologic dosages of folic acid (folate), pyridoxine (vitamin B_6), vitamin B_{12}, or betaine, although research is needed to establish that lowering homocysteine will reduce atherosclerotic morbidity and mortality (Duell and Malinow 1997). The strongest association is between folic acid and fasting homocysteine; folic acid is a substrate that has the potential to drive homocysteine metabolism (Verhoef et al. 1998). Workers who suggest folic acid supplementation recommend intake of at least 400 μg/day (Verhoef et al. 1998). We suggest 1 mg/day (in comparison, women with a previous pregnancy affected by a neural tube defect are advised to take 4 mg/day). According to NHANES II, 88% of American adults consume less than 400 μg/day (Subar et al. 1989). Humans cannot synthesize folic acid de novo; food sources rich in folic acid include liver, yeast, milk and milk products, green leafy vegetables, oranges, and bananas (Verhoef et al. 1998). It remains possible that an elevated homocysteine concentration is the marker and low folic acid the risk factor (Verhoef et al. 1998).

Very Low Fat Diets

Ornish et al. (1990) have argued that LDL-C lowering and angiographic benefit of the same degree achieved with drug therapy can be obtained with more intensive lifestyle changes than represented by the Step I or Step II Diet—for example, a very low fat vegetarian diet (<10% of energy intake as fat) accompanied by regular exercise and measures designed to promote psychologic health. Dietary modification of this degree, however, may pose nutritional hazards for some individuals and subgroups—for example, children, pregnant women, and the elderly—particularly if professional instruction is insufficient (Jones et al. 1998a). Other nutrient needs may be compromised by excessive restriction of fat intake, and in some individuals reduced-fat, high-carbohydrate diets result in potentially adverse metabolic changes, including decreased HDL-C and increased plasma TG concentrations (Schaefer et al. 1995). Cholesterol-lowering trials have shown that intensive dietary counseling consistent with the Step II Diet (≤30% of energy intake as fat) can halt the progression of coronary atherosclerosis and decrease the CHD event rate (Denke 1995). The AHA (Krauss et al. 1996) endorses the recommendation of the World Health Organization that the lower limit for total fat intake be 15% of calories (Food and Agriculture Organization 1994). Although people in Japan and China have low total fat intake and low rates of CHD, these populations are also very lean and highly active, which would tend to offset the adverse effects of increased HDL-C and decreased TG concentrations (Katan et al. 1997).

The Mediterranean Diet

Growing evidence supports the health benefits of the Mediterranean diet; evidence is stronger for CHD, but there is also benefit against some cancers

Table 15.3. KEY COMPONENTS OF THE MEDITERRANEAN DIET

- High intake of fruits, vegetables, legumes, and grains
  —Fresh fruit as typical dessert
- High ratio of monounsaturated to saturated fatty acids
  —Olive oil as principal source of fat
- Moderate consumption of milk and dairy products
  —Principally as cheese and yogurt
- Moderate consumption of fish and poultry
- Low intake of red meat and meat products
- Zero to four eggs consumed weekly
- Alcohol consumption at moderate levels
  —Typically with meals and mainly in the form of wine

Sources: Data from Trichopoulou and Lagiou 1997 and Willett et al. 1995.

(Trichopoulou and Lagiou 1997; Willett et al. 1995; Keys 1995; Nestle 1995). Although there are variants of the diet, typical components are those shown in Table 15.3. The diet is low in saturated fat (≤7–8%), and total fat intake in the region ranges from less than 25% to more than 35% of energy. The people of Crete, southern Italy, and other regions in which the diet developed were also, in the early 1960s, very physically active and infrequently obese (Willett et al. 1995). For Americans who wish to change their diet, this model may provide an attractive, palatable option. Ironically, with the trend toward world uniformity in diet, the Mediterranean lifestyle may be an endangered species in the regions where it originated (Nestle 1995).

Suggested Reading

Denke MA. Cholesterol-lowering diets: a review of the evidence. Arch Intern Med 1995;155:17–26.

Krauss RM, Deckelbaum RJ, Ernst N, et al. Dietary guidelines for healthy American adults: a statement for health professionals from the Nutrition Committee, American Heart Association. Circulation 1996;94:1795–1800.

National Cholesterol Education Program. Second report of the Expert Panel on Detection, Evaluation, and Treatment of High Blood Cholesterol in Adults (Adult Treatment Panel II). Circulation 1994;89:1329–1445. (Note: Softbound copies of the NCEP Second Report of the Expert Panel on Detection, Evaluation, and Treatment of High Blood Cholesterol in Adults [NIH publication no. 93-3095] may be obtained by writing the NHLBI Information Center, P.O. Box 30105, Bethesda, MD 20824-0105 [telephone 301-251-1222, fax 301-251-1223]. One copy is gratis.)

For practical implementation of lifestyle changes for the lay reader: DeBakey ME, Gotto AM Jr, Scott LW, et al. The new living heart diet. New York: Simon and Schuster, 1996.

Chapter 16

Other Lifestyle Changes and Major Modifiable Risk Factors

Health care workers play a key role in promoting risk reduction measures. Physicians have the opportunity and responsibility to promote smoking cessation and prevention, weight control, regular physical activity, blood pressure control, and management of the risk of diabetes mellitus, as highlighted in this chapter, as well as a heart-healthy diet as reviewed in Chapter 15. Although physicians may delegate to other members of the health care team the task of providing preventive services, the physician must set and support the agenda (Fletcher et al. 1996).

SMOKING CESSATION

Need for Improvement in Physician Intervention

Smoking cessation intervention by health care professionals is effective. In general, physician-based primary care interventions have yielded cessation rates of 10–20%, compared with a 1-year maintained cessation rate of only 4% in the general population (Agency for Health Care Policy and Research 1996a, 1996b). Intervention with patients who have already suffered a cardiac event yields particularly striking benefits (Ockene and Houston Miller 1997).

Yet recent surveys have described deficiencies among both primary care physicians and cardiologists in translating clinical recommendations to explicit guidance on how to quit smoking. In a large survey of primary care clinics in the United States, less than 50% of smokers had been advised to stop smoking (Kottke et al. 1997). In a similar survey, 92% of smokers had been asked about their smoking status, but only 60% had been given explicit instructions on how to quit and only 27% had been referred to a stop-smoking program (Woller et al. 1995). In the early 1990s, the American College of Cardiology's Subcommittee on the Implementation of Preventive Cardiology interviewed primary care physicians and cardiologists about why they did not provide preventive cardiology services to their patients. Typical replies from the two groups were, "When the cardiologist writes a letter describing LV function and coronary anatomy in detail but doesn't mention smoking, I'm led to believe smoking isn't important," and "I'm asked to treat an acute event. I don't want to interfere with the primary care physician's relationship with the patient." The confusion about responsibility should not happen and should not be an excuse for inaction (Kottke 1997). Kottke (1997) suggests that referring physicians include in their letter templates the statement shown in Figure 16.1.

Other barriers to physicians' providing smoking interventions include a belief that interventions are not effective; poor intervention skills; a belief that patients do not want intervention; and little time to fit intervention into practice, especially when reimbursement is not provided (Ockene and Houston Miller 1997). All these barriers can be overcome.

Difficulty of Quitting

For most people, three or more attempts are required to achieve smoking cessation (Tsoh et al. 1997). The CDC reports an overall annual cessation rate of 2.5% (Skaar et al. 1997). Data from the mid-1980s showed that after lung cancer surgery, 50% of patients continued to smoke; after laryngectomy, 40% continued; after an MI, 40% began to smoke again while still in the hospital (Stolerman and Jarvis 1995). Black American smokers have been described as more likely to try to quit smoking but less likely to succeed than white smokers (CDC 1993b). Their difficulty in quitting may be explained in part by higher serum concentrations of cotinine (the primary metabolite of nicotine, which is widely used as a marker for tobacco exposure) for the same level of cigarette smoking (Caraballo et al. 1998), a finding explained by both slower clearance of cotinine and higher intake of nicotine per cigarette in black smokers (Pérez-Stable et al. 1998).

Nicotine Addiction

The U.S. Surgeon General's office has deemed nicotine addictive (U.S. Department of Health and Human Services 1988); nicotine meets all the cri-

> I have advised the patient that abstinence from tobacco is the most important step that an individual can take to optimize health. My team has given the patient advice about how to become and remain a non-smoker. I would appreciate it if you would take the opportunity at each visit to reinforce any efforts that the patient makes to become and remain an exsmoker.

Figure 16.1. It is suggested that this statement be included in referring physicians' letter templates. (From Kottke 1997.)

Table 16.1. NICOTINE AS AN ADDICTIVE SUBSTANCE

- Produces brief, pleasurable psychoactive effects
- Use occurs despite known harmful effects
- Tolerance to both pleasurable and unpleasant effects develops during early use
- Tolerance is overcome with higher dosages
- Withdrawal symptoms occur with cessation of use

Source: Data from Gidding et al. 1994.

teria that define an addictive substance (Table 16.1) (Gidding et al. 1994). Degree of compulsion is central to adjudging a drug addictive or merely habit forming; that compulsive use is the norm in smoking is supported by patterns of use and the intractability of the habit (e.g., stable light smokers are uncommon; more than 50% of smokers light up within 30 minutes of morning awakening; 48% have not abstained for as long as 1 week during the most recent 5 years) (Stolerman and Jarvis 1995). Humans and animals of several species will self-administer intravenous nicotine; the behavior in humans appears to be motivated by both positive reinforcement (e.g., relaxation, reduced stress, reduced craving, improved cognitive function) and negative reinforcement (relief of nicotine withdrawal symptoms) (Benowitz 1996).

The most addictive delivery of nicotine appears to be through inhalation of cigarette smoke, which delivers nicotine to the brain in about 10–19 seconds via the arterial bloodstream (Benowitz 1996; Benowitz and Gourlay 1997). Peak venous concentrations after 1 cigarette are typically 5–30 ng/mL, and the elimination half-life is typically 2–3 hours (Benowitz and Gourlay 1997). Nicotine activates the release of neurotransmitters such as norepinephrine and dopamine in the CNS, and it elevates dopamine levels in areas of the brain associated with reinforcement of the effects of amphetamines, cocaine, and opiates (Hurt et al. 1997). Dopamine has a key role in reward signaling and addiction as well as movement (Stephenson 1996).

The occurrence of relatively intense effects on the CNS soon after exposure is ideal for behavioral reinforcement. In contrast, the slow release with transdermal nicotine yields little or no reinforcement (Benowitz 1996).

Risk for Beginning Smoking. Nearly all smokers begin smoking before the age of 18 years. Among risk factors for beginning smoking are use by other family members and friends, peer approval, low socioeconomic status, poor academic achievement, poor self-image, and susceptibility to influence of others and advertising images (Gidding et al. 1994).

Withdrawal Symptoms. Symptoms of nicotine withdrawal vary among individuals but in general are very unpleasant and often intolerable (Tsoh et al. 1997). They include anxiety, nervousness, irritability, insomnia, increased appetite, impaired concentration, and decreased heart rate. Typically, physical withdrawal symptoms last no more than 1 week (Danis and Seaton 1997).

Possible Synergy with Decreased Monoamine Oxidase B.   Fowler et al. (1996) recently demonstrated reduced monoamine oxidase (MAO) B in the brains of current smokers by using positron emission tomography (PET) and labeled L-deprenyl. The eight smokers averaged about 40% less MAO B than the eight nonsmokers or four former smokers. The enzyme MAO is involved in the degradation of biologically active monoamines (neurotransmitters such as dopamine, noradrenalin, and serotonin). Its B isozyme form is selective for the metabolic degradation of dopamine; inhibition of MAO B would increase the functional availability of dopamine (Glassman and Koob 1996). The findings of Fowler and colleagues suggest a synergistic effect between nicotine and reduced MAO B to boost dopamine concentrations even higher—in effect, making nicotine even more addictive (Stephenson 1996). The active ingredient in smoke responsible for the effect on MAO B concentrations is not known (Fowler et al. 1996; Glassman and Koob 1996).

MAO had been shown earlier to be reduced in the platelets of smokers, with return to normal on smoking cessation (Glassman and Koob 1996). In parkinsonism, which characteristically shows a reduction in dopamine function and loss of dopamine neurons, symptoms are reduced and progression may be slowed by administration of the MAO B inhibitor L-deprenyl (selegiline); on average, cigarette smoking may halve the risk for development of Parkinson's disease (Glassman and Koob 1996; Stephenson 1996).

Tobacco Industry Internal Documents.   It appears that, many years before the scientific community, the tobacco industry had a sophisticated understanding of nicotine pharmacology and knew that nicotine is addictive. Whereas the Brown and Williamson Tobacco Corporation (B&W) internal documents that came to light in 1994 revealed that B&W executives and scientists by the early 1960s considered nicotine addictive (Glantz et al. 1995, 1996), not until 1979 did the U.S. Surgeon General publish that same conclusion (U.S. Department of Health, Education, and Welfare 1979). In 1964, the original Surgeon General's report on smoking was mild in its condemnation of smoking; tobacco was described as habituating, not addictive (U.S. Public Health Service 1964). In his foreword to *The Cigarette Papers* (Glantz et al. 1996), C. Everett Koop (U.S. Surgeon General, 1981–1989) wrote, "I have often wondered how many people died as a result of the fact that the medical and public health professions were misled by the tobacco industry." Not until 1997 did any tobacco company admit that nicotine is addictive; that smoking causes lung cancer, heart disease, and emphysema; and that tobacco marketing targeted teenagers. These admissions were made by the Liggett Group in March 1997 in a lawsuit settlement (Broder 1997; Greenwald 1997).

Weight Gain

About 80% of people who quit smoking have attendant weight gain (NIH 1998). Weight gain is usually in the range of 2–5 kg (5–10 lb) (Tsoh et al.

1997; Williamson et al. 1991), but in 13% of women and 10% of men weight gain exceeds 12.7 kg (28 lb) (NIH 1998). Women have been reported to gain more weight than men, whether in absolute kilograms or as a percentage of body weight (Perkins et al. 1997). It is generally recommended that physicians be open about the possibility of weight gain, emphasizing that the risks of smoking far outweigh risks of moderate weight gain. It may be inadvisable to institute significant dietary restrictions immediately after a patient stops smoking (Tsoh et al. 1997). Nicotine gum, nicotine spray, or bupropion may in the short term reduce weight gain associated with smoking cessation (Hurt et al. 1997; Tsoh et al. 1997); this short-term effect may allay patients' initial anxiety about gaining weight.

In both sexes, the increase in weight appears to be due to increased caloric intake (average increase of 300–400 calories per day), primarily from snacking (calories increased 50% in men and 94% in women during smoking abstinence in one study). There is an inverse relation between nicotine intake and food consumption: Nicotine may lessen the unpleasant effects of food restriction, and eating may help attenuate some symptoms of nicotine withdrawal and negative affect. It is also possible that smoking and eating are competing sources of reinforcement (Perkins et al. 1997).

Guide for Clinicians

A smoking cessation guide for primary care physicians was developed by a panel convened by the Agency for Health Care Policy and Research (AHCPR) of the U.S. Public Health Service working with the CDC (Tables 16.2 and 16.3). The panel reviewed the smoking cessation literature and conducted a meta-analysis of the results of more than 300 randomized, controlled clinical trials published between 1975 and 1994; in each trial, follow-up was for at least 5 months after the quit date (Skaar et al. 1997).

The panel found a dose-response relation between intensity and duration of a treatment and its effectiveness. Even brief counseling sessions or simple words of encouragement (e.g., "I want you to quit. Will you let me arrange an appointment with a smoking cessation counselor?") can be effective, however. (Kottke 1997). Richards (1992) has noted that the words a physician chooses to discuss smoking with a patient should be considered no less a therapeutic agent than the pharmacologic agent that the physician prescribes. At least minimal intervention should be provided to every patient who smokes. Up to 2% of smokers will quit after a single routine consultation (Danis and Seaton 1997). Effectiveness of intervention did not differ according to the professional discipline of the provider (e.g., physician, nurse, dentist, psychologist). Person-to-person contact was a key determinant; self-help materials did not significantly improve cessation rates (Skaar et al. 1997).

The AHCPR panel recommended that patients be encouraged to use nicotine replacement therapy (NRT) except in special medical circum-

Table 16.2. SMOKING CESSATION: A GUIDE FOR PRIMARY CARE PHYSICIANS

1. Every smoker should be offered smoking cessation treatment at every office visit.
2. Every patient's tobacco use status should be recorded.
3. Cessation treatment even as brief as 3 minutes is effective.
4. The more intense the treatment, the more effective it is, ideally, 4–7 person-to-person sessions (≥20 or 30 minutes each) over 8 weeks.
5. Effective components of treatment include
   • Nicotine replacement
   • Social support
   • Skills training (how to resist cues to smoke): willpower is ineffective; need "skillpower"
6. Health care systems should be modified to identify and intervene with tobacco users at every visit.

Source: Data from Agency for Health Care Policy and Research 1996a, 1996b.

stances. Counseling sessions yielded higher cessation rates if they included general problem-solving/skills training and provider support (Skaar et al. 1996). Teachable skills of the greatest benefit are the ability to recognize situations that trigger smoking and the ability to plan to avoid the situation or substitute a behavior for smoking (Kottke 1997). Alcohol avoidance during the first few weeks is critical (Tsoh et al. 1997).

Cinciripini et al. (1995) reported a novel scheduled smoking procedure that yielded excellent cessation rates at 1 year: 44% with gradual reduction (vs. 18% gradual reduction alone) and 32% with abrupt cessation (vs. 22% abrupt cessation alone). Patients are instructed to smoke only at specific times, for example, 30 cigarettes in 15 hours (1 each 30 minutes), and missed cigarettes may not be accumulated. Although the approach requires confirmation and further research, the investigators suggest that physicians may wish to consider using it before the quit date or for patients who are not candidates for NRT.

Review of the risk of smoking with patients is important. In recent surveys of U.S. smokers, 56% failed to identify smoking cessation as a health priority (Ratner et al. 1995) and less than one-third of older smokers believed in a strong link between smoking and illness (Rubenstein 1991). Many of the older smokers attributed smoking-related symptoms to the natural aging process.

Numerous resources on the Internet provide information about smoking cessation; examples of organizations and their addresses are provided in Table 16.4. A selected list of patient education and counseling materials recommended by Hays et al. (1996) appears in Table 16.5.

Patients may ask about nonstandard approaches to smoking cessation, such as acupuncture (e.g., nasopuncture or auriculopuncture) or hypnosis. In methodologically sound studies of acupuncture in this application, cessa-

Table 16.3. HELPING YOUR PATIENTS QUIT SMOKING

Ask about tobacco use.
- Implement an officewide system that ensures that tobacco use status is obtained and recorded.
    Every patient
    Every office visit
- Include tobacco use in vital signs data collected.
    May place tobacco use stickers on charts
    May use computer reminder system

Advise every tobacco user to quit.
- Be clear.
    "I think it is important for you to quit smoking now, and I will help you."
- Speak strongly.
    "Quitting smoking is the most important thing you can do to protect your health."
- Personalize your advice.
    "You have already had a heart attack."
    "You know your children need you."

Assist with a quit plan.
Advise smoker to
- Set a quit date, ideally within 2 weeks.
- Inform friends, family, and coworkers of plan to quit, and ask for support.
- Remove cigarettes from home, office, and car.
- Review previous quit attempts.
- Anticipate challenges, including nicotine withdrawal.
    Avoid (e.g., smoke-filled bar)
    Cope (e.g., distraction, substitute behavior, positive self-talk, stress management)
    Escape (e.g., step outside, away from smokers)
Give advice on successful quitting.
- Total abstinence is essential: 95% who take one puff relapse.
- Drinking alcohol is strongly associated with relapse.
- Having other smokers in the household hinders quitting.
Encourage use of NRT.
- Both the patch and gum are effective.
- The nicotine patch may be easier to use in most clinical settings (fewer compliance problems).

Recommend intensive programs.
- Intensive programs are strongly correlated with success.
- Assessment information (e.g., comorbidity) is useful in counseling.
- Many different types of clinical workers are effective.
- Intensive programs should offer 4–7 sessions, each about 20–30 minutes, lasting at least 2 weeks.
- Counseling should offer problem-solving/skills training, and social support.
- Counseling should reinforce motivation and relapse prevention.
- Every smoker should be offered nicotine replacement therapy except when medically contraindicated.

Follow up.
Timing
- Make first contact within 2 weeks of quit date (preferably during week 1).
- Make second contact within first month.
- Initiate further follow-up as needed.

Actions
- Congratulate success.
- Ask for recommitment if there is a lapse.
- If lapse occurred, remind patient that it can be a learning experience; review circumstances and suggest alternative behaviors.
- Identify problems and anticipate challenges.

Prevent relapse.
- Congratulate, encourage, and stress the importance of remaining abstinent.
- Review the benefits of cessation.
- Review the patient's success in quitting.
- Inquire about problems encountered and offer suggestions.
- Anticipate problems.
- Discuss specific problems, such as
  Weight gain (typically 2–5 kg, or 5–10 lb)
  Negative mood/depression
  Prolonged nicotine withdrawal
  Lack of cessation support

Source: Data from Agency for Health Care Policy and Research 1996a, 1996b.

tion rates have been low and similar to those achieved with a placebo (Schwartz 1992). Meta-analyses as well have found lack of effectiveness (Law and Tang 1995; Ter Riet et al. 1990). Seven of eight studies using "correct" sites and "sham" sites showed no advantage with the "correct" sites (Schwartz 1992). Endorphin release has been hypothesized as a potential mechanism, but physiologic evidence for alleviation of withdrawal symptoms is lacking (Schwartz 1992). Effectiveness is also unproved for group or individual hypnosis for smoking cessation, and no trials have used biochemical markers

Table 16.4. SMOKING CESSATION: SOME WORLD WIDE WEB RESOURCES

Organization	Address
American Lung Association	http://www.lungusa.org
American Heart Association	http://www.amhrt.org
American Cancer Society	http://www.cancer.org
Tobacco Control Research Center	http://www.tobacco.neu.edu
Action on Smoking and Health	http://ash.org
Technical Assistance on the QuitNet	http://www.quitnet.org
Smoking Cessation Facts	http://www.kickbutt.org
CDC Prevention Guidelines	http://wwonder.cdc.gov
Smoking Cessation Resources	http://www.welltech.com/net_connect/smoke.html
Agency for Health Care Policy and Research	http://www.ahcpr.gov

Table 16.5. SELECTED PATIENT EDUCATION AND COUNSELING MATERIALS

Source	Publication(s)

National Cancer Institute
  Office of Cancer Communications,
  Bldg. 31, Room 10A24,
  Bethesda, MD 20892,
  1-800-4-CANCER
	Clearing the Air (NIH 92-1647)
	How to Help Your Patients Stop Smoking (NIH 90-3064)
	Why Do You Smoke? (NIH 83-1822)

Centers for Disease Control
  and Prevention
  Office on Smoking and Health,
  Rockville, MD 20857
	The Health Benefits of Smoking Cessation. A Report of the Surgeon General, 1990, at a Glance (CDC 90-8419)

American Heart Association
  7272 Greenville Avenue,
  Dallas, TX 75231-4596
	Children and Smoking: A Message to Parents
	How to Avoid Weight Gain When Quitting Smoking

American Cancer Society (Local Office), 1-800-ACS-2345	*The Most Often Asked Questions about Tobacco and Health and . . . the Answers* *Tobacco Free Young America Q & A: Questions and Answers for the Busy Practitioner*

American Medical Association
  Division of Health Science,
  515 North State Street,
  Chicago, IL 60610
	How to Help Patients Stop Smoking: Guidelines for Diagnosis and Treatment of Nicotine Dependence

American Lung Association (Local office)	*Freedom from Smoking for You and Your Family* *Freedom from Smoking for You and Your Baby* (kit) *Nicotine Addiction and Cigarettes*

W. R. Spence, M.D.
  HEALTH EDCO,
  Waco, TX 76702-1207
	The ABC's of Smoking (graphic photographs)
	Smokeless Tobacco: A Chemical Time Bomb (graphic photographs)

March of Dimes Birth Defects
  Foundation
  1275 Mamaroneck Ave.,
  White Plains, NY 10605
	Give Your Baby a Healthy Start: Stop Smoking

Source: Adapted from Hays et al. 1996; used with permission.

(Law and Tang 1995). Most studies have enrolled small numbers of patients, and only a few have included appropriate follow-up (Schwartz 1992).

Pharmacologic Smoking Aids

Use of tobacco has been controversial at least since its introduction to Europe soon after Columbus's voyages (Glantz et al. 1996). Most early European physicians accepted the Native American belief in tobacco's medicinal properties (A brief history of tobacco. CNN Interactive 1997). Yet King James I tried to stamp out the "Indian vice," and pamphleteers of the time warned that smoking caused a variety of diseases. British dandies with their elaborate smoking paraphernalia ("artillery") were known as "reeking gallants" "clowding the loathing ayr with foggie fume" (Dunhill 1954).

A variety of deterrents intended to help break the smoking habit have been available since before 1900, including preparations to create a disagreeable taste, mucosal irritation, dry mouth, or diminished sensory drive. Products containing the irritant lobeline (e.g., CigArrest, Nikoban) were popular sellers in the 1960s. (The contention that lobeline satisfies nicotine craving has not been supported.) In 1982, an FDA panel concluded that such products to date had been ineffective (Schwartz 1992). Many agents to help overcome nicotine withdrawal have been tested, among them sedatives, antidepressants, anticholinergics, tranquilizers, sympathomimetics, anticonvulsants, and nicotine replacements (Schwartz 1992). Agents recently tested include moclobemide, a reversible inhibitor of MAO A (Berlin et al. 1995), the antihypertensive agent clonidine (Robbins 1993), and the antianxiety agent buspirone (Robbins 1993).

The only FDA-approved pharmacologic smoking aids at present are nicotine replacement therapies (i.e., patch, polacrilex chewing gum, and spray) and sustained-release bupropion. Use of such aids is to accompany nonpharmacologic interventions. Such medications are approved as aids in smoking cessation; use in patients who do not want to quit but who must undergo a period of abstinence (e.g., airline pilots, hospitalized patients) is not an FDA-approved indication (Henningfield 1995).

Nicotine Replacement Therapy

Kerr in 1994, using criteria of efficacy, safety, cost-effectiveness, a large data base, and evidence of underuse, characterized NRT as one of eight underused therapies that could have a major impact on morbidity and mortality rates. On average, transdermal (patch), gum, and spray nicotine each double smoking cessation rates at 6–12 months compared with placebo (Benowitz 1996). Efficacy is well established for transdermal and gum nicotine; spray is more recently approved (Said et al. 1994).

NRT is believed to reduce withdrawal symptoms (Benowitz 1996; Skaar et al. 1997). It possibly reduces satisfaction from tobacco, perhaps as a consequence of desensitization of nicotinic receptors (Benowitz 1996). The effect of nicotine spray in increasing smoking abstinence may in part be through positive reinforcement (Benowitz 1996). Gum and patches take longer to produce peak nicotine blood concentrations and produce lower concentrations than cigarettes; time to peak concentration with nasal spray or inhaler delivery is intermediate between cigarettes and gum or a patch (Skaar et al. 1997).

Simply prescribing therapy does not constitute NRT; it is usually ineffective and may lead to inappropriate use. Essential elements of NRT are

Table 16.6. FAGERSTRÖM TEST FOR NICOTINE DEPENDENCE

Questions to smoker	Scoring			
	0	1	2	3
1. How soon in minutes do you smoke after morning awakening?	>60	30–60	6–30	≤5
2. Do you find it difficult to refrain in places where smoking is forbidden?	No	Yes		
3. Which cigarette would you most hate to give up?	Any other	1st in AM		
4. How many cigarettes do you smoke daily?	<10	11–20	21–30	≥31
5. Do you smoke more during the first hours after waking?	No	Yes		
6. Do you smoke when you are so ill that you are in bed most of the day?	No	Yes		

Note: A score ≥7 indicates a high degree of dependence.
Source: Adapted from Danis and Seaton 1997; used with permission.

diagnosis, rational dosing, appropriate instruction, and follow-up (Henningfield 1995).

Selection. Some authorities consider patches to be first-line NRT because of their effectiveness with even minimal (vs. intensive) nonpharmacologic therapy, because compliance is better than with gum (Haxby 1995), and because spray may be less well tolerated (Said et al. 1994). Patches are possibly more effective for smokers with lower dependence, whereas spray may have greater relative benefit in more dependent smokers (Benowitz 1996). Patches have little if any psychologic effect; subjective effects are moderate with gum and more intense with spray, in both cases less than with cigarette smoking (Benowitz 1996). The Fagerström test for nicotine dependence (Table 16.6), one of several such questionnaires that have been developed, may influence NRT selection and dosing (Danis and Seaton 1997). Level of dependence generally correlates with difficulty in achieving abstinence, severity of withdrawal symptoms, and speed of relapse (Henningfield 1995).

Some physicians may wish to consider providing patients with a sample kit of gum, patches, and spray, so that they may determine which delivery system is the most pleasing for them (Kottke 1997). Higher than standard doses of gum or patches have not been shown to increase abstinence rates in the long-term, nor has a combination of gum and patch (Skaar et al. 1997).

Cardiovascular Safety. Despite anecdotal reports of fatal and nonfatal MIs, worsened unstable angina, and stroke with patch use, reviews (Benowitz and Gourlay 1997; Gourlay 1994) and trials of transdermal nicotine (Joseph et al. 1996; Mahmarian et al. 1997; Working Group 1994) suggest that NRT does not increase the already elevated risk for CVD in smokers. Trials included smokers with CHD or other CVD.

Pharmacokinetic and pharmacodynamic considerations in the cardiovascular safety of nicotine have recently been well reviewed by Benowitz and Gourlay (1997). Among their conclusions are (1) NRT plus continued smoking yields plasma concentrations of nicotine not much greater than those before the quit attempt; (2) cigarette smoking results in more intense acute cardiovascular effects than same dose of nicotine by NRT; (3) cigarette smoking and transdermal nicotine appear to have similar overall hemodynamic effects; (4) the cardiovascular dose-response relation for nicotine is relatively flat, so that after a threshold, there is little effect besides higher blood concentrations; and (5) cardiovascular effects from smoking plus NRT appear similar to those from smoking alone.

Nevertheless, caution with NRT should be used if patients have experienced a recent MI, a recent cerebrovascular accident, arrhythmia, or severe or worsening angina pectoris, or if they have very high blood pressure or diabetes mellitus requiring insulin. Recommendations include stopping patch NRT if the patient is unable to stop smoking after 4 weeks because of the risk of nicotine overdose (symptoms include nausea and lightheadedness) (Tsoh et al. 1997). Physicians should consult product information for complete lists of contraindications and cautions, including noncardiovascular cautions.

Studies of transdermal and gum NRT have suggested no adverse effects on plasma lipid concentrations. In the Transdermal Nicotine Study, the lipid profile tended to normalize with the switch from smoking to the patch (Allen et al. 1994). In abstinent subjects, despite an increase in weight, HDL-C and total TG increased and LDL-C decreased.

Other Selected Safety Issues.   The risk:benefit ratio of NRT in pregnancy has not been quantified (Haxby 1995); nonpharmacologic methods should be tried first in pregnant or nursing women (Gourlay 1994). The risk:benefit ratio for gum or transdermal NRT during pregnancy appears to be favorable if efforts to quit have failed and the patient smokes more than 10 or 15 cigarettes per day (Henningfield 1995). Polacrilex gum carries an FDA Pregnancy Category C warning ("risk cannot be ruled out"), and transdermal nicotine carries a Pregnancy Category D warning ("positive evidence of risk").

Henningfield (1995) has reviewed other selected safety issues with NRT. Data have not been published on the safety of NRT in youths. Patients with a history of depression, anxiety disorder, or alcohol abuse require particularly careful monitoring and may benefit from referral to a specialist. Caffeine concentrations in blood may increase more than 250% on smoking cessation; symptoms of acute caffeine overdose may resemble those of nicotine withdrawal.

Nicotine Patch.   Depending on the patch, nicotine patches deliver 5–22 mg of nicotine over 16–24 hours. There is substantial development of tolerance (Benowitz 1996). Treatment for 6–8 weeks is required; longer treatment has not been demonstrated to increase efficacy, although it may be warranted if severe withdrawal symptoms persist (Tsoh et al. 1997). Generally, the maximum dose is recommended for patients who smoke 10–15 cigarettes (or more) per day. As treatment progresses, stepping down the dose may help patients through reaching goals and makes intuitive sense, although no empirical data exist to support this approach (Tsoh et al. 1997).

Patch use is begun on the quit date. The patch is applied to a nonsensitive, nonhairy, dry, and clean area (shaving may be necessary). Recommended sites are above the waist and below the neck; sites are rotated daily. Generally, each patch is worn for 24 hours, including while asleep unless otherwise directed. Applying a new patch before bedtime should be avoided (Tsoh et al. 1997). All NRT products must be disposed of with care to prevent access by children or pets. Nicotine patches can be a dermal irritant; after handling a patch, patients should wash their hands with water alone because nicotine absorption can be increased by soap.

The most common adverse effects of transdermal NRT are a short-term erythema (35%), pruritus (35%), and burning at the application site (35%). Other common side effects include insomnia and other sleep disturbances, headache, diarrhea, dyspepsia, and nervousness (Tsoh et al. 1997).

Nicotine Polacrilex Chewing Gum. The two standard dosing strengths of 2 and 4 mg of nicotine polacrilex chewing gum yield absorption of, respectively, 1 or 2 mg of nicotine over 20–30 minutes (Benowitz 1996). For most patients, 2 mg is the standard dose; providers may consider 4 mg in patients who smoke at least 20 cigarettes daily (Tsoh et al. 1997). Recommended use is for at least 1–3 months, although 15–20% of abstainers continue to use the gum for longer than 1 year (Tsoh et al. 1997). Patients tend gradually to cut down or discontinue use because of the gum's unpleasant taste or other side effects; empirical data are not available concerning decreasing gum use (Tsoh et al. 1997).

Nicotine gum is begun on the quit date. Patient instruction is important to reduce side effects, many of which arise from too-vigorous chewing (Benowitz 1996). The gum is not a candy gum, and the "chew and park" technique is used: chew the gum (5–10 times) until a "peppery" taste emerges, then park the gum between cheek and gum, repeating occasionally for about 30 minutes. The patient should avoid drinking while chewing the gum, especially acidic beverages such as coffee, soft drinks, and juices, and should avoid eating 15 minutes before and after chewing the gum. At least 1 or 2 pieces per hour should be used, not to exceed 30 pieces per day (Tsoh et al. 1997).

Common adverse effects include headache (20%), dyspepsia (12%), nausea (10%), increased salivation (3–9%), stomatitis (5%), aphthous stomatitis (5%), tooth disorders (4%), glossitis (3%), and hiccups (Fagerström and Tönnesen 1995; Williamson et al. 1991).

Nicotine Spray. As with other forms of NRT, nicotine spray is not begun until the quit date and is used as part of a comprehensive behavioral smoking cessation program. The usual dosing is 1–2 doses per hour to start (minimum, 8 doses daily; maximum, 5 doses hourly or 40 doses daily), where 1 dose equals 1 mg nicotine (2 sprays) (data for Nicotrol NS). Nicotine from nasal spray is absorbed very rapidly; 0.5 mg of 1 mg spray is absorbed systemically (Benowitz 1996). Use for longer than 6 months has not been assessed and is not recommended (*Physicians' Desk Reference* 1998).

Review of trials of patches and sprays showed similar quit rates; spray, however, was less well tolerated than transdermal nicotine (Said et al. 1994). Nasal irritation is almost universal (94%) during the first 2 days of use of nicotine spray but usually declines in frequency and severity with continued use. Other common side effects include watering eyes, runny nose, throat irritation, sneezing, coughing, and headache. All forms of NRT are contraindicated when there is known hypersensitivity or allergy to nicotine or another product component; nicotine nasal spray is also contraindicated in patients who have asthma or chronic nasal disorders such as allergy, rhinitis, nasal polyps, or sinusitis.

Bupropion

Sustained-release bupropion HCl tablets (Zyban; initially developed as an antidepressant, Wellbutrin) were approved by the FDA in May 1996 as the first non-nicotine prescription medication available for use as an aid in smoking cessation. The possibility of using antidepressant medication to assist in smoking cessation has been pursued for several reasons. Smokers are more than twice as likely as those who have never been smokers to have a history of major depression, and a history of depression is associated with reduced likelihood of stopping smoking (Aubin et al. 1996). Nicotine may act as an antidepressant in some smokers (Aubin et al. 1996; Glass 1990), and development of depression after smoking cessation may lead to relapse (Covey et al. 1990). The neurochemical effects of nicotine, such as release of dopamine, norepinephrine, and serotonin, resemble the effects of some antidepressant drugs (Benowitz 1996). Some other agents that have been tested in this application are doxepin, fluoxetine, serotonin uptake inhibitors, and nortriptyline (Edwards et al. 1989; Hurt et al. 1997; Sellers et al. 1987).

In a randomized trial of bupropion with long-term follow-up (Hurt et al. 1997), rates of smoking cessation at the end of 7 weeks of treatment were 19%, 29%, 39%, and 44% in the placebo and the 100-mg, 150-mg, and 300-mg bupropion groups ($P < .001$ for all drug groups vs. placebo). All patients ($N = 615$) also received brief counseling weekly during treatment and less often through 52 weeks. The respective cessation rates at 1 year were 12%, 20% ($P = .09$), 23% ($P = .02$), and 23% ($P = .01$). Smoking abstinence was determined by self-report confirmed by measurement of carbon monoxide in expired air. There was a significant dose-response relation at all follow-up periods. Among subjects who were continuously abstinent during treatment ($n = 103$), mean absolute weight gain was inversely associated with dose (gains of 2.9, 2.3, 2.3, and 1.5 kg in the respective groups). Enrollees could not have current depression, and no effects of treatment were observed on Beck Depression Inventory scores.

The mechanism by which bupropion enhances the ability of patients to abstain from smoking is unknown; the action is presumed to be mediated by noradrenergic mechanisms (which would affect nicotine withdrawal), dopaminergic mechanisms (which would affect areas of the brain having to do with reinforcement), or both (Hurt et al. 1997; *Physicians' Desk Reference* 1998). The drug is a relatively weak inhibitor of the neuronal uptake of dopamine, norepinephrine, and serotonin; it does not inhibit MAO (*Physicians' Desk Reference* 1998).

Treatment to accompany smoking cessation counseling is initiated while the patient is still smoking because approximately 1 week is required to reach steady-state blood concentrations of the drug; a target quit date is usually set for week 2. The usual and maximum dosage is 150 mg twice daily. Treatment should usually continue for 7–12 weeks, although the drug should probably be discontinued if significant progress toward quitting has not been made by week 7. Bupropion has been used beyond 12 weeks for depression, but its use for such lengths of time for smoking cessation has not been described. Dose tapering with discontinuation of bupropion for smoking cessation is not required (*Physicians' Desk Reference* 1998). Insomnia (31%) and dry mouth (11%) are the most common adverse effects. Both are generally mild and transient; reducing the dose may alleviate the effects. The most common effects leading to discontinuation have been shakiness and skin rash. Bupropion may be used with nicotine patches under physician supervision; the combination may increase blood pressure (*Physicians' Desk Reference* 1998).

Zyban is contraindicated in patients with a seizure disorder; patients treated with bupropion for another disorder; patients with a prior or current diagnosis of bulimia or anorexia nervosa; and patients being treated with an MAO inhibitor (at least 14 days should elapse after an MAO inhibitor is stopped). Zyban is not recommended for women who are pregnant or nursing (*Physicians' Desk Reference* 1998). Risk for seizure is approximately 0.1%. For smoking cessation, doses above 300 mg/day should not be used because of risk for seizure. Risk for seizure is dose dependent but is also increased by a variety of other factors (e.g., history of head trauma or seizure, CNS tumor, excessive use of alcohol, diabetes mellitus treated with oral hypoglycemics or insulin, and such concomitant medications as antipsychotics, antidepressants, and systemic steroids). Physicians should review full product information for complete prescribing information.

WEIGHT CONTROL

The first U.S. federal guidelines on the identification, evaluation, and treatment of overweight and obesity in adults were issued by the NIH in June 1998. A summary of the guidelines, which focus on the role of the primary care practitioner, is provided here. The overall strategy for evaluation and treatment is shown in the algorithm in Figure 16.2.

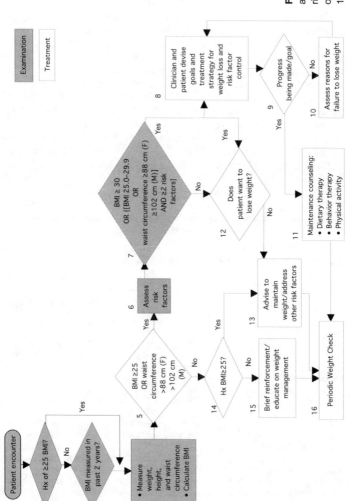

Figure 16.2. NIH evaluation and treatment algorithm for overweight and obesity in adults (NIH 1998).

Prevention of Overweight

Prevention of weight gain with aging among adults is a high priority, in particular given the difficulty of weight loss. To avoid such weight gain and the development of overweight and obesity, fundamental modifications in eating and exercise habits must be made as young adults progress toward middle age (Grundy 1998).

Assessment

Assessment for overweight and obesity entails evaluation of BMI, waist circumference, and risk factors for disorders associated with obesity (Tables 16.7–16.9). BMI should be determined in all adults; it should be reassessed in 2 years in those of normal weight. It is strongly correlated with total body fat content in adults, although some very muscular (i.e., not overfat) individuals may have a high BMI without health risks. Waist circumference is strongly associated with abdominal fat; excess abdominal fat is an independent predictor of disease risk. A waist circumference greater than 102 cm (40 in) in men or greater than 88 cm (35 in) in women signifies increased risk in those who are overweight or obese. Waist circumference cutpoints lose their incremental predictive power with a BMI of 35 kg/m^2 or higher. Overweight or obese patients are considered to be at higher risk at any risk level defined by other risk factors. Assessment of absolute risk entails summation of risk factors. These definitions of overweight and obesity and their risks supersede the Metropolitan Life Insurance Company definitions—which are related to body frame size and only to mortality (Eckel 1997)—historically used in the United States.

Table 16.7. NIH CLASSIFICATION OF OVERWEIGHT AND OBESITY IN ADULTS

Category	BMI (kg/m^2)[a]	Relative risk for disease[b] M ≤102 (40) F ≤88 (35)	M >102 (40) F >88 (35)
Underweight	<18.5		
Normal weight	18.5–24.9		
Overweight	25.0–29.9	Increased	High
Obesity			
Class I	30.0–34.9	High	Very high
Class II	35.0–39.9	Very high	Very high
Class III = extreme obesity	≥40.0	Extremely high	Extremely high

[a]Nonmetric conversion formula = [weight (lb)/height (in)^2] × 704.5.
[b]Risk for type 2 diabetes mellitus, hypertension, and CVD according to body weight and waist circumference. Increased waist circumference can also indicate risk in individuals of normal weight.
Source: NIH 1998.

Table 16.8. CONSIDERATIONS IN ESTIMATING ABSOLUTE RISK FOR MORBIDITY AND MORTALITY FROM OVERWEIGHT AND OBESITY IN ADULTS

Absolute risk	Factors*
Very high	Established atherosclerotic disease, Type 2 diabetes mellitus, or Sleep apnea
High	≥3 CVD risk factors: cigarette smoking, hypertension, high-risk LDL-C, low HDL-C, fasting plasma glucose 110–125 mg/dL, family history of premature CHD, age ≥45 years for men and ≥55 years for women
Additional incremental risk	Physical inactivity, or Plasma TG >200 mg/dL

*Also consider other obesity-related disorders as well as end organ damage in hypertension.
Source: Data from NIH 1998.

Some would consider the NIH cutpoints liberal. Grundy (1998), for example, considers BMIs of 25.0–26.9, 27.0–30.9, and 31.0 kg/m^2 or higher to indicate borderline (moderate) obesity, obesity, and marked obesity. He notes that moderate obesity, because of its high prevalence, is responsible for

Table 16.9. BMI FOR SELECTED HEIGHTS AND WEIGHTS

Height in cm (in)	Body weight in kg (lb)		
	BMI 25	BMI 27	BMI 30
147 (58)	54 (119)	59 (129)	65 (143)
150 (59)	56 (124)	60 (133)	67 (148)
152 (60)	58 (128)	63 (138)	69 (153)
155 (61)	60 (132)	65 (143)	72 (158)
158 (62)	62 (136)	67 (147)	74 (164)
160 (63)	64 (141)	69 (152)	77 (169)
163 (64)	66 (145)	71 (157)	79 (174)
165 (65)	68 (150)	73 (162)	82 (180)
168 (66)	70 (155)	76 (167)	84 (186)
170 (67)	72 (159)	78 (172)	87 (191)
173 (68)	74 (164)	80 (177)	89 (197)
175 (69)	77 (169)	83 (182)	92 (203)
178 (70)	79 (174)	85 (188)	94 (207)
180 (71)	81 (179)	87 (193)	98 (215)
183 (72)	83 (184)	90 (199)	100 (221)
185 (73)	86 (189)	93 (204)	103 (227)
188 (74)	88 (194)	95 (210)	106 (233)
191 (75)	91 (200)	98 (216)	109 (240)
193 (76)	93 (205)	100 (221)	112 (246)

Source: NIH 1998.

most obesity-related disorders in the United States. The European Athero-sclerosis Society defines desirable body weight as a BMI of 20.1–25.0 kg/m^2 in men and 18.7–23.8 kg/m^2 in women (International Task Force 1993).

Assessment before intervention includes reasons and motivation for weight reduction, history of successful and unsuccessful attempts, social support, patient understanding of risk, attitude toward physical activity, ability to engage in physical activity, time availability, and financial con-siderations. The health care provider needs to heighten the patient's motivation for weight loss and to prepare him or her for treatment, including enumeration of the hazards of overweight/obesity and the ben-efits of weight loss (see Chapter 11). Long-term success is more likely when there is a cognitive shift from focusing on weight to focusing on health (Foreyt 1997). Individuals need to become aware of their eating behavior and exercise habits (Grundy 1998).

Treatment

The most successful strategies for weight loss are calorie reduction, increased physical activity, and behavior therapy designed to improve eat-ing and physical activity habits (Table 16.10). Management also entails instituting measures to control accompanying risk factors. Drug therapy and surgery for weight loss may be considered in selected patients. Patients using nonprescription drugs for weight loss that have not been approved for that purpose should be advised that adverse effects in some cases could be serious and that efficacy is unproved (Popovich and Wood 1997). The AHA has noted that experience of the surgeon and type of operation pre-dict outcome of weight reduction surgery, and that in general Roux-en-Y gastric bypass is superior to gastric plication (Eckel 1997; Consensus Devel-opment Panel 1992). There is considerable hope that the next 10 years will bring better treatments for obesity, in particular in the pharmacologic arena (Finer 1997; Campfield et al. 1998).

Treatment approaches, including weight loss programs, should be tai-lored to the needs of individual patients or patient groups. Lost weight will usually be regained unless a weight maintenance program of dietary therapy, physical activity, and behavior therapy is continued indefinitely. The AHA notes that, except for those treated surgically, less than 5% of obese patients may maintain their reduced weight at 4 years (Eckel 1997). Smoking cessa-tion entails weight gain in about 80% of quitters, and the weight gain is resistant to most interventions. Nevertheless, smoking cessation should be advocated regardless of baseline weight; see "Weight Gain" under "Smoking Cessation," above. The significance of weight cycling (repeated loss and regaining of large amounts of weight) remains unclear because of inade-quate data; until further findings are available, concerns about weight cycling should serve to increase emphasis on long-term maintenance of weight loss and prevention of obesity but not to discourage weight loss (Daly et al. 1996).

Very low calorie diets (maximum of 800 kcal/day) produce greater ini-tial weight losses than low-calorie diets, but weight loss is not different

Table 16.10. NIH RECOMMENDATIONS FOR WEIGHT LOSS IN ADULTS

- **Most successful strategies:**
  Calorie reduction—Reducing dietary fat intake without reducing calorie intake will not lead to weight loss; however, reducing dietary fat intake is a practical way to reduce calories. In dietary fat reduction, priority should be given to reduction of saturated fatty acids (SFAs; low SFA intake is needed even in individuals of normal weight to help prevent atherosclerosis).
  Increased physical activity—Patients should engage in moderate physical activity, progressing to ≥30 minutes on most or preferably all days of the week. Exercise enables preferential loss of fat with preservation of lean tissue and may suppress the appetite. Significant weight loss should not be expected with exercise alone without calorie restriction.
  Behavior therapy—Designed to improve eating and physical activity habits. Specific behavior therapy strategies include self-monitoring, stress management, stimulus control, problem solving, contingency management, cognitive restructuring, and social support. Many self-help and commercial diet programs are available. However, commercial programs often use "crash diets," which are almost always unsuccessful.
- **Initial goal:** Reduce body weight by ~10% from baseline value, an amount that reduces obesity-related risk factors. With success, if warranted, further weight loss may be attempted.
- **Time line:** 6 months of therapy for a 10% reduction in body weight, with a weight loss of 0.5–1.0 kg (1–2 lb) per week (calorie deficit of 500–1,000 kcal/day).
- **Weight maintenance:** A priority after the first 6 months of weight loss therapy. Rate of weight loss usually declines and weight plateaus after 6 months because of reduced energy expenditure at the lower weight.
- **Drug therapy:** Lifestyle therapy should be tried for at least 6 months before consideration of physician-prescribed drug therapy. Weight loss drugs approved by the FDA for long-term use may be tried as part of a comprehensive weight loss program that includes dietary therapy and physical activity in carefully selected patients (BMI >30 kg/m^2 without additional risk factors; BMI >27 kg/m^2 with ≥2 other risk factors) who have been unable to lose weight or maintain weight loss with conventional nondrug therapies. Disorders considered important enough to warrant drug therapy at a BMI of 27.0–29.9 kg/m^2 are hypertension, dyslipidemia, CHD, type 2 diabetes, and sleep apnea. Drug therapy may also be used during the weight maintenance phase of treatment. Drug safety and effectiveness beyond 1 year of total treatment have not been established.
- **Surgery:** Weight loss surgery is an option for carefully selected patients with clinically severe obesity: BMI >40 kg/m^2, or BMI >35 kg/m^2 with comorbid conditions, when less invasive methods have failed and the patient is at high risk for obesity-associated illness. Lifelong medical surveillance after surgery is required.
- **Nonparticipants:** Overweight or obese patients who do not wish to lose weight or who are not candidates for weight loss treatment should be counseled on strategies to avoid further weight gain.
- **Older patients:** Age alone should not preclude weight loss treatment in older adults. Management should be guided by careful evaluation of potential risks and benefits.

Source: NIH 1998.

between the two approaches after 1 year (NIH 1998). Very low calorie diets must contain sufficient high-quality protein and adequate vitamins, minerals, and electrolytes to minimize cardiac complications and loss of lean tissue. Adverse outcomes and effects of severe calorie restriction include sudden cardiac death, gallstones, fatigue, weakness, orthostatic dizziness, constipation, diarrhea, nausea, headache, cold intolerance, menstrual irregularities, peripheral neuropathy, and hyperuricemia (Daly et al. 1996).

Physiology of Weight Loss

Daly et al. (1996) provided a précis of the physiology of weight loss. Energy expenditure must exceed energy intake for weight loss to occur. Humans ingest energy as carbohydrates (4 kcal/g), protein (4 kcal/g), fat (9 kcal/g), or alcohol (7 kcal/g). In sedentary individuals, resting metabolic rate accounts for 50–60% of energy expenditure and the thermic effects of food and physical activity each account for about 20%. Energy may also be lost as heat; this facultative thermogenesis, which is driven by the sympathetic nervous system and regulated in part by insulin and thyroid hormone, allows dissipation of excess calories and varies significantly interindividually. When calorie intake is markedly reduced, facultative energy expenditure is decreased to preserve energy, a response that accounts in part for the diminishing weight loss with duration of very low calorie diets.

INCREASED PHYSICAL ACTIVITY

Recommendations issued by a number of authorities, including the AHA (Fletcher et al. 1996, Fletcher 1997), the U.S. Surgeon General (1996), and the CDC and American College of Sports Medicine (Pate et al. 1995), reflect a growing body of evidence that links regular moderate physical activity to CVD risk reduction and other health benefits. However, about 40% of Americans are predominantly sedentary (Harris et al. 1989), and the trend is toward decreasing physical activity with aging (CDC 1993a). Regular aerobic physical activity plays a role in both primary and secondary prevention of CVD. Individuals of all ages should be physically active, and the exercise routine should include both aerobic and resistance activities.

Every patient's customary physical activity level should be assessed by his or her physician and should be an integral part of the medical history. The physician, with the support of nurses, physical and occupational therapists, exercise scientists, and other health professionals, should prescribe and give advice about physical activity with individual patient needs and capabilities in mind (Fletcher et al. 1996, 1997). Risks of a sedentary lifestyle should be emphasized. The foremost consideration in selecting the level of exercise is the individual's overall health status. Medical evaluation, including exercise testing, is needed for some individuals (see later), although not for an apparently healthy individual less than 40 years of age who has no coronary risk factors and who plans to begin only a moderate-intensity activity program (Fletcher 1996, 1997).

Most benefit against CVD mortality can be achieved through moderately intense activity. It is best that the activity be performed for at least 30–60 minutes four to six times per week or 30 minutes on most days of the week (Fletcher et al. 1996, 1997). Frequency, duration, and intensity should be individualized to personal satisfaction, mode, and progression. Exercise should include aerobic activities such as bicycling (stationary or routine), swimming, and other active recreational/leisure sports. A readily accessible form of exercise for achieving aerobic fitness is brisk, regular walking. The exercise program should additionally include resistive exercises, performed two to three times weekly using free weights or standard equipment (Fletcher et al. 1996, 1997).

Even low-intensity activities performed daily can confer some health benefit. Patients who meet the daily standards may derive additional health and fitness benefit by becoming more active or including more vigorous activity (NIH Consensus Development Panel 1996). A factor to consider is the prior activity level of the individual. For example, it is unrealistic to instruct a completely sedentary patient to exercise for 30 minutes three times a week at 60–70% of maximal capacity; a more gradual approach is advisable (Paffenbarger and Lee 1996).

Physicians also need to provide systematic follow-up of physical activity prescriptions. The greatest challenge may be maintenance of the exercise program; the physician should attempt to identify barriers to the patient's integration of exercise into the usual lifestyle and daily routine (Paffenbarger and Lee 1996) (Table 16.11).

Potential risks of physical activity can be reduced by medical evaluation, risk stratification, supervision, and education. Individuals with a known or suspected cardiovascular, respiratory, metabolic, orthopedic, or neurologic disorder should consult their physician before undertaking or significantly increasing physical activity (Fletcher et al. 1996). Middle-aged or older sedentary individuals with symptoms of CVD should seek medical advice as well. Physicians should give advice according to recommended guidelines (Fletcher et al. 1995; Pina et al. 1995; Balady et al. 1994; American Association of Cardiovascular and Pulmonary Rehabilitation 1990; Parmley et al. 1986). Exercise testing can be an important basis for appropriate prescription of physical activity. Medically supervised exercise programs are recommended in some cases; bias against women in referral to cardiac rehabilitation has been described and should be avoided (Fletcher et al. 1996) (see Chapter 18). Recommendations for cardiovascular screening, staffing, and emergency policies at health fitness facilities are also available (Balady et al. 1998).

Secondary Prevention

In secondary prevention (Fletcher et al. 1997), walking is recommended for early activity unless the individual can attend supervised classes where other activities can be provided. Walking should at first be limited, then gradually increase to 5–10 minutes of continuous movement. As long as

Table 16.11. FACTORS THAT INFLUENCE MOTIVATION FOR AND ABILITY TO SUSTAIN PHYSICAL ACTIVITY

The individual
- Perceives a net benefit
- Chooses an enjoyable activity
- Feels competent doing the activity
- Feels safe doing the activity
- Can easily access the activity on a regular basis
- Can fit the activity into the daily schedule
- Feels that the activity does not generate financial or social costs that he or she is unwilling to bear
- Experiences a minimum of negative consequences, such as injury, loss of time, negative peer pressure, and problems with self-identity
- Is able to address issues of competing time demands successfully
- Recognizes the need to balance the use of labor-saving devices (e.g., automobiles, power lawn mowers) and sedentary activities (e.g., watching television, playing computer games, "surfing the web") with activities that involve a higher level of physical exertion

Source: NIH Consensus Development Panel 1996; used with permission.

healing of a sternal incision is not stressed or impaired, active but nonresistive range of motion of upper extremities is also well tolerated. Emphasis in the first 2 weeks after MI or CABG is offsetting the effects of bed rest or former periods of inactivity. Activity should increase when the patient's condition is stable, as determined by ECG, vital signs, and symptomatic standards. Precautions include awareness of chest discomfort, faintness, and dyspnea. Initial activities need to be supervised.

Exercise testing is required in secondary prevention before a physical activity program is begun. Symptom-limited exercise testing is often performed as soon as the patient's condition has stabilized (as early as 2–6 weeks after the coronary event). If echocardiography, angiography, or other studies are not indicated, a regular conditioning program can be initiated with a careful prescription of activity based on results of the exercise test. For purposes of conditioning, large-muscle group activities should be performed for at least 20–30 minutes at least three to four times weekly; activities should be preceded by warm-up and followed by cool-down. Supervised group sessions are recommended initially. In motivated, low-risk individuals who understand the basic principles of exercise training, unsupervised home programs are acceptable (Fletcher et al. 1997).

The Physically Disabled

Atherosclerotic disease is a common killer among people with spinal cord injuries (Bauman et al. 1992; Ragnarrson 1993). Susceptibility to CHD risk factors is worsened by a potential for progressive physical inactivity, continued high rates of smoking, and the potential for a progressive increase in BMI (Zigler et al. 1998). Many individuals become obese during the chronic phase of spinal cord injury, and reduced lean body mass and increased body fat have been demonstrated in disabled individuals even without apparent obesity (Ragnarsson 1993). The lipid profile determines part of the CHD risk; HDL-C is significantly reduced in disabled persons in association with a lack of physical activity (Bauman et al. 1992). In a cross-sectional study in subjects older than 80 years, HDL-C strongly discriminated between the free living and the disabled (Zuliani et al. 1997).

Many of the changes resulting from a sedentary lifestyle in some disabled persons, including some with spinal cord injury, can be reversed with appropriate endurance exercise programs (Ragnarsson 1993). In a randomized, controlled trial in physically disabled men with CHD and functional use of two or more extremities, including an arm, home exercise training and dietary instruction significantly increased HDL-C and improved peak exercise performance (Fletcher et al. 1994). Physical exercise may also improve mood and self-image in disabled individuals (Ragnarsson 1993). Clinicians need to be educators of disabled patients and their family members and caregivers to enable lifelong management of wellness (Zigler et al. 1998).

BLOOD PRESSURE CONTROL

The NHBPEP of the NHLBI issued the sixth report of the JNC (JNC VI) in November 1997 (NIH 1997). The purpose of the report is to provide guidance for primary care clinicians. Although a summary of the guidelines, including full workup and drug selection, is beyond the scope of this manual, components of risk factor stratification and recommended lifestyle interventions are summarized in Tables 16.12–16.16. As with any CHD risk factor, prevention must be emphasized: As discussed in Chapter 11, risk increases in a continuous relation to rising SBP and DBP, including in the ranges now defined as normotensive. Reducing the CVD complications of uncontrolled hypertension requires at the outset (1) accurate determination of blood pressure, preferably both in and out of the office; (2) recognition of causes of secondary hypertension, so that their treatment may obviate lifelong antihypertensive drug therapy; (3) assessment of target organ damage; and (4) detection and management of concomitant risk factors (Kaplan 1995). Because of the large physiologic variation in blood pressure, repeated measurement on several separate occasions is required to establish the usual blood pressure level. For a brief discussion of the risk of LVH, see Chapter 11. Some considerations in managing patients with concomitant hypertension and dyslipidemia are provided in Chapter 21.

In addition to the individual approach highlighted here, modifying lifestyles in populations can have a major protective effect against elevated blood pressure and CVD risk. Hypertension is a particular problem among African Americans (see Chapter 20).

Table 16.12. JNC VI CLASSIFICATION OF BLOOD PRESSURE IN ADULTS (≥18 YEARS)

Category	SBP (mm Hg)		DBP (mm Hg)
Optimal[a]	<120	and	<80
Normal	<130	and	<85
High normal	130–139	or	85–89
Hypertension[b]			
Stage 1	140–159	or	90–99
Stage 2	160–179	or	100–109
Stage 3	≥180	or	≥110

Note: Applies to those who are not taking antihypertensive drugs and who are not acutely ill. When SBP and DBP fall into different categories, the higher category is used. Risk stratification also requires assessment of target organ damage and other risk factors (see Table 16.14).
[a]Evaluate unusually low readings for clinical significance.
[b]Based on the average of ≥2 readings taken at each of ≥2 visits after the initial screening.
Source: NIH 1997.

Lifestyle Modifications

Lifestyle modifications proved effective in the treatment of hypertension are weight loss, moderation of alcohol intake, increased physical activity, and sodium restriction. Modifications with less well-proved benefit include increased intakes of potassium, calcium, and magnesium (see Table 16.16). Increased intakes of fiber and fish oil may also be helpful

Table 16.13. JNC VI RECOMMENDATIONS FOR FOLLOW-UP ON THE BASIS OF INITIAL BLOOD PRESSURE MEASUREMENTS IN ADULTS

Initial blood pressure (mm Hg)[a]		Recommended follow-up[b]
Systolic	Diastolic	
<130	<85	Recheck in 2 years.
130–139	85–89	Provide advice about lifestyle changes, and recheck blood pressure in 1 year.
140–159	90–99	Provide advice about lifestyle changes, and confirm blood pressure within 2 months.
160–179	100–109	Evaluate or refer to source of care within 1 month.
≥180	≥110	Evaluate or refer to source of care immediately or within 1 week depending on clinical situation.

[a]If SDP and DBP are in different categories, proceed according to the higher risk category (shorter time of follow-up).
[b]Modify according to history of blood pressure values, target organ damage, and presence of other risk factors (see Table 16.14).

Table 16.14. COMPONENTS OF JNC VI CARDIOVASCULAR RISK STRATIFICATION IN PATIENTS WITH HYPERTENSION

Major risk factors	Target organ damage/clinical CVD
Smoking	Heart disease: LVH, angina pectoris, prior MI, prior coronary revascularization, heart failure
Dyslipidemia	
Diabetes mellitus	Stroke or TIA
Age >60 years	Nephropathy
Male or post-menopausal	PVD
Family history of premature CVD	Retinopathy

Source: NIH 1997.

Table 16.15. JNC VI RISK STRATIFICATION AND TREATMENT

	Risk group A	Risk group B	Risk group C
Risk group definition			
Organ damage,* clinical CVD,* diabetes mellitus	*No for all 3*	*No for all 3*	*Yes for ≥1*
Other risk factors*	*No*	*≥1*	*Yes or no*
Intervention			
High-normal blood pressure	Lifestyle	Lifestyle	Drug therapy if heart failure, renal insufficiency, or diabetes mellitus
Stage 1 hypertension	Lifestyle up to 12 months	Lifestyle up to 6 months; consider drug therapy if multiple risk factors	Drug therapy
Stage 1 or 2 hypertension	Drug therapy	Drug therapy	Drug therapy

Goal: Blood pressure <140/90 mm Hg (in diabetes mellitus <130/85 mm Hg; in renal disease ≤130/85 mm Hg, or ≤125/75 mm Hg with proteinuria >1 g per 24 hours)

Note: Lifestyle changes must be maintained when drug therapy is given. For drug selection, see JNC VI guidelines.
*See Table 16.14.
Source: Modified in format from NIH 1997.

Table 16.16. LIFESTYLE MODIFICATIONS FOR PREVENTION AND MANAGEMENT OF HYPERTENSION

Effective means
- Lose weight if overweight.
  - —See "Weight Control" in this chapter.
  - —Loss of as little as 4.5 kg (10 lb) reduces blood pressure in many hypertensives.
  - —Weight loss enhances the effectiveness of antihypertensive medication.
  - —Weight loss improves other CHD risk factors.
- Limit daily alcohol intake.
  - —No more than 1 fl oz (30 mL) ethanol (~2 drinks) or
  - —No more than 0.5 fl oz (15 mL) ethanol (~1 drink) for women and lighter-weight men.

    1 drink = 1 can (12 fl oz) beer (360 mL)

               5 fl oz nonfortified wine (150 mL)

               3 fl oz fortified wine (sherry, port, marsala, Madeira) (90 mL)

               1 fl oz 100-proof liquor (30 mL)

               1.5 fl oz 80-proof liquor (45 mL)
  - —Excessive alcohol intake can cause resistance to antihypertensive medication and is a risk factor for stroke.
  - —Abrupt withdrawal from heavy alcohol use can lead to significant hypertension, which will recede within several days.
- Increase aerobic physical activity.
  - —Engage in moderate activity 30–45 minutes most days of the week.
  - —Sedentary individuals are at 20–50% greater risk for the development of hypertension than their physically active counterparts.
  - —See also "Increased Physical Activity" in this chapter.
- Reduce daily sodium intake.
  - —To ≤2,400 mg sodium (lower when renal disease is present).
  - —Sensitivity of blood pressure to sodium intake varies interindividually; in general, those with hypertension or diabetes, African Americans, and older individuals are more sensitive to sodium.
  - —Moderately decreased sodium intake may also enable reduced dosages of antihypertensive medications, reduce diuretic-induced potassium wastage, protect from osteoporosis and renal stones, and possibly induce LVH regression.
  - —Processed food accounts for >75% of sodium intake in the U.S. diet.
  - —Foods high in sodium include cured meats, pickled foods, cheese, convenience foods, bread (several servings), and soy sauce.
  - —Consumers should be alert to sodium-containing compounds added to foods, such as salt, baking powder, baking soda, and monosodium glutamate. One-fourth teaspoon salt contains 533 mg sodium.

Less well-proved means
- Maintain adequate daily intake of dietary potassium.
  - —Daily intake needed is ~3,500 mg.
  - —High potassium intake may improve blood pressure in hypertensive patients and may protect against the development of hypertension.
  - —Preferably from fresh fruits, vegetables, and beans. Good sources include white, pinto, lima, kidney, and baked beans; lentils; baked potatoes; yogurt; tomato juice; cantaloupe; orange juice; apricots; bananas; milk; spinach; and brussels sprouts.

—Additional potassium may be needed from potassium-containing salt substitutes, potassium supplements, or potassium-sparing diuretics if hypokalemia occurs during diuretic therapy. Use with caution in some (e.g., renal insufficiency, ACE inhibitor use, angiotensin II receptor blocker use).
- Maintain adequate daily intake of dietary calcium and magnesium for general health.
  —Low calcium intake is associated with increased risk for hypertension, and increased intake may lower blood pressure in some patients with hypertension, although usually minimally. Good sources of calcium include dairy products, especially yogurt and milk, as well as tofu and canned salmon with bones. NIH recommendations for daily calcium intake are as follows:

  Men: 1,000 mg for ages 25–65
  1,500 mg for age >65

  Women: 1,000 mg for ages 25–50 and for ages 51–65 with ERT
  1,500 mg for age >65 and for ages 51–65 without ERT

  —Evidence suggests an association of magnesium intake with blood pressure, but data do not yet support a benefit from increased intake. Good sources of magnesium include tofu, almonds, halibut, wheat germ, peanuts, and spinach. Recommended dietary allowances of magnesium are as follows:

  Males: 270, 400, and 350 mg for ages 11–14, 15–18, ≥19 years
  Females: 280, 300, and 280 mg for ages 11–14, 15–18, ≥19 years

For general cardiovascular health
- Stop smoking.
  —Smoking may blunt the benefit of antihypertensive therapy.
  —See "Smoking Cessation" in this chapter.
- Reduce intake of saturated fat and cholesterol.
  —See Chapter 15.

Sources: Modified from NIH 1997 with information from *The new living heart diet* by DeBakey et al. 1996.

(Whelton et al. 1996). High dosages of omega-3 fatty acids may decrease blood pressure, but blood pressure appears to be insensitive to the ratio of saturated to unsaturated fatty acids. Data do not support efficacy for carbohydrate, garlic, or onion content in the diet or for relaxation therapy (NIH 1997). Caffeine acutely increases blood pressure, as does smoking.

Drug Therapy

Meta-analyses of randomized, controlled clinical trials have shown antihypertensive pharmacotherapy to have benefit against stroke, CHD events, heart failure, progression of renal disease, progression to more severe hypertension, and all-cause mortality (Psaty et al. 1997; Moser and Herbert 1996). Beta-blockers and diuretics have been shown to reduce mortality in hypertension (Sleight 1996). For drug selection and use, see the JNC VI guidelines.

Compliance

Maximizing compliance is an important part of therapy. Techniques include maintaining awareness of noncompliance, establishing a goal of therapy to have minimal or no adverse effects, educating patients about hypertension, asking patients to measure blood pressure at home, maintaining contact with patients, keeping care inexpensive and simple, encouraging lifestyle changes, integrating pill taking into daily routines, prescribing medications according to pharmacologic principles (favoring long-acting formulations), being willing to stop unsuccessful therapy and try another approach, anticipating adverse effects and adjusting therapy to prevent or minimize them, continuing to add effective and tolerated drugs in a stepwise fashion, encouraging a positive attitude about achieving goals, and considering using nurse case management (NIH 1997).

MANAGING THE RISK OF DIABETES MELLITUS

In the United States, practice guidelines for the assessment and management of diabetes mellitus are the province of the ADA (1998a). Treatment of diabetes mellitus to reduce risk for clinical sequelae consists of a multiple risk factor approach, including medical nutrition therapy, increased physical activity, weight reduction when indicated, and the use of oral glucose-lowering agents and/or insulin, with careful attention to other CVD risk factors (ADA 1998b). Intervention must be vigorous. The ADA practice guidelines now include recommendations for the management of dyslipidemia in diabetes; these recommendations are synopsized in Chapter 21. CHD benefit in diabetic patients from the use of statin therapy for lipid lowering as secondary prevention has been demonstrated in post hoc analyses of the 4S and CARE data sets. As noted in Table 16.15, the blood pressure goal in diabetes should be less than 130/85 mm Hg. Lifestyle modification is particularly important because of high complication and failure rates in diabetic patients after interventions such as CABG and PTCA (Barzilay et al. 1994; The Bypass Angioplasty Revascularization Investigation Investigators 1996).

New Diagnostic Cutpoints

As highlighted by Peters (1998), epidemiologic studies have shown that diabetes is undiagnosed in 50% of individuals who have the disease (Harris et al. 1987). Most patients with type 2 diabetes mellitus were undiagnosed for 4–7 years; at diagnosis, 20% have retinopathy, 9% have neuropathy, 8% have nephropathy, and the prevalence of macrovascular complications is similar to that in patients with diabetes not newly diagnosed (Engelgau et al. 1995). Therefore, the ADA in 1997 developed new criteria for diagnosing diabetes (Table 16.17). The key changes are the lowering of the fasting plasma glucose cutpoint for diagnosis of diabetes to 126 mg/dL, the addition of a category of impaired fasting glucose, and the suggestion that oral glucose tolerance tests are not necessary for the diagnosis of diabetes in routine clinical practice (Peters 1998). Which patients to screen is essentially unchanged.

Table 16.17. COMPARISON OF CURRENT AND PREVIOUS ADA CUTPOINTS FOR DIAGNOSING DIABETES

	Venous plasma glucose concentration (mg/dL)	
	Current criteria	Old criteria
Fasting value		
Normal	**<110**	<115
Impaired fasting glucose	**110–125**	NA
Diabetes	**≥126**	≥140
2-Hour value (after 75 g glucose)		
Normal	**<140**	Same
Impaired glucose tolerance	**140–199**	Same
Diabetes	**≥200**	Same
Random value with symptoms of diabetes		
Diabetes	**≥200**	Same

Authors' note: Regardless of HgbA$_{1c}$, fasting glucose >110 mg/dL (and perhaps even >90 mg/dL) confers high risk for macrovascular disease (see text).
Source: Peters 1998; used with permission.

Risk of Insulin Resistance

The ADA and clinicians accept use of glycosylated hemoglobin (HgbA$_{1c}$) as a measure of tissue glycation and risk for diabetic complications. The ADA target for HgbA$_{1c}$ is 7%; about 63% of patients with a fasting plasma glucose value of 126 mg/dL or higher will have a normal HgbA$_{1c}$ value (4.3–6.3%), and only 7% will have a value higher than 7% (Peters 1998). But whereas the patients with normal HgbA$_{1c}$ are likely at fairly low risk for microvascular complications, they do not have normal glucose tolerance. They have significant insulin resistance, and their risk for macrovascular disease is very high. Management of their CHD risk factors must be aggressive, and they should be monitored for worsening of glycemic status (Peters 1998). Evidence supports risk for macrovascular disease at even slight elevations of fasting plasma glucose (Haffner et al. 1990; Meigs et al. 1998). Lifestyle changes to reduce the risk for macrovascular disease will also likely help prevent progression of insulin resistance and diabetes. Regardless of the HgbA$_{1c}$ level, fasting glucose of more than 110 mg/dL (and perhaps even >90 mg/dL) confers high risk for macrovascular disease (Peters 1998).

Suggested Reading

Smoking Cessation
Agency for Health Care Policy and Research. Smoking cessation. Clinical Practice Guideline No. 18. AHCPR publication no. 96-0692. Rockville, MD: U.S. Department of Health and Human Services, 1996. (Available:

http://www.ahcpr.gov/clinic/smokepcc.htm, or telephone 1-800-358-9295, or write AHCPR Publications Clearinghouse, P.O. Box 8547, Silver Spring, MD 20907.)

Agency for Health Care Policy and Research. Smoking cessation: a guide for primary care clinicians. AHCPR publication no. 96-0693. Rockville, MD: U.S. Department of Health and Human Services, 1996. (Available: see previous entry.)

Benowitz NL, Gourlay SG. Cardiovascular toxicity of nicotine: implications for nicotine replacement therapy. J Am Coll Cardiol 1997;29:1422–1431.

Gidding SS, Morgan W, Perry C, et al. Active and passive tobacco exposure: a serious pediatric health problem. A statement from the Committee on Atherosclerosis and Hypertension in Children, Council on Cardiovascular Disease in the Young, American Heart Association (review). Circulation 1994;90:2581–2590.

Glantz SA, Barnes DE, Bero L, et al. Looking through a keyhole at the tobacco industry: the Brown and Williamson documents. JAMA 1995;274:219–224.

Glantz SA, Slade J, Bero LA, et al. The cigarette papers. Berkeley, CA: University of California Press, 1996. (Available: http://www.library.ucsf.edu/tobacco/cigpapers.)

Hays JT, Hurt RD, Dale LC. Smoking cessation. In: Manson JE, Ridker PM, Gaziano JM, Hennekens CH, eds. Prevention of myocardial infarction. New York: Oxford University Press, 1996:99–129.

Henningfield JE. Nicotine medication for smoking cessation (review). N Engl J Med 1995;333:1196–1203.

Kottke TE. Managing nicotine dependence (editorial). J Am Coll Cardiol 1997;30:131–132.

Ockene IS, Houston Miller N, for the American Heart Association Task Force on Risk Reduction. Cigarette smoking, cardiovascular disease, and stroke. A statement for healthcare professionals from the American Heart Association. AHA medical/scientific statement. Circulation 1997;96:3243–3247. (Available: http://www.amhrt.org.)

Skaar K, Tsoh J, Cinciripini P, et al. Current approaches in smoking cessation. Curr Opin Oncol 1996;8:434–440.

Tsoh JY, McClure JB, Skaar KL, et al. Smoking cessation 2: components of effective intervention. Behav Med 1997;23:5–13.

Weight Control

National Institutes of Health. Clinical guidelines on the identification, evaluation, and treatment of overweight and obesity in adults. Bethesda, MD: National Institutes of Health, 1998. (Available at http://www.nhlbi.nih.gov/nhlbi, or telephone 301-251-1222, or write the NHLBI Information Center, P.O. Box 30105, Bethesda, MD 20824-0105.)

Increased Physical Inactivity

Fletcher GF. How to implement physical activity in primary and secondary prevention: a statement for healthcare professionals from the Task Force on Risk Reduction, American Heart Association. AHA medical/scientific statement. Circulation 1997;96:355–357.

Fletcher GF, Balady G, Blair SN, et al. Statement on exercise. Benefits and recommendations for physical activity programs for all Americans. A statement for health professionals by the Committee on Exercise and Cardiac
Rehabilitation of the Council on Clinical Cardiology, American Heart
Association. Circulation 1996;94:857–862.

Paffenbarger RS Jr, Lee I-M. Exercise and fitness. In: Manson JE, Ridker PM,
Gaziano JM, Hennekens CH, eds. Prevention of myocardial infarction.
New York: Oxford University Press, 1996:172–193.

Ragnarrson KT. The cardiovascular system. In: Whiteneck GG, Charlifue SW,
Gerhart KA, et al., eds. Aging with spinal cord injury. New York: Demos
Publications, 1993;73–92.

U.S. Surgeon General. Physical activity and health. Washington, DC: U.S.
Department of Health and Human Services, 1996.

Blood Pressure Control

National Institutes of Health. The sixth report of the Joint National Committee on Prevention, Detection, Evaluation, and Treatment of High Blood
Pressure. NIH publication no. 98-4080 (November 1997). Bethesda, MD:
National Institutes of Health, 1997. (Available from the NHLBI Information Center, P.O. Box 30105, Bethesda, MD 20824-0105; telephone 301-
251-1222; fax 301-251-1223.)

For practical implementation of lifestyle changes for the lay reader: DeBakey
ME, Gotto AM Jr, Scott LW, et al. The new living heart diet. New York:
Simon and Schuster, 1996.

Managing the Risk of Diabetes Mellitus

American Diabetes Association. Clinical practice recommendations. Diabetes
Care 1998;21(suppl 1) (full issue). (Available: http://www.diabetes.org.)

Peters AL. New criteria for the diagnosis of diabetes and the relationship to
macrovascular disease. Prev Cardiol 1998;(Spring):57–59.

Chapter 17

Lipid-Regulating Drugs and Low-Density Lipoprotein Apheresis

LIPID-REGULATING DRUGS

Four classes of lipid-regulating drugs are available in the United States: HMG-CoA reductase inhibitors (statins), bile acid sequestrants (resins), nicotinic acid (niacin), and fibric acid derivatives (fibrates). Each class offers a favorable risk:benefit ratio and has well-defined effects on the major lipid fractions (Table 17.1). It is of great interest that, as is discussed in Chapter 10, there is growing evidence that benefits of the drugs extend beyond their effects on lipid concentrations alone.

The available pharmacologic options allow drug therapy to be tailored to the specific lipid abnormality of an individual patient: Lipid-regulating drug therapy is not a "one size fits all" intervention (Farmer and Gotto 1996). Lipid-regulating drugs may be given as drug monotherapy, or as combination drug therapy, particularly in mixed dyslipidemias or severe hypercholesterolemia; either approach is always used in addition to lifestyle intervention. In many cases, combination drug therapy increases the effectiveness of lipid-regulating therapy and may allow lower dosages, the latter potentially decreasing side effects and cost and improving compliance. For example, adding low-dose resin therapy to a given dosage of statin therapy may enable a greater reduction of LDL-C than would simply doubling the dosage of the statin (Dujovne 1997). Oral estrogens, which usually decrease LDL-C and increase HDL-C, each by about 10–15%, may be considered for treatment of dyslipidemia in postmenopausal women (see Chapter 18), although they do not have an FDA indication for lipid regulation. Oral estrogens may also increase plasma TG, in particular when hypertriglyceridemia is already present.

NCEP recommendations for drug selection in adults are shown in Table 17.2. ADA recommendations for drug selection in diabetic adults are shown in Table 21.2. The priority of the NCEP guidelines is LDL-C reduction. Some authorities, such as the European Atherosclerosis Soci-

Table 17.1. EFFECTS OF DRUG CLASSES ON MAJOR PLASMA LIPID VALUES

	Statins	Resins	Niacin	Fibrates
LDL-C				Variable
HDL-C				
TG (VLDL)		No change or may increase		

Table 17.2. NCEP RECOMMENDATIONS FOR SELECTION OF LIPID-REGULATING AGENTS IN ADULTS

Disorder[a]	Single agent	Combination Agents	Potential interaction
LDL-C[b]	Resin, statin, niacin	Resin + statin	Resin may decrease statin absorption (should separate by several hours)
		Resin + niacin	
		Statin + niacin	Possible increased risk for myopathy or liver dysfunction
LDL-C + TG	Niacin, statin, fibrate	Niacin + statin	Possible increased risk for myopathy or liver dysfunction
		Statin + fibrate	Increased potential for myopathy with CK elevation (particularly careful monitoring and instruction of patient required)
		Niacin + resin	
		Niacin + fibrate	
TG	Niacin, fibrate	Niacin + fibrate	

Note: The ADA's recommendations for selection of lipid-regulating drugs in adult diabetic patients are shown in Table 21.2. Niacin has a relative contraindication in diabetes.
[a]When low or reduced HDL-C is present, drugs may also be selected on the basis of their effectiveness in raising HDL-C. In general, drug therapy is not recommended for isolated low HDL-C in patients who do not have known atherosclerotic disease.
[b]Oral estrogens may be considered in postmenopausal women (see Chapter 18).
Source: Data from NCEP 1994.

Table 17.3. SELECTED POSSIBLE DRUG AND FOOD INTERACTIONS WITH LIPID-LOWERING AGENTS

Agent(s)	Manifestation(s)
HMG-CoA reductase inhibitors	
Fibric acid derivatives, immunosuppressant agents, erythromycin, azole antifungals, cimetidine, methotrexate, mibefradil, grapefruit juice	Myopathy, rhabdomyolysis
Nicotinic acid	Elevations in liver enzymes; possible muscle necrosis
Coumarin anticoagulants	Prolongation of prothrombin time
Bile acid sequestrants	Reduced statin absorption
Bile acid sequestrants	
Thiazide diuretics, digitalis glycosides, beta-blockers, coumarin anticoagulants, exogenous thyroid hormones, gemfibrozil, statins, oral hypoglycemic agents (sulfonylureas), NSAIDs	Binding and delayed or decreased absorption of interactive agents
Nicotinic acid	
HMG-CoA reductase inhibitors	Elevations in liver enzymes; possible muscle necrosis
Aspirin (high dosage)	Increased concentration of nicotinic acid in circulation
Uricosuric agents (sulfinpyrazone)	Decreased efficacy of interactive agents
Drugs that adversely affect hepatic structure or function	Hepatocellular necrosis
Antihypertensive agents	Possible potentiation of antihypertensive effects
Fibric acid derivatives	
HMG-CoA reductase inhibitors, cyclosporine	Myopathy, rhabdomyolysis
Warfarin-type anticoagulants	Increased anticoagulant activity
Bile acid sequestrants, possibly antacids	Binding and decreased absorption of fibrate

Note: See labeling instructions of manufacturers regarding safety.
Source: Based in part on data from Farmer and Gotto 1994.

ety (International Task Force 1992), consider nicotinic acid as a single agent to be of limited usefulness because of problems with tolerability.

Because hypercholesterolemia is a chronic condition that requires long-term or even life-long therapy, tolerability and safety as well as cost (see "Cost-Effectiveness of Lowering Low-Density Lipoprotein Cholesterol" in Chapter 13) are central issues in the selection of pharmacologic therapy. Many patients who require lipid-regulating drugs will also at some time require concomitant medications. Drug interactions (Table 17.3) can compromise safety and efficacy, as well as increase costs of therapy because of the need for additional patient visits.

In a meta-analysis of controlled clinical trials of lipid-lowering drug therapy, Gould et al. (1998) found that for each 10% reduction in TC, CHD mortality risk would be decreased 15% and all-cause mortality risk would be decreased 11%. The rate of reduction in CHD mortality or all-cause mortality risk with increasing net decrease in TC was the same for statins and nonstatins. Statins reduced mortality risks more than other currently available drug classes because of their more effective reduction of cholesterol concentration.

Each of the four available drug classes is discussed in some detail below, although the physician must also read the manufacturers' product information sheets. Also discussed are probucol, which is no longer marketed in the United States, and fish oil supplementation, which should be considered a drug therapy.

When to Consider Drug Therapy: Four questions that should be considered before beginning lipid-regulating drug therapy (see Chapter 12) (Stone 1996b) are: (1) Is the workup complete? (2) Has the LDL-C goal (or have other lipid goals) been determined? (3) Has dietary and lifestyle instruction been given? (4) Does the selection of drug therapy match the lipid disorder and the risk for CHD (or risk for pancreatitis)?

Monitoring Drug Therapy: After the initiation of drug therapy, a full fasting lipoprotein profile should be obtained at 4–6 weeks and at 3 months. If the lipid goal is achieved, the patient should be seen every 4 months, or more frequently when drugs requiring closer follow-up are used, for monitoring of lipid response and adverse effects as well as for further counseling. Long-term monitoring should be at 4- to 6-month intervals. Nonfasting TC may provide a useful surrogate for LDL-C in long-term monitoring in some cases, but a full fasting lipoprotein profile is required at least annually and when therapy is changed or reaching a goal is to be verified.

UNDERUSE

Major discrepancies remain between current clinical practice and the guidelines laid down by the NCEP. Lipid-lowering drug therapy is underused, and physicians should be more diligent in applying this proved therapy (Gotto 1997). According to estimates based on phase 2 NHANES III data (1991–1994), only 1.4 million, or 6.6%, of 21.1 million American adults eligible for cholesterol-lowering drug therapy are receiving such therapy (Hoerger et al. 1998). The treatment rate is higher for secondary prevention (14%, or 0.8 of 5.5 million) than for primary prevention (4%, or 0.6 of 15.7 million), although it is still abysmally low. Sixty-five percent of diet- or drug-eligible adults are receiving no therapy of any kind. The NHLBI's fourth national survey found that among patients with CHD, only 27% had been prescribed dietary therapy and 29% drug therapy (NHLBI Cholesterol Awareness Surveys 1995).

Table 17.4. TACTICS FOR ENHANCING COMPLIANCE WITH LIPID-LOWERING THERAPEUTIC REGIMENS

Tactic	Examples/notes
Teach the patient to take the treatment regimen.	Instructions should be simple and concise but complete.
Help the patient identify ways to remember doses.	Tailor doses to daily rituals. Send reminders.
Develop reinforcers of compliance.	Keep a chart of lipid responses. Provide continuing encouragement.
Anticipate common problems and teach patients how to manage them.	Teach the patient how to minimize side effects.
Involve a family member or friend in the patient's therapy program.	Develop an advocate for the patient's welfare.
Establish a supportive relationship with the patient.	Listen carefully and respond in an open, nonjudgmental manner.
Make compliance important by asking about it.	Develop an approach that is encouraging, not condemnatory.
Provide ongoing education and updates about the patient's illness and treatment.	Incorporate new data and the patient's increasing level of understanding. Be on guard for misinformation the patient has received from the media, friends, or other sources.
Provide individualized services for patients who continue to be noncompliers.	Assess barriers: Physical—e.g., poor vision, forgetfulness Access—e.g., transportation, income, time Attitude—e.g., fatalism Therapy—e.g., complexity, side effects Social—e.g., family instability Faulty health perceptions—e.g., denial, looks to symptoms to prompt treatment

Source: Gotto et al. 1995; used with permission. Data from NCEP 1994.

In a chart review study by Harnick et al. (1998) of patients with CHD treated at a New York City hospital clinic or cardiology private practice (representing different socioeconomic classes), fewer than 50% of patients had had a lipid profile obtained within 12 months of treatment, and among those with a lipid profile, LDL-C exceeded 100 mg/dL in 78%. Individual physician behavior, not practice setting, was the most important determinant of quality of care. Percentages of patients with lipid values determined ranged from 0% to 83%, and drug treatment ranged from 10% to 88%, by individual physician.

Failure to reach NCEP goals in patients under treatment has been described in a number of surveys (Harris et al. 1998; Schrott et al. 1997). Marcelino and Feingold (1996) in a 1-year retrospective study of 90 patients prescribed statin monotherapy at a Veterans Administration Medical Center attributed failure to reach LDL-C goals in large measure to inadequate treatment by physicians. Nearly all the patients were given drug at a low dosage (and fewer than half were adequately monitored for hepatotoxicity). It is important to remember, however, that any reduction in elevated cholesterol appears to be associated with some benefit: In general, each 1% decrease in plasma cholesterol decreases CHD risk by at least 2–3% (Manson et al. 1992) (see also Chapter 11). Further studies are needed to determine the reasons underlying physician nonadherence to national guidelines.

Patient compliance is also inadequate, and intensified efforts need to be made by health care professionals to increase compliance (Table 17.4). In particular, more detailed counseling is needed to achieve compliance with nicotinic acid and the resins. In typical populations in the United States and Canada, only 52% of surviving patients who had been prescribed lipid-lowering pharmacotherapy were still taking a lipid-lowering agent 5 years later (Avorn et al. 1998). The odds ratio for good persistence was about twice as high for statins compared with other drugs; in particular, it was better than for bile acid sequestrants. Roberts (1996) has described even lower compliance rates with lipid-lowering drug therapy: about a 50% drug quit rate in the first year, and compliance of only 25% after 2 years.

HMG-CoA REDUCTASE INHIBITORS

The HMG-CoA reductase inhibitors, or statins, are newly established front-line therapy for hypercholesterolemia, and they have captured the market for cholesterol-lowering drugs. They are the most effective drugs available for lowering LDL-C, with clinical benefit unequivocally demonstrated not only for CHD mortality but also for all-cause mortality rate, and they have excellent records of safety and tolerability. William Roberts, MD, editor of the *American Journal of Cardiology*, has said that the statins are to athero-sclerosis what penicillin was to infectious disease (Roberts 1996).

Mevastatin (compactin), the first HMG-CoA reductase inhibitor developed, but one that was never marketed, was isolated from *Penicillium citrinum*. Lovastatin, simvastatin, and pravastatin are also fungal derivatives: Simvastatin, which is semisynthetic, is an analogue of lovastatin, and pravastatin, first discovered in the urine of animals administered mevastatin, is a purified metabolite of mevastatin (Lennernäs and Fager 1997; Bradford et al. 1994; Frishman and Rapier 1989; Plosker and McTavish 1995; Haria and McTavish 1997). Fluvastatin, atorvastatin, and cerivastatin are all purely synthetic (Plosker and Wagstaff 1996; Lea and McTavish 1997; Bischoff et al. 1997) (Table 17.5). In chemical structure, each statin has a moiety that resembles hydroxymethylglutaric acid, which may be present in an open (hydroxy acid) form, which is readily active, or in a closed (lactone) form (Figure 17.1; see Table 17.5). Ring opening of the inactive lactones (lactone prodrugs) occurs at alkaline pH or in the liver (Sirtori et al. 1991). Lovastatin will be the first HMG-CoA reductase inhibitor to lose its patent protection in the United States, in 2001.

**Table 17.5. BIOCHEMICAL AND PHARMACOKINETIC
CHARACTERISTICS OF HMG-CoA REDUCTASE INHIBITORS**

Agent	Gener-ation	Derivation	FDA approval	Form given	Solubility	Major CYP-3A4 metab.	Half-life (hr)
Atorva-statin	4	Synthetic	1997	Active	Lipo-philic	✓	13–16
Ceriva-statin	4	Synthetic	1997	Active	Hydro-philic	✓	2–3
Fluva-statin	3	Synthetic	1993	Active	Hydro-philic		0.5
Lova-statin	1	Fungal derivative	1987	Prodrug	Lipo-philic	✓	2–3
Prava-statin	1	Fungal derivative	1991	Active	Hydro-philic		1
Simva-statin	2	Semi-synthetic	1991	Prodrug	Lipo-philic	✓	2–3

Source: Adapted from Dujovne 1997; used with permission.

Cholestin, a product promoted as a dietary supplement intended to affect plasma cholesterol concentrations, was deemed an unapproved drug by the FDA in May 1998. Derived from red yeast rice, it has some efficacy because it contains lovastatin. As is the case for nicotinic acid (see later), patients may believe that Cholestin may be taken without physician supervision. Unsupervised use of such a preparation should not be condoned.

Mechanisms

HMG-CoA reductase catalyzes the conversion of HMG to mevalonate, the rate-limiting step in cholesterol biosynthesis. All the statins are reversible competitive inhibitors of HMG-CoA reductase. Pharmacologic inhibition of HMG-CoA reductase causes a decrease in cholesterol synthesis, which leads to transcriptionally up-regulated production of HMG-CoA reductase and cell surface LDL receptors, resulting in an increased rate of removal of LDL particles from plasma (Ma et al. 1986).

The drugs are designed to be hepatoselective. Typically, more than three-fourths of the body's cholesterol pool is of endogenous origin, and two-thirds is produced in the liver (Brown and Goldstein 1986). Inhibition of peripheral cholesterol synthesis would be more likely to lead to adverse drug effects (Hamelin and Turgeon 1998). Different processes explain the hepatoselectivity, including first-pass uptake for lovastatin, simvastatin, and fluvastatin and active carrier-mediated uptake for pravastatin (Hamelin and Turgeon 1998). Greater hepatoselectivity tends to be observed with the less lipophilic compounds; however, pharmacokinetic data on the statins in

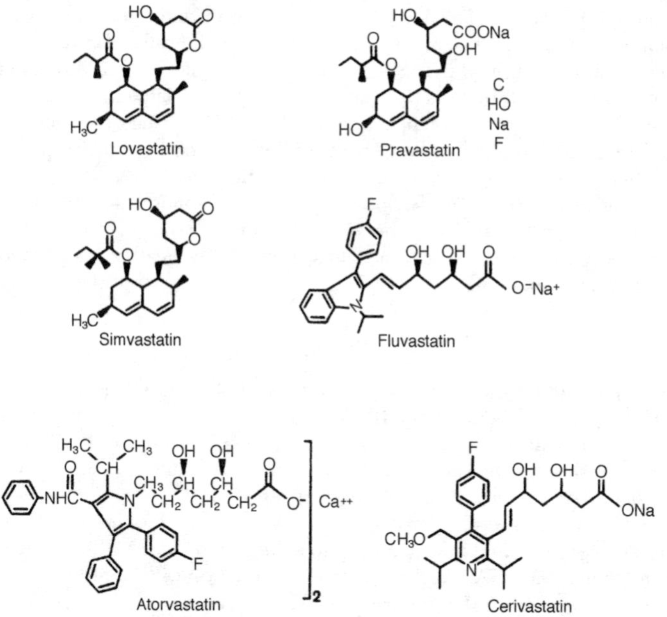

© 1997 Current Opinion in Lipidology

Figure 17.1. Chemical structures of the HMG-CoA reductase inhibitors. (From Dujovne 1997; used with permission.)

humans remain incomplete, and reported findings are confusing regarding different degrees of liver selectivity claimed for different statins (Lennernäs and Fager 1997). Atorvastatin is lipophilic but, because of extensive hepatic metabolism through first-pass mechanisms, has high hepatic selectivity (Lea and McTavish 1997).

It has been speculated that the statins may decrease plasma TG through increased uptake of VLDL particles by the up-regulated LDL (apo B/E) receptors or that the blocked cholesterol biosynthesis makes less cholesterol available for VLDL production and secretion (Bakker-Arkema et al. 1996). In a placebo-controlled crossover study in 13 normolipidemic men, simvastatin therapy decreased the hepatic secretion rate of VLDL apo B by 46% but did not change its fractional catabolism (Watts et al. 1997).

As discussed in Chapter 10, a variety of studies have suggested possible statin benefit through pathways other than changes in plasma lipid concentrations—for example, alterations in cell proliferation, vascular reactivity, clotting mechanisms and rheologic parameters, and lipoprotein composition and oxidation. Available data do not support differences among the statins in this regard, however (Scott 1997). Unlike simvastatin or fluvastatin, pravastatin does not inhibit SMC proliferation and migration in vitro and in vivo (Corsini et al. 1998), a difference that has been related to pravastatin's hydrophilicity and lack of penetration of cells. Many such changes have been reported to occur within just a few weeks or months of the beginning of therapy. Most studies have failed to show effects on LDL particle size or composition (Scott 1997). The possibility of immunomodulating properties has been of particular interest because of findings of reduced transplant vasculopathy and increased survival with statin use after heart transplantation (see Chapter 9).

Efficacy

All the statins produce substantial reductions in LDL-C with lesser but significant beneficial effects on HDL-C and plasma TG.

Reductions in LDL-C range from 15% to 60% (Dujovne 1997). Individual responses, however, can be highly variable, and response is best evaluated on a patient-by-patient basis (Dujovne 1997). Resistance may be great in patients with heterozygous FH, who usually require coprescription of a second lipid-lowering drug to achieve sufficient LDL-C lowering (Shepherd 1995a). After maximal LDL-C reduction with statin therapy at 2–3 weeks, there is a slow increase in LDL-C with prolonged use in a small subset of patients (Tikkanen 1996; Rubinstein and Weintraub 1995). This "statin escape" phenomenon is relatively small compared with other lipid-lowering agents and, anecdotally, may be most likely in patients with reduced dietary compliance and marked weight gain (Tikkanen 1996).

Atorvastatin has been reported to have greater efficacy in LDL-C reduction than milligram-equivalent doses of simvastatin, pravastatin, lovastatin, or fluvastatin (Jones et al. 1998b). As monotherapy, it reduces LDL-C up to 60% (Nawrocki et al. 1995). Results have suggested that the greater efficacy of atorvastatin may be due to more prolonged inhibition of HMG-CoA reductase, presumably reflecting longer residence of atorvastatin or its metabolites in the liver (Naoumova et al. 1997). Atorvastatin, 80 mg/day, achieved an additional 31% decrease in LDL-C concentration both before and after LDL apheresis in patients with homozygous FH (Marais et al. 1997), apparently through marked inhibition of cholesterol synthesis and decreased rate of production of LDL-C, and a 54% decrease in heterozygous FH (Naoumova et al. 1996). A 31% decrease in LDL-C in homozygous FH was also achieved with expanded-dose simvastatin (160 mg/day) (Raal et al. 1997).

Statin therapy increases HDL-C by 5–10%, but responses vary (Schectman and Hiatt 1996). TG reduction usually ranges from 10% to 20% (NCEP 1994), although in hypertriglyceridemia, atorvastatin has reduced TG 26–46% (Bakker-Arkema et al. 1996).

It has been suggested that atorvastatin may offer monotherapy drug treatment of patients with combined hyperlipidemia and provide a well-tolerated alternative to nicotinic acid in isolated hypertriglyceridemia

(McKenney et al. 1998). It has been argued that atorvastatin reduces TG through its more pronounced inhibitory effect on cholesterol synthesis (Bakker-Arkema et al. 1996). It could also be argued that all statins are qualitatively similar, so that other statins would similarly reduce TG if given at high enough dosages (Lea and McTavish 1997). An analysis of pooled study results has suggested that dose-dependent reductions of 22–45% can be obtained with all the statins when fasting TG exceeds 250 mg/dL, but that there is not a significant or dose-dependent response when TG is below 150 mg/dL (Stein and Laskarzewski. 1998). Because tests of statin therapy for hypertriglyceridemia have been published only since 1996 (Stein and Laskarzewski. 1998), additional direct data are needed.

Clinical Trial Findings

There is ample evidence from randomized, placebo-controlled trials that the statins benefit the clinical consequences and pathology of atherosclerotic disease. In the 4S (simvastatin), CARE, WOSCOPS, LIPID (pravastatin), and AFCAPS/TexCAPS (lovastatin) trials (see Chapter 12), statin therapy has been shown to reduce significantly the incidence of CHD in patients with and without CHD and the all-cause mortality rate in patients with CHD. In addition, meta- and subgroup analyses have shown significant reductions in risk for stroke (see Chapter 12). Antiatherogenicity has been demonstrated in trials in which angiographic monitoring was used, such as FATS, CCAIT, Post-CABG (lovastatin), MAAS (simvastatin), REGRESS, PLAC I (pravastatin), and LCAS (fluvastatin) (see Chapter 10).

Safety and Tolerability

Many patient-years of use have established the safety of this class of lipid-lowering drug. The most important adverse effects of statin therapy are hepatotoxicity and myopathy, which both are unusual and only rarely require drug cessation.

Mild, asymptomatic increases in serum transaminase values have been observed in about 2–5% of patients (Hamelin and Turgeon 1998). Increases are dose related and often transient; transaminase values normalize after drug discontinuation without permanent liver damage. Small increases may represent altered lipid metabolism, since the effect is observed with most other lipid-altering agents (Hamelin and Turgeon 1998). Elevation of alanine or aspartate transaminase to three times the upper limit of normal (or higher) is very uncommon; if it occurs and persists, it is recommended that statin therapy be withdrawn.

Myopathy associated with an increase in muscle enzymes is rare, as is progression to frank rhabdomyolysis, a condition that can be life threatening. Much more common are muscle aches and arthralgia of variable severity, reported in up to 10% of patients, but often difficult to attribute to drug therapy. There is apparently little correlation between degree of CK elevation and severity of symptoms (Hamelin and Turgeon 1998; Scott

1997; Shepherd 1995b). The potential for a statin to produce myositis is dose dependent and perhaps related to extent of lipid lowering because the effect is reversible with mevalonate administration (Dujovne 1997). Occurrence of skeletal muscle abnormalities is most common when there is renal insufficiency or concomitant therapy with certain drugs, including cyclosporine, erythromycin, gemfibrozil, fenofibrate, and itraconazole (Hamelin and Turgeon 1998; Farmer and Gotto 1994) (see also "Interactions"). Patients should be advised to report promptly any unexplained tenderness, weakness, or pain in muscles, particularly if accompanied by malaise or fever. If marked CK elevation is found or myopathy is diagnosed or suspected, statin therapy should be discontinued.

Statins are very well tolerated. The most common complaints are gastrointestinal in nature (heartburn, abdominal pain, diarrhea, constipation, flatulence), followed by headache and rash (Hamelin and Turgeon 1998; Garnett 1995) and reports of sleep disturbances. Such effects are uncommon and rarely severe enough to require interruption of therapy. A 3-year, placebo-controlled, randomized trial showed no mood disturbances with cholesterol lowering by statin therapy (simvastatin) (Wardle et al. 1996). Statin therapy in the elderly is well tolerated and associated with no reduction in quality in life (Santanello et al. 1997).

Data are insufficient to validate claims for differences in side effect profiles among the statins (Scott 1997). The hydrophilic statins do not cross the blood-brain barrier and possibly give rise to fewer CNS side effects such as insomnia (Garnett 1996).

Statins are contraindicated in active or chronic liver disease or unexplained persistent elevations of serum transaminases. They should not be given to pregnant or lactating women and should not be used in women of childbearing potential unless contraception is fully satisfactory. They should be withheld in patients experiencing an acute or serious condition predisposing them to the development of renal failure secondary to rhabdomyolysis (e.g., sepsis, hypotension, major surgery, trauma, uncontrolled epilepsy, or severe metabolic, endocrine, or electrolyte disorders).

Interactions

Coadministration of HMG-CoA reductase inhibitors and other drugs or compounds whose metabolism involves cytochrome P450 3A4 (CYP3A4) can increase the potential for myopathy and CK elevation, since inhibition of a statin's metabolism can result in its higher peak or steady-state concentration in plasma (Dujovne 1997). Such drugs and compounds include but are not limited to fibric acid derivatives (see also "Fibric Acid Derivatives," later), immunosuppressant agents, erythromycin, azole antifungals, cimetidine, methotrexate, and grapefruit juice (Dujovne 1997; Farmer and Gotto 1994; Garnett 1995; Kantola et al. 1998). As discussed in Chapter 21 (see "Patients with Concomitant Dyslipidemia and Hypertension"), mibefradil has been withdrawn from the U.S. market because of concerns about its interaction with other drugs whose metabolism involves CYP3A4.

Susceptibility to interaction with CYP3A4 inhibitors varies among the statins: For example, lovastatin and simvastatin are very susceptible to interaction with itraconazole, whereas interaction between itraconazole and pravastatin or fluvastatin may be minor or may not occur (Kantola et al. 1998). CYP3A4 plays an important role in the biotransformation of lovastatin, simvastatin, atorvastatin, and cerivastatin, but other enzymes are primarily responsible for the metabolism of pravastatin and fluvastatin (Kantola et al. 1998; Boberg et al. 1997). The interaction of grapefruit juice and drugs results in the main from a reduction of first-pass metabolism in the small intestine, where grapefruit juice selectively down-regulates CYP3A4 (Kantola et al. 1998). Thus, important interactions with grapefruit juice are limited to drugs with low systemic bioavailability because of first-pass gut metabolism (Miller and Spence 1998). Grapefruit juice has been shown to increase greatly serum concentrations of lovastatin, which has a systemic bioavailability of only about 5% (Kantola et al. 1998). Miller and Spence (1998) speculate that it is likely that differences among statins with respect to potential for interaction with fibrates may also be importantly affected by systemic bioavailability.

Statins may also potentially interact with coumarin anticoagulants, so that prothrombin time is prolonged, and with nicotinic acid, leading to elevations in liver enzymes and possible muscle necrosis (Farmer and Gotto 1994). Bile acid resins can decrease the absorption of statins. In three lovastatin-treated patients receiving pectin or oat bran, LDL-C rose, perhaps because of decreased absorption of lovastatin (Garnett 1995).

Dosage

The statins are all administered as tablets, given once daily except for high-dose fluvastatin (80 mg given in divided doses) and lovastatin (may be given in divided doses). Atorvastatin may be administered at any time of day without regard to meals; other statins are administered in the evening or at bedtime (Table 17.6), without regard to food, except for lovastatin, which should be taken with a meal. Cholesterol biosynthesis is greatest at night and during the early morning hours (Plosker and McTavish 1995). Recommended starting daily doses and daily dose ranges are shown in Table 17.6. Cerivastatin is effective at dosages about 100 times lower than those for the other statins; its affinity for HMG-CoA reductase inhibition is about 100 times greater than that of lovastatin (Dujovne 1997). Phase III trials of the comparative efficacy of 0.4- and 0.8-mg cerivastatin are under way.

Dose-response appears to be nonlinear: Schectman and Hiatt (1996) reviewed published data on fluvastatin, lovastatin, pravastatin, and simvastatin and found that lower dosages captured most of the expected efficacy, without a proportional increase in effectiveness with dosage.

Monitoring

In addition to lipid monitoring for response, liver function values should be periodically monitored before and during treatment. Liver function

Table 17.6. DOSAGES OF HMG-CoA REDUCTASE INHIBITORS

Agent	Trade name	Standard daily starting (mg)*	Range (mg)	Time of day	With meals?
Atorvastatin	Lipitor	10	10–80	Anytime	With or without
Cerivastatin	Baycol	0.3		Evening	With or without
Fluvastatin	Lescol	20–30	20–80	Bedtime	With or without
Lovastatin	Mevacor	20	10–80	Evening	With
Pravastatin	Pravachol	10 or 20	10–40	Bedtime	With or without
Simvastatin	Zocor	5–10	5–40	Evening	With or without

*The lowest starting daily dose (in the case of cerivastatin, the 0.2-mg tablet) should be used in patients with significant renal or hepatic impairment and in the elderly.
Source: Data from *Physicians' Desk Reference* 1998.

testing every 6 weeks for the first 3 months, every 8 weeks for the remainder of the first year, and about every 6 months thereafter is recommended. Monitoring is particularly important if there are abnormal liver function test values or substantial use of alcohol (Gotto et al. 1995). Fatty liver, which is frequently present in patients with severe hyperlipidemia, often leads to fluctuation of alanine transaminase values, confounding monitoring. CK may be elevated in up to 30% of such patients before the initiation of drug therapy, making a diagnosis of drug-induced myositis more equivocal (Dujovne 1997).

BILE ACID SEQUESTRANTS

The bile acid sequestrants, or resins, have a long-established record of safe and effective clinical use. Resins available in the United States are cholestyramine (LoCholest, Questran, Prevalite) and colestipol (Colestid).

Mechanisms

At the simplest level, these anion exchange resins nonspecifically bind bile acids (which are cholesterol rich) in the gut, increasing the bile salts' fecal excretion and interrupting their enterohepatic recirculation, which has a major impact on lipid and lipoprotein metabolism in the liver (Shepherd 1989; Moore et al. 1968). With resin treatment, daily intestinal loss of bile acids is 2–3 g, whereas it normally seldom exceeds 1 g (Sirtori et al. 1991). The decrease in bile acid reabsorption leads to an increased flux of intrahepatic cholesterol into the production of bile acids secondary to increased activity of 7α-hydroxylase, the rate-limiting enzyme of bile acid synthesis. The subsequent decrease in intrahepatic cholesterol results in increased expression of high-affinity LDL receptors on liver cell membranes (Shepherd et al. 1980); this effect is responsible for the increased removal of LDL particles from plasma. The decrease in intrahepatic cholesterol also causes an increase in cholesterol synthesis within the hepatocyte as the result of increased activity of HMG-CoA reductase, thereby blunting the long-term effectiveness of bile acid resin monotherapy (Farmer and Gotto 1996). It is believed that the increase in hepatic cholesterol biosynthesis is accompanied by parallel increases in hepatic VLDL synthesis and secretion, which is responsible for the plasma TG increases that can occur with resin use (Illingworth 1988; Brunzell et al. 1973).

Efficacy

Cholestyramine, 4–24 g/day, or colestipol, 5–30 g/day, typically lowers LDL-C by 15–30% and may increase HDL-C by 3–5% (Farmer and Gotto 1996; NCEP 1994). Although plasma TG concentration is usually not affected, a marked increase occasionally occurs, primarily in patients who are hypertriglyceridemic before therapy. The apparent increase in the synthesis of VLDL, with saturation of the clearance mechanism, can occur in familial hypertriglyceridemia, remnant hyperlipidemia, and some cases of familial combined and common hyperlipidemia (Anonymous 1988). Resin use may be considered if plasma TG is only slightly raised; very high LDL-C can sometimes give this picture, since LDL particles contain 10–15% TG (Anonymous 1988). Response to resin therapy in individual patients is quite variable (NCEP 1994).

Clinical Trial Findings

Clinical benefit of resin therapy has been demonstrated in randomized trials in patients both with and without CHD. In the Lipid Research Clinics Coronary Primary Prevention Trial (LRC-CPPT), conducted in hypercholesterolemic men without known CHD, cholestyramine significantly reduced the incidence of MI or CHD death by 19%, new-onset angina by 20%, and new positive exercise stress tests by 25% (Lipid Research Clinics Program 1984a, 1984b). Need for CABG was reduced by 21%, although the reduction was not statistically significant. Evidence of clinical benefit in secondary prevention was documented in the FATS regression trial (see Chapter 10), in which colestipol combined with either lovastatin or nicotinic acid significantly reduced by 75% the incidence of cardiovascular events, and in the STARS regression trial, in which cholestyramine was used to enhance dietary therapy.

Safety and Tolerability

The bile acid resins have proved for many years to be very safe drugs. They are essentially not absorbed during transit through the gastrointestinal tract; therefore, there is little or no systemic toxicity. However, the use of bile acid sequestrants is limited by poor tolerability and by drug interactions. Gastrointestinal complaints, including constipation, bloating, epigastric fullness, indigestion, nausea, and flatulence, are frequent (NCEP 1994; Farmer and Gotto 1996). In the LRC-CPPT, although 24 g/day cholestyramine in packets was prescribed, the average daily dose taken was only about 14 g, and a significant percentage of patients were unable to take the drug at all. Sixty-eight percent of the patients reported gastrointestinal symptoms, although side effects greatly diminished as the study continued. In a health maintenance organization primary care setting, bile acid resins were discontinued in 41% of patients by 1 year (Andrade et al. 1995).

Because patients may object to the sandy, gritty taste of the powders or granules, some may prefer resin tablets (Insull et al. 1995), which were developed to improve compliance but are theoretically unlikely to reduce gastrointestinal side effects (Dujovne 1997). Constipation may be minimized by the use of stool softeners and increased fluid intake (Table 17.7); combination therapy with psyllium has been suggested to allow reduced resin dosage and to improve tolerability (Spence et al. 1995b). Occasionally, mild and usually transient increases in serum concentration of liver enzymes occur with resin use (NCEP 1994). Cholestyramine is among medications reported to cause rare pharmacobezoars (Stack and Thomas 1995).

The resins are absolutely contraindicated in complete biliary obstruction, in familial type III hyperlipidemia, and when fasting TG exceeds 500 mg/dL. There is a relative contraindication when fasting TG exceeds 200 mg/dL (NCEP 1994; Gotto et al. 1995; *Physicians' Desk Reference* 1998). Resins must be used with great care in diabetic patients with gastrointestinal autonomic neuropathy because they may produce constipation or even fecal impaction (Gotto et al. 1995). Orange-flavored Colestid contains phenylalanine and should not be used in patients with phenylketonuria.

Interactions

Bile acid resins can nonspecifically bind coadministered oral drugs, among them coumarin anticoagulants (warfarin), digitalis glycosides, exogenous thyroid hormones, thiazide diuretics, oral hypoglycemic agents (sulfonylureas), statins, gemfibrozil, and nonsteroidal anti-inflammatory drugs (NSAIDs) (Farmer and Gotto 1994, 1996; NCEP 1994; Johnson et al. 1994; Davies 1998). Interactions are generally avoidable by administering the drugs at different times: resins should be administered 1 hour after or 4 hours before susceptible agents to ensure absorption of the latter into the plasma compartment. When a resin and a statin are prescribed together, the resin can be given with the evening meal and the statin at bedtime. Colestipol has been reported to decrease absorption of gemfibrozil, an effect eliminated by a 2-hour separation (Forland et al. 1990). Decreased absorption of fat-soluble vitamins and folic acid has been reported with prolonged high doses of resins (NCEP 1994; Farmer and Gotto 1994); an increased bleeding tendency may be associated with vitamin K deficiency. Folic acid supplementation is usual in pediatric patients (Expert Panel 1992).

Table 17.7. SUGGESTIONS FOR INCREASING PALATABILITY AND TOLERABILITY OF BILE ACID RESINS

- Start at a low dosage, and increase the dosage only gradually.
- Split doses (usually taken two times per day).
- Resin granules and powders should always be mixed with water or another fluid, or a highly fluid food such as applesauce or soup, to avoid inhalation or gastrointestinal distress. Skim milk may be appealing. Mixing should be done slowly to avoid excess foaming. Refrigeration may improve the taste.
- Resin tablets should always be taken with water or another fluid.
- A resin should be taken before or with meals; if only one dose is taken, it should be taken with the heaviest meal.
- The same number of doses should be taken each day. A missed breakfast dose should be taken at lunch, a missed lunch dose at dinner, a missed dinner dose with an evening snack (low fat), but the patient should not try to catch up on doses between days.
- Individual patients may find one powder/granule resin more palatable than another. Some patients may prefer tablets, or tablets may provide an option when patients are traveling or eating out.
- Constipation may be relieved by increasing intake of fluid and dietary fiber or commercial products containing fiber such as psyllium, as well as by exercise.
- Bloating or gas may be relieved by trying to avoid swallowing air while taking the resin mixture.
- Any side effect symptoms should lessen with time.
- To avoid discoloration, erosion, or decay of the teeth, a resin should not be sipped or held in the mouth; good oral hygiene needs to be maintained.

Sources: Based in part on data from NCEP 1994 and *Physicians' Desk Reference* 1998.

Among the drugs whose absorption may be reduced or delayed by cholestyramine are phenylbutazone, warfarin, thiazide diuretics, propranolol, tetracycline, penicillin G, phenobarbital, thyroid hormones, estrogens and progestins, digitalis preparations (*Physicians' Desk Reference* 1998), troglitazone (Young et al. 1998), valproic acid (Malloy et al. 1996), mycophenolic acid (Mignat 1997), diclofenac (Davies and Anderson 1997), sulindac (Davies and Watson 1997), fluvastatin (Smith et al. 1993), and simvastatin (Nakai et al. 1996). Also, cholestyramine enhances the elimination of some acidic drugs through interruption of their enterohepatic cycling (e.g., piroxicam and tenoxicam); such an interaction may result in clinically significant loss of NSAID efficacy (Johnson et al. 1994). Cholestyramine can be used to enhance the biliary excretion of methotrexate (Furst 1995). Some drugs with which colestipol has been reported to interact are propranolol, chlorothiazide (even when given 1 hour before), tetracycline, furosemide, penicillin G, hydrochlorothiazide, digitalis preparations (*Physicians' Desk Reference* 1998), diclofenac (Davies and Anderson 1997), hydrocortisone (Nekl and Aron 1993), and, as noted above, gemfibrozil.

Dosage

A packet or scoopful of cholestyramine (powder) contains 4 g drug; the usual daily dose of cholestyramine is 4–16 g (maximum 24 g). A packet or scoopful of colestipol (granules) contains 5 g drug; the usual daily dose of colestipol is 5–20 g (maximum 30 g) (NCEP 1994; *Physicians' Desk Reference* 1998). Colestid tablets (micronized colestipol) each contain 1 g drug (*Physicians' Desk Reference* 1998). The tablets are swallowed whole with water (at least 4 fluid ounces, or 120 mL, per tablet). Tablets appear to provide equal efficacy at equivalent dosages to colestipol granules (Insull et al. 1995) and may be preferred by some patients or provide an additional option when patients are traveling or eating out. Because the tablets are large, higher doses may not be practicable. The tablets are calorie free; light preparations of resin powders or granules contain sweeteners such as aspartame and sorbitol (see product information for complete ingredients).

Bile acid resins have a nonlinear dose-response relation and retain most of their effectiveness at lower dosages (Schectman and Hiatt 1996). In one study, increasing the dosage from 8 to 16 g/day increased the reduction in LDL-C only from 27% to 31% (Angelin and Emarsson 1981). Lower dosages are often surprisingly effective (LaRosa 1989). As small a dose as 2–3 scoops daily reduces LDL-C by 15–25%. Higher dosages are associated with poor long-term compliance rates because of gastrointestinal side effects (Schectman and Hiatt 1996).

Monitoring

In addition to lipid monitoring for response, a complete blood count should be obtained once yearly (Gotto et al. 1995).

NICOTINIC ACID

Nicotinic acid, or niacin, is a water-soluble B complex vitamin that is widely distributed in plant and animal foods, including the rich sources of meat, fish, and cereals (1–40 mg/100 g), as well as coffee beans after roasting (about 40 mg/100 g) (van den Berg 1997). Niacin deficiency was nearly endemic in some populations relying on maize as their staple food (van den Berg 1997). The vitamin at pharmacologic doses, when it becomes a drug, has been used since 1955 as a lipid-lowering agent (Gibbons et al. 1995). The drug is available as immediate-release (crystalline) and sustained-release (slow- or extended-release) preparations. Nicotinamide, which is sometimes referred to as niacin, does not affect lipid concentrations (NCEP 1994).

Mechanisms

The mechanisms of the effects of nicotinic acid on lipid concentrations are not well understood. One hypothesis is that the drug inhibits lipolysis in adipose tissue; decreased transport of FFAs to the liver could reduce VLDL production. Another hypothesis suggests that the drug may directly inhibit the hepatic synthesis or secretion of apo B–containing lipoproteins (Tatò et al. 1998).

Efficacy

Nicotinic acid is unique among approved lipid-lowering agents in improving all major lipid parameters, and it is the most inexpensive of these drugs (Gotto 1998). At 2–3 g/day, nicotinic acid (crystalline) very effectively reduces LDL-C (20–30%) and TG (35–55%) and increases HDL-C (20–35%), and is effective in the treatment of hypercholesterolemia, mixed hyperlipidemia, and low HDL-C (McKenney et al. 1994). It also reduces alimentary lipemia, Lp[a], and small, dense LDL (Crouse 1996) as well as plasma fibrinogen (Johansson et al. 1997), although the clinical significance of these changes is not established. Nicotinic acid reduces risk for CHD events, as shown by the Coronary Drug Project; however, a reduction of total mortality rate (11% vs. placebo) as seen at follow-up 9 years after termination of that trial (Canner et al. 1986) requires support from additional clinical trial data (Tatò et al. 1998). In the CLAS, FATS, and UCSF-SCOR trials, use of nicotinic acid in combination drug therapy was associated with reduced coronary lesion progression (see Chapter 10).

Safety and Tolerability

Nicotinic acid is generally not well tolerated, although new preparations may improve tolerability. Suggestions for improving tolerability are listed in Table 17.8. Adverse effects include flushing, itching of the skin, gastrointestinal irritation, elevated transaminases, hyperglycemia, and hyperuricemia; all effects are usually reversible after discontinuation. More severe liver toxicity and even fulminant hepatic failure have been reported but are rare (Tatò et al. 1998). Also uncommon but potentially severe are myopathic changes and reversible cystic maculopathy (Brown 1995). Acanthosis nigricans is rare (International Task Force 1993), as is worsening angina in patients with unstable angina (McKenney and Hawkins 1995). Liver damage usually presents as markedly increased transaminases, jaundice, and the histologic finding of centrilobular cholestasis and parenchymal necrosis. Recently, however, Tatò et al. (1998) reported three cases in which markedly decreased TC and LDL-C resulted from hepatotoxicity from crystalline nicotinic acid. Therefore, a marked reduction in LDL-C may suggest generalized liver toxicity; if liver function test results confirm toxicity, the drug should be discontinued. It appears that higher dosages of nicotinic acid are associated with greater risk for toxicity (Schectman and Hiatt 1996).

Contraindications include hypersensitivity, liver disease/jaundice, peptic ulcer disease, significant glucose intolerance/diabetes mellitus (relative contraindication), severe hypotension, gallbladder disease, inflammatory bowel disease, arterial hemorrhaging, and hyperuricemia (Brown 1995).

Table 17.8. SUGGESTIONS FOR INCREASING TOLERABILITY OF NICOTINIC ACID

- Initiate therapy at low dosages.
- Premedicate with 325 mg aspirin (preferably enteric coated) or 200 mg ibuprofen 30 minutes before nicotinic acid is taken, to relieve prostaglandin-mediated symptoms.
- Nicotinic acid should be taken with meals—with or just after breakfast (or lunch) and dinner is suggested; a (low-fat) snack is recommended with (once-nightly) Niaspan.
- Hot liquids, alcohol, and spicy foods should be avoided immediately after a dose.
- The patient should not take more than the prescribed dose during 1 day (should not try to catch up on missed doses).
- The patient may wish to reduce the dosage if symptoms are intolerable, then return to the higher dosage when the symptoms have lessened or disappeared.
- The patient should understand that tolerance to the symptoms may develop.

Sources: Data from NCEP 1994 and Brown 1995.

Interactions

Isolated cases of rhabdomyolysis have been reported with combined lova-statin and nicotinic acid (Reaven and Witztum 1988). Although the incidence is low, nicotinic acid can cause hepatic necrosis and, thus, should not be used with drugs that adversely affect hepatic structure or function (Farmer and Gotto 1994). There is a possible potentiation of antihypertensive agents, and interaction with uricosuric agents (sulfinpyrazone) can yield decreased efficacy of the interactive drugs (Farmer and Gotto 1994). Stockley (1994) has compiled other rare drug interactions with nicotinic acid, including an increase in its serum concentrations with concomitant high-dosage aspirin administration (1 g orally) (Ding et al. 1989) and an isolated report of delirium and lactic acidosis in a nicotinic acid recipient who had drunk about 1 L of wine (Schwab and Bachhuber 1991). The side effects of nicotinic acid may be worsened by concomitant use of cyclosporine and prednisone (Valantine and Schroeder 1997).

Differences Among Preparations

Variations in efficacy and safety among different preparations of nicotinic acid remain controversial; more studies are required to assess safety among different sustained-release preparations (Dujovne 1997). Sustained-release preparations ameliorate the itching and flushing. However, liver toxicity has been reported to be more common with slow-release nicotinic acid (McKenney et al. 1994; Crouse 1996). Some authorities have recommended restriction of use of slow-release preparations, with administration only to patients who can be carefully monitored by experienced health professionals (McKenney et al. 1994).

Sustained-release nicotinic acid in about one-half the dosage of immediate-release nicotinic acid gives equivalent LDL-C reduction, but slow-release preparations may be less effective in reducing TG or raising HDL-C (Brown 1995). Effects on plasma TG appear to be similar between slow-release and crystalline nicotinic acid (McKenney et al. 1994).

Vasodilatory side effects occur in up to 100% of patients given immediate-release nicotinic acid; about 25% of patients in clinical trials had to discontinue use because of such side effects (McKenney at al. 1994). In a series of 110 well-instructed patients seen in everyday clinical practice, 43% of patients given crystalline nicotinic acid and 42% of those given slow-release drug had to discontinue treatment because of side effects, some of them after treatment for 1 or 2 years (Gibbons et al. 1995). Side effects in that series were fairly similar between crystalline and slow-release preparations (18 and 12 reports of flushing, 20 and 19 abnormal liver function tests, 11 and 10 cases of elevated serum glucose, 15 and 5 cases of elevated uric acid, 10 and 15 reports of abdominal pain).

Extended-release nicotinic acid (Niaspan, given once daily) appears to be similar to immediate-release nicotinic acid in efficacy (LDL-C reduced up to 17%, TG reduced up to 35%, HDL-C increased up to 26%), but with an improved tolerability and safety profile (78% fewer flushing episodes, <1% of patients discontinuing Niaspan because of serum transaminase elevations) (data on file, Kos Pharmaceuticals, Inc.). Full safety monitoring, as with any nicotinic acid preparation, is required. Efficacy appeared to be enhanced in women. Niaspan should not be substituted for equivalent dosages of immediate-release nicotinic acid; it should be initiated at a low dosage (Niaspan prescribing information).

Dosage

Crystalline nicotinic acid is usually given at 1.5–3.0 g/day (maximum 6 g/day) and slow-release nicotinic acid at 1–2 g/day (maximum 2 g/day) (NCEP 1994). Therapy with extended-release tablets (Niaspan), taken at bedtime after a low-fat snack, must be initiated with the titration starter pack (which starts with 375 mg once daily); daily dosage should not be increased more than 500 mg in any 4-week period. The recommended maintenance dosage is 1–2 g once daily at bedtime (Niaspan package insert, rev. 08/97). Extended- or slow-release nicotinic acid preparations must not be substituted for equivalent dosages of crystalline nicotinic acid; therapy must be initiated at low dosages, then titrated to the desired response.

Lipid effects of nicotinic acid appear to be dose dependent (Kreisberg 1994). Increases in HDL-C occur at a lower dosage (1.5 g/day crystalline) than reductions in LDL-C (>1.5 g/day) (Crouse 1996). Many physicians may begin at a dosage that is too high and increase the dosage too quickly. A starting dosage of crystalline nicotinic acid might be 100 mg three times a day, with 1.5 g/day reached after 4–6 weeks (Kreisberg 1994). Available data from dose-response studies of nicotinic acid suggest that fairly low dosages can achieve most of the effect of raising HDL-C; higher dosages are necessary for substantial LDL-C reduction (Schectman and Hiatt 1996).

Monitoring

Careful education, supervision, and monitoring are needed in all patients taking nicotinic acid. Self-medication should be discouraged. Because nicotinic acid is a vitamin and can be purchased without a prescription, many people believe it may be taken without physician supervision (Gibbons et al. 1995). The FDA has issued guidance stating its opposition to the sale of over-the-counter products for the treatment of hypercholesterolemia (FDA 1997). Approved agents (Niacor, Niaspan, Nicolar, Slo-Niacin) are recommended for optimum safety and efficacy (Dujovne 1997).

Risk for significant harm from adverse events is reduced by baseline determinations and follow-up of plasma glucose, serum uric acid, and serum transaminase and alkaline phosphatase. Testing should be done at 6- to 8-week intervals after a change in dosage and every 6 months when the dosage is stable. A change in symptoms also requires testing (Brown 1995). Monitoring costs are similar to those with other lipid-lowering agents (Brown 1995).

Acipimox

A number of derivatives and analogues of nicotinic acid have been developed in an effort to overcome its problems. The derivative acipimox is used in many countries but not in the United States. It is slightly less potent than nicotinic acid but is better tolerated and shows a better side effect profile, including no ill effects on glucose metabolism (Fogari et al. 1997). Acipimox at low dosages (250 mg three times a day) can effectively reduce cholesterol and TG (Fattore and Sirtori 1991), although its effectiveness as a single agent may be variable according to the type of dyslipidemia present (Hoogerbrugge et al. 1997). It attenuated hypertriglyceridemia in type 2 diabetes without perturbation of insulin sensitivity and glycemic control (Shih et al. 1997).

FIBRIC ACID DERIVATIVES

Clofibrate was the first fibric acid derivative described, in 1962; adverse effects were seen and more potent analogues were developed given a better understanding of structure-function relations (Davignon 1994; Illingworth 1991). Subsequent drugs include gemfibrozil, fenofibrate, bezafibrate, ciprofibrate (Figure 17.2), and long-acting forms of gemfibrozil, fenofibrate, and bezafibrate. Clofibrate, the prototype, is a derivative of chlorphenoxy-isobutyric acid; whereas gemfibrozil may not be of the fibric acid derivative class by a strictly chemical definition, it is always classified as a fibrate. Clofibrate (Atromid-S and generic) remains available in the United States but is rarely used here; the other fibrates available in this country are immediate-

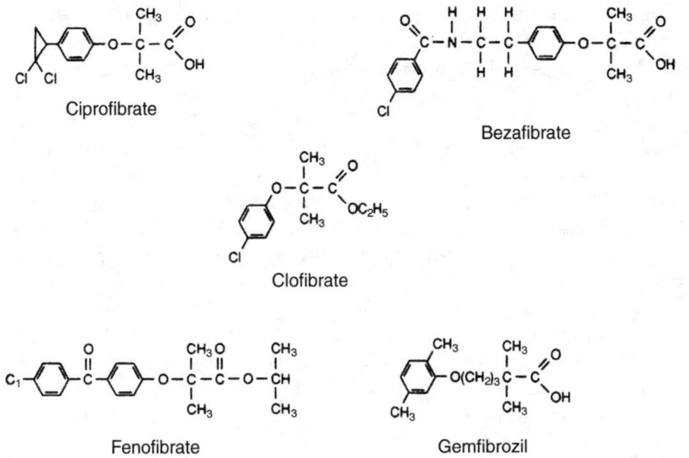

Figure 17.2. Chemical structures of the fibrates. Clofibrate, the parent compound, is rarely used in the United States. Bezafibrate and ciprofibrate are not available in the United States. (From Shepherd 1993; used with permission.)

acting gemfibrozil (Lopid and generic) and the long-acting form of fenofibrate (TriCor), produced through micronization. Marketing clearance for micronized fenofibrate was granted by the FDA in February 1998. Bezafibrate and ciprofibrate are available in other countries.

Mechanisms

Although the mechanisms of fibrate action remain incompletely understood, there is evidence that both enhanced catabolism of TGRLs—possibly through stimulation of LPL and/or hepatic lipase activity—and reduced secretion of VLDL contribute to the lipid-lowering effect (Schoonjans et al. 1996; Davignon 1994; Shepherd 1993; Miller and Spence 1998). A lipase-stimulating mechanism may also contribute to the effect of marked improvement in postprandial lipoprotein clearance (Miller and Spence 1998). Data are conflicting, perhaps reflecting patient group, regarding whether LDL catabolism may be increased or decreased by fibrates (Miller and Spence 1998).

There have recently been significant advances in the understanding of fibrate action at the molecular level. The peroxisome proliferator–activated receptor (PPAR), a member of the nuclear hormone receptor family, has been shown to be responsive to fibrates (Haubenwaller et al. 1995; Staels et al. 1995; Hertz et al. 1995). It is believed that the factor controls a number of genes, including apo C-III. PPAR also alters the synthesis of LPL (Auwerx et al. 1996). Activation of PPAR leads to decreased apo C-III mRNA in the liver, reduced plasma concentrations of apo C-III, and enhanced clearance of chylomicrons and VLDL (Packard 1998). Also, PPARs partially mediate the inductive effects of fibrates on HDL-C concentration by regulating the transcription of apo A-I and apo A-II (Schoonjans et al. 1996). Stabilization of LDL receptor mRNA has recently been suggested to be a novel mode of action of gemfibrozil (Goto et al. 1997). Thus, although fibrates have been shown to have other actions such as reducing fibrinogen concentrations, altering platelet reactivity, altering factor VIIc, and improving plasma viscosity (Scott 1997), it is likely that antiatherosclerotic effects are mediated largely through effects on plasma lipoproteins (Havel 1997).

The long-acting forms of gemfibrozil and bezafibrate are similar to their parent compounds in pharmacokinetic properties. Among the fibrates, immediate-release fenofibrate has the lowest and most variable bioavailability; micronization makes fenofibrate almost 100% bioavailable and reduces the dose-to-dose variability in absorption (Miller and Spence 1998).

Efficacy

The major effects of fibrates are to lower plasma TG and increase HDL-C, both substantially. TG may be decreased 20–50%, and HDL-C may be increased 10–30% (Spencer and Barradell 1996; Adkins and Faulds 1997; Farmer and Gotto 1996). There have been case reports of paradoxical decreases in HDL-C with fenofibrate, ciprofibrate, and bezafibrate (Collinson et al. 1996; Capps 1994). The effect on LDL-C is variable; marked decreases can occur in a subset of responders, and marked increases can occur in a subset of nonresponders. The paradoxical and sustained increase in LDL-C may occur in particular when TG is significantly lowered; care should be taken to identify any nonresponders early in the treatment process (Davignon 1994). However, since fibrate-induced reductions in plasma TG increase mean LDL particle size and enhance LDL clearance through the LDL receptor (Shepherd 1993; Spencer and Barradell 1996), it may be inappropriate to make predictions of the CHD risk associated with the LDL increases (Shepherd 1995b). Reductions in TG, LDL-C, and apo B may be somewhat greater in women than in men, and the response in both sexes may vary according to phenotype (Spencer and Barradell 1996; Adkins and Faulds 1997). A nonresponder to one fibrate may respond to another fibrate (Davignon 1994). Some dissimilarities among the drugs in this class may allow exploitation of their nonclass effects (Davignon 1994; Sirtori et al. 1992).

Fibrates are particularly useful in patients with combined hyperlipidemia or hypertriglyceridemia; type IIb hyperlipidemia with elevated LDL-C and TG and reduced HDL-C; and type III, IV, or V hyperlipidemia. In type III hyperlipidemia, they yield marked reductions in plasma of remnant lipoproteins and regression of xanthomas (Gotto et al. 1995). They do not appear to alter carbohydrate tolerance in diabetic patients

(ADA 1993), and some studies have suggested improved glucose tolerance (Spencer and Barradell 1996; Goa et al. 1996).

Clinical Trial Findings

In the primary prevention Helsinki Heart Study, conducted in dyslipidemic men, gemfibrozil therapy over 5 years reduced CHD incidence by 34% compared with placebo (Frick et al. 1987). Subsequent analyses of the Helsinki data showed the greatest CHD benefit in patients with type IIb hyperlipidemia (Manninen et al. 1988), and more specifically in patients with an LDL-C:HDL-C ratio greater than 5 and TG greater than 200 mg/dL (71% risk reduction) (Manninen et al. 1992) and overweight patients (78% risk reduction in those with BMI >26 kg/m^2, TG ≥200 mg/dL, and HDL-C <42 mg/dL) (Tenkanen et al. 1995). The overweight subjects often had clustered risk factors. Whereas the World Health Organization (WHO) Cooperative Study (WHO Principal Investigators 1978, 1980, 1984), a primary prevention trial of clofibrate, did demonstrate reduction of CHD events (20%), a significantly higher all-cause mortality rate in the drug group relegated clofibrate to a minor role in the United States. The results of the WHO trial have remained controversial for these 20 years. There were more cholecystectomies among the WHO trial clofibrate recipients, although more recently developed fibrates have not been generally shown to increase gallstones.

The nonblinded Stockholm Ischemic Heart Disease Secondary Prevention Study randomized men and women with a history of MI to therapy with clofibrate plus nicotinic acid or to a control group. After 5 years, significant changes in the drug group included reductions in CHD mortality rate (36%) and total mortality rate (26%). Retrospective subset analysis showed the decrease in CHD mortality to be directly related to the decrease in TG. The reduction in CHD death rate was 60% in drug recipients in whom TG decreased at least 30%, and significant benefit occurred only in patients whose baseline TG was greater than 130 mg/dL (Carlson and Rosenhamer 1988).

Results have recently become available from randomized, placebo-controlled trials supporting angiographic improvement of atherosclerosis with fibrate therapy (see Chapter 10). In BECAIT, bezafibrate therapy in young MI survivors slowed progression of coronary lesions and dramatically reduced coronary events (from 11 to 3) (Ericsson et al. 1996). Gemfibrozil therapy in LOCAT retarded coronary lesion progression and the formation of graft lesions after CABG in men with average LDL-C and low HDL-C (Frick et al. 1997). In smaller prospective trials without placebo control, fenofibrate therapy was associated with angiographic benefit in minor coronary narrowings in hypercholesterolemic patients (Hahmann et al. 1991), and gemfibrozil treatment slowed ultrasound progression of early carotid atherosclerosis in asymptomatic hyperlipidemic diabetic subjects (Migdalis et al. 1997).

Also, fibrate therapy has yielded regression of xanthomas in heterozygous FH (Rouffy et al. 1988) and familial type III hyperlipidemia (Kuo et al. 1988).

Safety and Tolerability

Although most evidence suggesting any increase in mortality with lipid-lowering therapy has proved inconsequential (Law et al. 1994), some doubts have continued to be expressed about the safety of use of the fibrates in low-risk patients (Gould et al. 1995). Unlike the situation with the statins, clinical trial evidence to support improvement in overall survival is not yet available for the fibrates. However, with the exception of clofibrate, it may be viewed that the margin of safety for the fibrates is well enough established to support their use in patients at high risk for CHD (Durrington 1997).

The fibrates are generally well tolerated. Side effects are fairly uncommon and include upper gastrointestinal disturbances, headache, anxiety, fatigue, vertigo, sleep disorders, myalgia, loss of libido, and alopecia (Davignon 1994). As noted, increased lithogenicity of bile has been reported with clofibrate (Coronary Drug Project Research Group 1975) but has not been conclusively demonstrated with other agents in this class. Occurrence of reversible myopathy with elevation of CK appears to be a class effect (Davignon 1994); although it is rare, it can lead to life-threatening rhabdomyolysis. Myopathy usually appears within 2 months of the start of therapy but has been reported after as long as 2 years of treatment (Shepherd 1995b). It is more likely to occur when renal function is impaired, hypoalbuminemia is present, or (see also below) an HMG-CoA reductase inhibitor is given concomitantly (Davignon 1994). Although the excretion of fibrates is largely renal, they generally do not accumulate except in patients with severe renal failure (Miller and Spence 1998). Limited data are available on the long-term tolerability of micronized fenofibrate, but findings from a large 3-month study show gastrointestinal side effects to be most common; elevations of serum transaminase and CK have been reported rarely (Adkins and Faulds 1997).

Fibrates have an absolute contraindication in hepatic or severe renal dysfunction (including primary biliary cirrhosis) and pre-existing gallbladder disease (Gotto et al. 1995). Fibrates need to be avoided in diabetic nephropathy (Durrington 1994). There are no adequate, well-controlled studies of their effects during pregnancy (*Physicians' Desk Reference* 1998). The drugs should not be used by nursing mothers.

Interactions

The principal reasons for drug interactions with the fibrates are (1) very high plasma protein binding, primarily to albumin, and (2) the requirement of cytochrome P450 3A4 (CYP3A4) for fibrate metabolism (Miller and Spence 1998).

Potentiation of the effects of warfarin-type oral anticoagulants is particularly important; warfarin may be displaced from albumin, so that prothrombin times are prolonged and the risk for bleeding is increased. On institution of fibrate therapy, anticoagulant dosage should be reduced by about one-third and prothrombin time should be monitored frequently (Davignon 1994); patients must be alerted to the importance of careful compliance. Bezafibrate, which is 95% protein bound, may interact with warfarin by increasing the affinity of the receptor sites for coumarins rather than through displacement of warfarin (Beringer 1997). Clofibrate and possibly other fibrates can displace oral hypoglycemic agents (including metformin, tolbutamide, and glyburide) from albumin; monitoring for hypoglycemia is recommended in cases of concomitant therapy (Miller and Spence 1998).

Lovastatin-gemfibrozil, simvastatin-gemfibrozil, pravastatin-gemfibrozil, atorvastatin-gemfibrozil, simvastatin-bezafibrate, pravastatin-bezafibrate, and simvastatin-fenofibrate are among the combinations for which myopathic complications have been reported (Shepherd 1995b; Tal et al. 1997; Duell et al. 1998). Most cases have occurred during lovastatin-gemfibrozil therapy (Spencer and Barradell 1996). However, Shepherd (1995b), from a review of clinical trials in which a statin was combined with a fibrate, estimated a rate of myopathic complications of only 1%, with no cases of a severe nature. Although the risk is not great, patients should be warned about it and carefully monitored. The relative myotoxicity of each of the fibrates, alone or combined with a statin, is unknown, as is the exact mechanism for the fibrate-statin interaction (Miller and Spence 1998). Both classes of agents require CYP3A4 for metabolism, although a study by Spence et al. (1995a) showed no change in fluvastatin or gemfibrozil pharmacokinetics during combination therapy (see "HMG-CoA Reductase Inhibitors," earlier).

Myotoxicity with combined use of a fibrate and cyclosporine, which is also metabolized by CYP3A4, has been much less frequently reported than with a statin plus cyclosporine (Miller and Spence 1998). As noted in the above section on statins, many other compounds are metabolized by or inhibit CYP3A4, for example, erythromycin, ketoconazole, felodipine, and grapefruit juice. Because important interactions with grapefruit juice are limited to drugs that have low bioavailability (Spence 1997), the fibrates, which are highly bioavailable, are considered unlikely to be affected (Miller and Spence 1998).

Absorption of fibrates may be decreased when bile acid resins, and possibly antacids, are coadministered (Spencer and Barradell 1996; Stockley 1994). No interaction between colestipol and gemfibrozil was seen when the time between administration of the drugs was 2 hours (Forland et al. 1990).

Dosage

The recommended dosage of immediate-release gemfibrozil is 1,200 mg administered in two divided doses 30 minutes before the morning and evening meals (*Physicians' Desk Reference* 1998). A daily dose of 900–1,500 mg may be used (Spencer and Barradell 1996). Micronized fenofibrate is usually begun at 67 mg (one capsule) once daily with a meal; it is increased sequentially as needed. The maximum daily dose is three 67-mg capsules, once daily (TriCor package insert). The recommended dosage of clofibrate is 2 g daily in divided doses (*Physicians' Desk Reference* 1998).

Immediate-release fenofibrate is given as 300 mg daily in divided doses (Adkins and Faulds 1997). The recommended dosage of bezafibrate is 400 mg once daily as a sustained-release tablet; 200 mg two or three times daily as a standard tablet may also be used (Goa et al. 1996). Ciprofibrate is given at 100 mg daily (Gotto et al. 1995).

Monitoring

In addition to lipid monitoring for response, liver enzymes should be monitored after the initiation of fibrate therapy and at 4- to 6-month intervals thereafter. Periodic blood counts are recommended for the first 12 months (Gotto et al. 1995).

PROBUCOL

Probucol was developed about 40 years ago as a potent industrial antioxidant; it is chemically related to beta-hydroxytoluene (Sirtori et al. 1991; Dujovne 1997). It protects LDL and Lp[a] from oxidation (Naruszewicz et al. 1992) and promotes endogenous antioxidants (Singal et al. 1997). In the early 1970s probucol was introduced as a weak cholesterol-lowering agent, advocated in part because of good tolerability (Kuzuya and Kuzuya 1993), and it has been used for many decades around the world. Side effects are few and mild, most commonly gastrointestinal effects (diarrhea, loose stools, flatulence, nausea) that typically resolve after a few months of treatment (Zimetbaum et al. 1990; Gotto et al. 1995). However, probucol was voluntarily removed from the U.S. market in 1995, in part because of concerns about safety. A potentially serious adverse effect of the drug is prolongation of the QT interval, and serious ventricular arrhythmias have been reported (Gotto et al. 1995).

Probucol lowers TC and LDL-C by 10–20% and also lowers HDL-C by about 30% (Franceschini et al. 1994). Effects on plasma TG are usually neutral. The drug's HDL-C effect, which has not been associated with increased CHD risk (Zimetbaum et al. 1990), may be through increased reverse cholesterol transport; probucol increases CETP activity and decreases HDL particle size. The mechanisms for probucol's lipid effects are not entirely understood, although cholesterol lowering appears to be independent of the LDL receptor because probucol lowers LDL-C even in patients with homozygous FH, who lack functional LDL receptors. In those patients, probucol is extremely effective in promoting regression of tendinous and cutaneous xanthomas, an effect that, interestingly, has been related to the drug's HDL-C lowering effect but not to its LDL-C lowering effect (Franceschini et al. 1994; Zimetbaum et al. 1990; Olsson and Yuan 1996).

In various animal models probucol improved atherosclerotic lesion progression, perhaps related to its antioxidant properties. However, in the 3-year Probucol Quantitative Regression Swedish Trial (PQRST), in which femoral atherosclerosis was monitored by angiography in hypercholesterolemic patients, probucol did not induce regression (Walldius et al. 1994). The trial was a test of the lipid lowering but not the LDL oxidation hypothesis. Recently, there has been heightened interest in probucol because of its possible effect against restenosis and its improvement of acetylcholine-induced coronary vasodilation (see Chapters 9 and 10), as well as promise from animal studies for improvement of diabetic cardiomyopathy (Kaul et al. 1996) and for prevention of adriamycin cardiomyopathy (Singal et al. 1997).

Probucol's best use in lipid lowering is probably in combination with other drugs, particularly a bile acid resin or statin, in patients with hypercholesterolemia (Gotto et al. 1995). Probucol is administered in tablets, usually at 500 mg twice daily, which is the maximum dosage. Absorption is improved when the drug is taken with a meal (Gotto et al. 1995). The drug is highly lipophilic and tends to accumulate in adipose tissue (Sirtori et al. 1991). ECG monitoring is required before and periodically during use. Probucol is contraindicated in patients with an abnormally long QT interval, with evidence of recent or progressive myocardial damage, with findings suggestive of serious ventricular arrhythmia, or with unexplained syncope or syncope of cardiovascular origin (Gotto et al. 1995). Possible interactive agents include androgens, progestins, beta-blockers, clofibrate, and other agents that lower HDL-C (possible amplification of HDL-C reduction), as well as group Ia antiarrhythmic agents, tricyclic antidepressants, and phenothiazines (possible amplification of corrected QT interval prolongation) (Farmer and Gotto 1994).

FISH OIL SUPPLEMENTATION

Seafood is a rich source of the omega-3 polyunsaturated fatty acids eicosapentaenoic acid (EPA) and docosahexaenoic acid (DHA), and at high dosages (≥ 4 g/day) fish oils substantially reduce plasma TG, in particular when hypertriglyceridemia is marked. The mechanism may involve decreased hepatic secretion of VLDL, enhanced VLDL turnover, and increased catabolism of chylomicrons (reduced postprandial lipemia). TG lowering is not seen with plant sources of omega-3 fatty acids (soybeans and canola oil are rich sources of alpha-linolenic acid). Fish oil supplementation may have a role in the treatment of severe hypertriglyceridemia (in particular the chylomicronemia of type V hyperlipidemia) resistant to other therapies (Stone 1996a). The TG lowering effects appear to be sustainable as long as therapeutic doses are given (Harris 1996). In modest (but not usually in severe) hypertriglyceridemia, TG lowering with fish oils can lead to increases in LDL-C (Stone 1996a). Whether fish oil supplementation is appropriate in diabetic patients requires further investigation (see Chapter 21).

General usage of fish oil supplementation is not recommended, and it is not known if long-term ingestion has adverse effects (NCEP 1994). Potential side effects of fish oil capsules (Stone 1996a) include nosebleeds, easy bruising, and gastrointestinal upsets. The capsules can increase calorie intake and hence weight gain. Some preparations contain added cholesterol, and some that are not well refined may contain pesticides. There are concerns about certain decreased immune response parameters (uncertain significance), and with some preparations there is vitamin A and vitamin D toxicity. Furthermore, fish oils may be hard to take because of a fishy odor, although highly purified forms offer benefit in this regard. Four grams of purified fish oil (85% omega-3 fatty acids) given daily provided a median reduction of plasma TG of 39% and a 6% elevation of HDL-C (Pownall et al. in press).

Benefit in CHD risk is not established. Posited nonlipid beneficial effects are numerous, including an improved coagulation profile (effects on bleeding time are additive to those of aspirin), small decreases in blood pressure in hypertensive patients, and anti-inflammatory effects (Stone 1996a). There is increasing evidence that omega-3 fatty acids have a strong antiarrhythmic effect (Leaf and Kang 1997; Albert et al. 1998). Fish oil supplementation, which should be viewed as a drug therapy, is to be distinguished from fish consumption (see "Polyunsaturated Fatty Acids" in Chapter 15).

LOW-DENSITY LIPOPROTEIN APHERESIS

Plasmapheresis for hypercholesterolemia was first reported as a last-resort treatment by de Gennes et al. in 1967; the first systematic clinical trial, of plasma exchange, was reported by Thompson et al. in 1975 (Bosch 1996). Experience since has shown LDL apheresis, a procedure for specifically removing apo B–containing lipoproteins from the blood, to be safe, effective therapy for treatment of severe hyperlipidemia. LDL apheresis was approved by the FDA in 1996 for use in patients who despite diet and maximum tolerated drug therapy have LDL-C higher than 300 mg/dL in the absence of CHD and higher than 200 mg/dL when CHD is present. The procedure is usually performed in regional centers. A patient registry has been established to monitor prospectively clinical outcome and adverse effects.

The most commonly used systems of LDL apheresis have been those utilizing immunoadsorption columns, dextran sulfate cellulose columns, and heparin precipitation. With each of these techniques, Richter et al. (1996) found a single treatment to reduce LDL-C 120–150 mg/dL and Lp[a] 52–65%. There was a small reduction in HDL-C concentration (a dilutional effect), which returned to normal within 24 hours. With heparin precipitation, VLDL-C and VLDL-TG values declined 45–55%. Apheresis is the most effective therapeutic modality for reducing the plasma Lp[a] concentration (Hajjar and Nachman 1996). With dextran sulfate adsorption, Olbricht (1996) notes that one treatment per week is enough in most patients to reduce LDL-C to 100–150 mg/dL. In a 5-year experience with automated dextran sulfate adsorption apheresis in 49 patients with FH (Gordon et al. 1998), mean lipid reduction per procedure was 76% for LDL-C, 14% for HDL-C, 49% for TG, and 69% for Lp[a] in homozygotes; reductions were similar in heterozygotes. Adverse events occurred in 142 (3.6%) of 3,902 procedures, about half of the events accounted for by hypotension (easily treated by slowing the blood flow rate or by infusing saline), nausea/vomiting, or flushing. Adverse events lessened as workers became more experienced with the procedure. Experience has shown that antihypertensive drugs need to be withheld immediately before LDL apheresis in patients at risk for hypotension. Hypotension can be severe in patients taking an ACE inhibitor (Gordon and Saal 1996).

LDL apheresis can stabilize coronary atherosclerosis in most patients with refractory hypercholesterolemia, as seen in trials such as the LDL Apheresis Regression Study (Tatami et al. 1992) and the LDL Apheresis Atherosclerosis Regression Study (LAARS) (Kroon et al. 1996a) (see also Chapter 10). In LAARS, apheresis plus medication also yielded functional improvement. Recent data have supported prevention of restenosis after PTCA (Daida et al. 1994; Adachi et al. 1995) and prevention of graft vessel disease after heart transplantation (Jaeger et al. 1997) or induction of its regression (Park et al. 1997). Apheresis may be useful in improving symptoms and stenoses in PVD (Kroon et al. 1996b; Uno et al. 1995; Sato and Agishi 1996). Improved endothelial vasodilation as measured by forearm blood flow has been demonstrated in hypercholesterolemic patients (Tamai et al. 1997). Possible mechanisms for benefit beyond LDL-C lowering have included decreased blood viscosity, reduction of plasma fibrinogen, improved coronary microcirculation, alterations in immune function, and decreased LDL oxidation (Gordon and Saal 1996; Schuff-Werner 1997; Napoli et al. 1997).

Treatment options, alone or combined with LDL apheresis, for severe refractory hypercholesterolemia include liver transplantation (Bilheimer et al. 1984), portacaval shunt (McNamara et al. 1983), plasmapheresis (Thompson et al. 1975), partial ileal bypass surgery (Buchwald 1963; Buchwald et al. 1990), and gene therapy (Grossman et al. 1994; Brown et al. 1994); the last is a number of years away from routine clinical application (Gordon and Saal 1996). As noted in the discussion of lipid-lowering drugs above, substantial additional lowering of LDL-C in patients with homozygous FH who were undergoing apheresis has been achieved with high-dose atorvastatin (Marais et al. 1997).

Suggested Reading

Noncompliance

Gotto AM Jr. The case for aggressive lipid regulation (review). Hosp Pract (Off Ed) 1997;32:145–149.

Hoerger TJ, Bala MV, Bray JW, et al. Treatment patterns and distribution of low-density lipoprotein cholesterol levels in treatment-eligible United States adults. Am J Cardiol 1998;82:61–65.

LaRosa JC. Cholesterol agonistics. Ann Intern Med 1996;124:505–508.

Drug Selection

Farmer JA, Gotto AM Jr. Choosing the right lipid-regulating agent: a guide to selection (review). Drugs 1996;52:649–661.

National Cholesterol Education Program. Second report of the Expert Panel on Detection, Evaluation, and Treatment of High Blood Cholesterol in Adults (Adult Treatment Panel II). Circulation 1994;89:1329–1445.

Drug Interactions

Farmer JA, Gotto AM Jr. Antihyperlipidaemic agents: drug interactions of clinical significance (review). Drug Safety 1994;11:301–309.

Garnett WR. Interactions with hydroxymethylglutaryl–coenzyme A reductase inhibitors (review). Am J Health Syst Pharm 1995;52:1639–1645.

Miller DB, Spence JD. Clinical pharmacokinetics of fibric acid derivatives (fibrates). Clin Pharmacokinet 1998;14:156–162.

HMG-CoA Reductase Inhibitors

Desager J-P, Horsmans Y. Clinical pharmacokinetics of 3-hydroxy-3-methylglutaryl-coenzyme A reductase inhibitors. Clin Pharmacokinet 1996;31:348–371.

Dujovne CA. New lipid lowering drugs and new effects of old drugs (review). Curr Opin Lipidol 1997;8:362–368.

Grundy SM. Consensus statement: role of therapy with "statins" in patients with hypertriglyceridemia. Am J Cardiol 1998;81(4A):1B–6B.

Lea AP, McTavish D. Atorvastatin: a review of its pharmacology and therapeutic potential in the management of hyperlipidaemias (review). Drugs 1997;53:828–847.

Lennernäs H, Fager G. Pharmacodynamics and pharmacokinetics of the HMG-CoA reductase inhibitors: similarities and differences. Clin Pharmacokinet 1997;32:403–425.

Shepherd J. Fibrates and statins in the treatment of hyperlipidaemia: an appraisal of their efficacy and safety. Eur Heart J 1995;16:5–13.

Bile Acid Sequestrants

Anonymous. Bile acid sequestrants and hyperlipidaemia (review). Lancet 1988;1:220–221.

LaRosa J. Review of clinical studies of bile acid sequestrants for lowering plasma lipid levels. Cardiology 1989;76(suppl 1):55–64.

Shepherd J. Mechanism of action of bile acid sequestrants and other lipid-lowering drugs (review). Cardiology 1989;76(suppl 1):65–74.

Nicotinic Acid

Brown WV. Niacin for lipid disorders: indications, effectiveness, and safety (review). Postgrad Med 1995;98:185–189.

Crouse JR III. New developments in the use of niacin for treatment of hyperlipidemia: new considerations in the use of an old drug (review). Coron Artery Dis 1996;7:321–326.

Dujovne CA. New lipid lowering drugs and new effects of old drugs (review). Curr Opin Lipidol 1997;8:362–368.

Gotto AM Jr. The new cholesterol education imperative and some comments on niacin. Am J Cardiol 1998;81:492–494.

Tatò F, Vega GL, Grundy SM. Effects of crystalline nicotinic acid-induced hepatic dysfunction on serum low-density lipoprotein cholesterol and lecithin cholesteryl acyl transferase. Am J Cardiol 1998;81:805–807.

Fibric Acid Derivatives

Adkins JC, Faulds D. Micronised fenofibrate: a review of its pharmacodynamic properties and clinical efficacy in the management of dyslipidaemia (review). Drugs 1997;54:615–633.

Davignon J. Fibrates: a review of important issues and recent findings. Can J Cardiol 1994;10(suppl B):61B–71B.

Durrington P. Statins and fibrates in the management of diabetic dyslipidemia (editorial). Diabetic Med 1997;14:513–516.

Fruchart JC, Brewer HB Jr, Leitersdorf E. Consensus for the use of fibrates in the treatment of dyslipoproteinemia and coronary heart disease. Eibrate Consensus Group (review). Am J Cardiol 1998;81:912–917.

Miller DB, Spence JD. Clinical pharmacokinetics of fibric acid derivatives (fibrates). Clin Pharmacokinet 1998;14:156–162.

Shepherd J. Fibrates and statins in the treatment of hyperlipidaemia: an appraisal of their efficacy and safety. Eur Heart J 1995;16:5–13.

Spencer CM, Barradell LB. Gemfibrozil: a reappraisal of its pharmacological properties and place in the management of dyslipidaemia (review). Drugs 1996;51:982–1018.

Probucol

Franceschini G, Werba JP, Calabresi L. Drug control of reverse cholesterol transport (review). Pharmacol Ther 1994;61:289–324.

Olsson AG, Yuan XM. Antioxidants in the prevention of atherosclerosis (review). Curr Opin Lipidol 1996;7:374–380.

Zimetbaum P, Eder H, Frishman W. Probucol: pharmacology and clinical application (review). J Clin Pharmacol 1990;30:3–9.

Fish Oil Supplementation

Stone NJ. Fish consumption, fish oil, lipids, and coronary heart disease. AHA medical/scientific statement. Circulation 1996;94:2337–2340.

Low-Density Lipoprotein Apheresis

Gordon BR, Kelsey SF, Dau PC, et al., for the Liposorber Study Group. Long-term effects of low-density lipoprotein apheresis using an automated dextran sulfate cellulose adsorption system. Am J Cardiol 1998;81:407–411.

Gordon R, Saal SD. Current status of low density lipoprotein-apheresis for the therapy of severe hyperlipidemia (review). Curr Opin Lipidol 1996;7:381–384.

REFERENCES

Adachi H et al. Artif Organs 1995;19:1243–1247.

Adkins JC, Faulds D. Drugs 1997;54:615–633.

Agency for Health Care Policy and Research. Smoking cessation. Clinical practice guideline No. 18. AHCPR publication no. 96-0692. Rockville, MD: U.S. Department of Health and Human Services, 1996a.

Agency for Health Care Policy and Research. Smoking cessation: a guide for primary care clinicians. AHCPR publication no. 96-0693. Rockville, MD: U.S. Department of Health and Human Services, 1996b.

Albert CM et al. JAMA 1998;279:23–28.

Allen SS et al. for the Transdermal Nicotine Study Group. Prev Med 1994;23:190–196.

American Association of Cardiovascular and Pulmonary Rehabilitation. Guidelines for cardiac rehabilitation programs. Champaign, IL: Human Kinetics Publishers, 1990.

American Diabetes Association. Diabetes Care 1993;16(suppl 2):106–112.

American Diabetes Association. Diabetes Care 1998a;21(suppl 1) (full issue).

American Diabetes Association. Diabetes Care 1998b;21(suppl 1):S23–S31.

Anderson JW et al. N Engl J Med 1995;333:276–282.

Andrade SE et al. N Engl J Med 1995;332:1125–1131.

Angelin B, Emarsson K. Atherosclerosis 1981;38:33–38.

Anonymous. Lancet 1988;1:220–221.

Ascherio A, Willett WC. Am J Clin Nutr 1997;66(suppl):1006S–1010S.

Aubin HJ et al. Encephale 1996;22:17–22.

Auwerx J et al. Atherosclerosis 1996;124(suppl):S29–S37.

Avorn J et al. JAMA 1998;279:1458–1462.

Bakker-Arkema RG et al. JAMA 1996;275:128–133.

Balady GJ et al. Circulation 1994;90:1602–1610.

Balady GJ et al. Circulation 1998;97:2283–2293.

Barzilay JI et al. Am J Cardiol 1994;74:334–339.

Bauman WA et al. Paraplegia 1992;30:697–703.

Bell LP et al. Am J Clin Nutr 1990;52:1020–1026.

Benowitz NL. Annu Rev Pharmacol Toxicol 1996;36:597–613.

Benowitz NL, Gourlay SG. J Am Coll Cardiol 1997;29:1422–1431.

Beringer TR. Postgrad Med J 1997;73:657–658.

Berlin I et al. Clin Pharmacol Ther 1995;58:444–452.

Bilheimer BW et al. N Engl J Med 1984;311:1658–1664.

Bischoff H et al. Atherosclerosis 1997;135:119–130.

Boberg M et al. Drug Metab Dispos 1997;25:321–331.

Bosch T. Artif Organs 1996;20:414–419.

Bradford RH et al. Am J Cardiol 1994;74:667–673.

Brewster AC et al. Am J Clin Nutr 1966;19:255–259.

A brief history of tobacco. CNN Interactive, 1997. Available at: http://www.cnn.com.

Broder JM. New York Times. March 21, 1997.

Brown MS, Goldstein JL. Science 1986;232:34–47.

Brown MS et al. Nat Genet 1994;7:349–350.

Brown WV. Postgrad Med 1995;98:185–189.

Brownell KD, Cohen LR. Behav Med 1995;20:155–164.

Brunzell JD et al. J Clin Invest 1973;52:1578–1585.

Buchwald H. Circulation 1963;28:649.

Buchwald H et al. N Engl J Med 1990;323:946–955.

Burr ML. J R Soc Health 1995;115:217–219.

Burr ML et al. Lancet 1989;2:757–761.

The Bypass Angioplasty Revascularization Investigation (BARI) Investigators. N Engl J Med 1996;335:217–235.

Campfield LA et al. Science 1998;280:1383–1387.

Canner PL et al. J Am Coll Cardiol 1986;8:1245–1255.

Capps N. Lancet 1994;344:684–685.

Caraballo RS et al. JAMA 1998;280:135–139.

Carlson LA, Rosenhamer G. Acta Med Scand 1988;223:405–418.

Centers for Disease Control and Prevention. MMWR CDC Surveill Summ 1993a;42:576–590.

Centers for Disease Control and Prevention. MMWR Morb Mortal Wkly Rep 1993b; 42:504–507.

Cinciripini PM et al. J Consult Clin Psychol 1995;63:388–399.

Collinson PO et al. Ann Clin Biochem 1996;33:159–161.

Consensus Development Panel. Am J Clin Nutr 1992;55(2 suppl):615S–619S.

Constant J. Clin Cardiol 1997;20:420–424.

Coronary Drug Project Research Group. JAMA 1975;231:360–381.

Corsini A et al. J Cardiovasc Pharmacol 1998;31:773–778.

Covey LS et al. Compr Psychiatry 1990;31:350–354.

Criqui MH. Clin Chim Acta 1996;246:51–57.

Crouse JR III. Coron Artery Dis 1996;7:321–326.

Daida H et al. Am J Cardiol 1994;73:1037–1040.

Daly PA et al. In: Manson JE et al., eds. Prevention of myocardial infarction. New York: Oxford University Press, 1996:203–240.

Danis PG, Seaton TL. Am Fam Phys 1997;55:1207–1214.

Davies NM. Clin Pharmacokinet 1998;34:101–154.

Davies NM, Anderson KE. Clin Pharmacokinet 1997;33:184–213.

Davies NM, Watson MS. Clin Pharmacokinet 1997;32:437–459.

Davignon J. Can J Cardiol 1994;10(suppl B): 61B–71B.

DeBakey ME et al. The new living heart diet. New York: Simon and Schuster, 1996.

de Gennes JL et al. Soc Med Hôpital Paris 1967;118:1377–1387.

Denke MA. Arch Intern Med 1995;155:17–26.

Desager J-P, Horsmans Y. Clin Pharmacokinet 1996;31:348–371.

Diaz MN et al. N Engl J Med 1997;337:408–416.

Ding RW et al. Clin Pharmacol Ther 1989;46:642–647.

Dreon DM, Krauss RM. In: Lusis AJ et al., eds.

Molecular genetics of coronary heart disease and stroke. Basel: Karger, 1992;325–349.

Duell PB, Malinow MR. Curr Opin Lipidol 1997;8:28–34.

Duell PB et al. Am J Cardiol 1998;81:368–369.

Dujovne CA. Curr Opin Lipidol 1997;8:362–368.

Dunhill AH. The gentle art of smoking. New York: Putnam, 1954.

Durrington PN. Hyperlipidaemia: diagnosis and management, 2nd ed. London: Butterworth–Heinemann, 1994.

Durrington P. Diabetic Med 1997;14:513–516.

Eckel RH for the Nutrition Committee. Circulation 1997;96:3248–3250.

Edwards NB et al. Am J Psychiatry 1989;146:373–376.

Engelgau MM et al. Diabetes Care 1995;18:1606–1618.

Ericsson C-G et al. Lancet 1996;347:849–853.

Erkelens W, Brunzell JD. J Hum Nutr 1980;34:370–375.

Expert Panel on Blood Cholesterol Levels in Children and Adolescents. Pediatrics 1992;89:525–584.

Fagerström KO, Tönnesen Ph. Wien Med Wochenschr 1995;145:77–82.

Farmer JA, Gotto AM Jr. Drug Safety 1994;11:301–309.

Farmer JA, Gotto AM Jr. Drugs 1996;52:649–661.

Fattore PC, Sirtori CR. Curr Opin Lipidol 1991;2:43–47.

Finer N. Br Med Bull 1997;53:409–432.

Fletcher BJ et al. Am J Cardiol 1994;73:170–174.

Fletcher GF. Circulation 1997;96:355–357.

Fletcher GF et al. Circulation 1995;91:580–615.

Fletcher GF et al. Circulation 1996;94:857–862.

Fogari R et al. Int J Clin Pharmacol Ther 1997;35:61–64.

Food and Agriculture Organization. Fats and oils in human nutrition: report of a Joint Expert Consultation (WHO.FAO). FAO Paper 57. Geneva: World Health Organization, 1994.

Food and Drug Administration. Guidance for industry: OTC treatment of hypercholesterolemia. Rockville, MD: U.S. Department of Health and Human Services, 1997.

Food and Drug Administration. FDA Talk Paper: FDA determines Cholestin to be an unapproved drug. May 20, 1998. Rockville, MD: U.S. Department of Health and Human Services, 1998.

Foreyt JP. Hosp Pract (Off Ed) 1997;32:123–124, 128, passim.

Forland SC et al. J Clin Pharmacol 1990;30:29–32.

Fowler JS et al. Nature 1996;379:733–736.

Franceschini G et al. Pharmacol Ther 1994;61:289–324.

Frick MH et al. N Engl J Med 1987; 317:1237–1245.

Frick MH et al. Circulation 1997;96:2137–2143.

Frishman WH, Rapier RC. Med Clin North Am 1989;73:437–448.

Furst DE. Br J Rheumatol 1995;34(suppl 2):20–25.

Garnett WR. Am J Health Syst Pharm 1995;52:1639–1645.

Garnett WR. Am J Cardiol 1996;78(suppl 6A):20–25.

Gibbons LW et al. Am J Med 1995;99:378–385.

Gidding SS et al. Circulation 1994;90:2581–2590.

Glantz SA, Parmley WW. Circulation 1991;83:1–12.

Glantz SA et al. JAMA 1995;274:219–224.

Glantz SA et al. The cigarette papers. Berkeley, CA: University of California Press, 1996.

Glass RM. JAMA 1990;264:1583–1584.

Glassman AH, Koob GF. Nature 1996;379:677–678.

Goa KL et al. Drugs 1996;52:725–753.

Gordon R, Saal SD. Curr Opin Lipidol 1996;7:381–384.

Gordon BR et al. Am J Cardiol 1998;81:407–411.

Goto D et al. Arterioscler Thromb Vasc Biol 1997;17:2707–2712.

Gotto AM. N Engl J Med 1991;324:912–913.

Gotto AM Jr. Hosp Pract (Off Ed) 1997;32:145–149.

Gotto AM Jr. Am J Cardiol 1998;81:492–494.

Gotto AM Jr et al. The ILIB lipid handbook for clinical practice: blood lipids and coronary heart disease. Houston: International Lipid Information Bureau, 1995.

Gould AL et al. Circulation 1995;91:2274–2282.

Gould AL et al. Circulation 1998;97:946–952.

Gourlay S. Med J Aust 1994;160:152–159.

Greenwald J. Time. March 31, 1997.

Grossman M et al. Nat Genet 1994;6:335–341.

Grundy SM. Am J Clin Nutr 1997;66(4 suppl): 988S–990S.

Grundy SM. Am J Clin Nutr 1998;67(suppl):563S–572S.

Grundy SM et al. Circulation 1997a;95: 1683–1685.

Grundy SM et al. Circulation 1997b;95:2329–2331.

Haffner SM et al. JAMA 1990;263:2893–2898.

Hahmann HW et al. Am J Cardiol 1991;67:957–961.

Hajjar KA, Nachman RL. Annu Rev Med 1996;47:423–442.

Hamelin BA, Turgeon J. Trends Pharmacol Sci 1998;19:26–37.

Haria M, McTavish D. Drugs 1997;53:299–336.

Harnick DJ et al. Am J Cardiol 1998;81:1416–1420.

Harris DE et al. Am J Cardiol 1998;81:929–933.

Harris MI et al. Diabetes 1987;36:523–534.

Harris SS et al. JAMA 1989;261:3590–3598.

Harris WS. Curr Opin Lipidol 1996;7:3–7.

Haubenwaller S et al. J Lipid Res 1995;36:2541–2551.

Havel RJ. Circulation 1997;96:2113–2114.

Haxby DG. Am J Health Syst Pharm 1995;52:265–281.

Hays JT et al. In: Manson JE et al., eds. Prevention of myocardial infarction. New York: Oxford University Press, 1996:99–129.

Heady JA et al. Lancet 1992;340:1405–1406.

Hegsted DM et al. Am J Clin Nutr 1965;17:281–295.

Henningfield JE. N Engl J Med 1995;333:1196–1203.

Hertz R et al. J Biol Chem 1995;270:13470–13475.

Illingworth DR. In: Rifkind BM, ed. Drug treatment of hyperlipidemia. New York: Marcel Dekker, 1991:103–139.

Hoerger TJ et al. Am J Cardiol 1998;82:61–65.

Hoogerbrugge N et al. J Intern Med 1997;241:151–155.

Howard BV, Kritchevsky D. Circulation 1997;95:2591–2593.

Hurt RD et al. N Engl J Med 1997;337:1195–1202.

Hyson DA, Mueller W. Prev Cardiol 1998;Spring:60.

Illingworth DR. Drugs 1988;36(suppl 3):63–71.

Insull W Jr et al. Atherosclerosis 1995;112:223–235.

International Task Force. Nutr Metab Cardiovasc Dis 1992;2:113–156.

International Task Force for the Prevention of Coronary Heart Disease. Guidelines of the European Atherosclerosis Society. London: Current Medical Literature, 1993.

Jaeger BR et al. Circulation 1997;96(9 suppl):II-154–II-158.

Johansson JO et al. J Cardiovasc Risk 1997;4:165–171.

Johnson AG et al. Int J Clin Pharmacol Ther 1994;32:509–532.

Jones PH et al. In: Alexander RW et al., eds. Hurst's The heart, arteries and veins, 9th ed. New York: McGraw-Hill, 1998a:1553–1581.

Jones P et al. for the CURVES Investigators. Am J Cardiol 1998b;81:582–587.

Joseph AM et al. N Engl J Med 1996;335:1792–1798.

Kantola T et al. Clin Pharmacol Ther 1998;63:397–402.

Kaplan NM. J Hypertens 1995;13(suppl 2):S1–S5.

Katan MB et al. N Engl J Med 1997;337:563–566.

Kaul N et al. Mol Cell Biochem 1996;160/161:283–288.

Kern F Jr. N Engl J Med 1991;324:896–899.

Kerr CP. Am Fam Phys 1994;50:1497–1504.

Key TJ et al. BMJ 1996;313:775–779.

Keys A et al. Metabolism 1965;14:776–787.

Keys A. Am J Clin Nutr 1995;61(suppl):1321S–1323S.

Kottke TE. J Am Coll Cardiol 1997;30:131–132.

Kottke TE et al. Mayo Clin Proc 1997;72:515–523.

Krauss RM et al. Circulation 1996;94:1795–1800.

Kreisberg RA. Am J Med 1994;97:313–316.

Kromhout D. JAMA 1998;279:65.

Kroon AA et al. Circulation 1996a;93:1826–1835.

Kroon AA et al. Ann Intern Med 1996b;125:945–954.

Kuo PT et al. Am Heart J 1988;116:85–90.

Kuzuya M, Kuzuya F. Free Radic Biol Med 1993;14:67–77.

LaRosa J. Cardiology 1989;76(suppl 1):55–64.

Law M, Tang JL. Arch Intern Med 1995;155:1933–1941.

Law MR et al. BMJ 1994;308:373–379.

Lea AP, McTavish D. Drugs 1997;53:828–847.

Leaf A, Kang JX. Curr Opin Lipidol 1997;8:4–6.

Lennernäs H, Fager G. Clin Pharmacokinet 1997;32:403–425.

Lichtenstein AH. Circulation 1997;95:2588–2590.

Lipid Research Clinics Program. JAMA 1984a;251:351–364.

Lipid Research Clinics Program. JAMA 1984b;251:365–374.

Ma PTS et al. Proc Natl Acad Sci U S A 1986;83:8370–8374.

Mahmarian JJ et al. J Am Coll Cardiol 1997;30:125–130.

Malloy MJ et al. Int J Clin Pharmacol Ther 1996;34:208–211.

Manninen V et al. JAMA 1988;260:641–651.

Manninen V et al. Circulation 1992;85:37–45.

Manson JE et al. N Engl J Med 1992;326:1406–1416.

Marais AD et al. J Lipid Res 1997;38:2071–2078.

Marcelino JJ, Feingold KR. Am J Med 1996;100:605–610.

McCann BS et al. J Am Diet Assoc 1990;90:1408–1414.

McKenney JM, Hawkins DW, eds. Handbook on the management of lipid disorders. Springfield, NJ: National Pharmacy Cholesterol Council, 1995.

McKenney JM et al. JAMA 1994;271:672–677.

McKenney JM et al. Am J Med 1998;104:137–143.

McNamara DJ et al. Proc Natl Acad Sci U S A 1983;80:564–568.

Meigs JB et al. Ann Intern Med 1998;128:524–533.

Messena M, Erdman JW Jr, eds. J Nutr 1995;125(suppl):567s–808s.

Meyers DG et al. Arch Intern Med 1996;156:925–935.

Migdalis IN et al. Int Angiol 1997;16:258–261.

Mignat C. Drug Safety 1997;16:267–278.

Miller DB, Spence JD. Clin Pharmacokinet 1998;14:156–162.

Moore RB et al. J Clin Invest 1968;47:1664–1671.

Moser M, Herbert PR. J Am Coll Cardiol 1996;27:1214–1218.

Nagata C et al. J Nutr 1998;128:209–213.

Nakai A et al. Biol Pharm Bull 1996;19:1231–1233.

Naoumova RP et al. Atherosclerosis 1996;119:203–213.

Naoumova RP et al. J Lipid Res 1997;38:1496–1500.

Napoli C et al. Am Heart J 1997;133:585–595.

Naruszewicz M et al. Metab Clin Exp 1992;41:1225–1228.

National Cholesterol Education Program. Circulation 1994;89:1329–1445.

National Heart, Lung, and Blood Institute (NHLBI) Cholesterol Awareness Surveys. Presented at the Cholesterol Awareness Surveys Press Conference; December 4, 1995; Bethesda, MD.

National Institutes of Health. The sixth report of the Joint National Committee on Prevention, Detection, Evaluation, and Treatment of High Blood Pressure. NIH publication no. 98-4080 (November 1997). Bethesda, MD: National Institutes of Health, 1997.

National Institutes of Health. Clinical guidelines on the identification, evaluation, and treatment of overweight and obesity in adults. Bethesda, MD: National Institutes of Health, 1998.

Nawrocki JW et al. Arterioscler Thromb Vasc Biol 1995;15:678–682.

Nekl KE, Aron DC. Ann Pharmacother 1993;27:980–981.

Nestle M. Am J Clin Nutr 1995;61(suppl): 1313S–1320S.

NIH Consensus Development Panel on Physical Activity and Cardiovascular Health. JAMA 1996;276:241–246.

Ockene IS, Houston Miller N for the American Heart Association Task Force on Risk Reduction. Circulation 1997;96:3243–3247.

Olbricht CJ. Artif Organs 1996;20:332–335.

Olsson AG, Yuan XM. Curr Opin Lipidol 1996;7:374–380.

Ornish D et al. Lancet 1990;336:129–133.

Packard CJ. Eur Heart J 1998;19(suppl A): A62–A65.

Paffenbarger RS Jr, Lee I-M. In: Manson JE et al. Prevention of myocardial infarction. New York: Oxford University Press, 1996:172–193.

Park JW et al. J Heart Lung Transplant 1997;16:290–297.

Parmley WW. J Am Coll Cardiol 1986;7:451–453.

Pate RR et al. JAMA 1995;273:402–407.

Pearson TA. JAMA 1994;272:967–968.

Pearson TA. Circulation 1996;94:3023–3025.

Pérez-Stable EJ et al. JAMA 1998;280:152–156.

Perkins KA et al. J Subst Abuse Treat 1997;14:173–182.

Peters AL. Prev Cardiol 1998;Spring:57–59.

Physicians' desk reference, ed. 52. Montvale, NJ: Medical Economics Company, 1998.

Pina IL et al. Circulation 1995;91:912–921.

Plosker GL, McTavish D. Drugs 1995;50:334–363.

Plosker GL, Wagstaff AJ. Drugs 1996;51:433–459.

Plotnick GD et al. JAMA 1997;278:1682–1686.

Popovich NG, Wood OB. J Am Pharm Assoc (Wash) 1997;NS37:31–39, 56.

Potter SM. Curr Opin Lipidol 1996;7:260–264.

Pownall HJ. J Lipid Res 1994;35:2105–2113.

Pownall HJ et al. Atherosclerosis, in press.

Psaty BM et al. JAMA 1997;277:739–745.

Raal FJ et al. Atherosclerosis 1997;135:249–256.

Ragnarrson KT. In: Whiteneck GG et al., eds. Aging with spinal cord injury. New York: Demos Publications, 1993:73–92.

Ratner PA et al. Prev Med 1995;24:389–395.

Reaven P, Witztum JL. Ann Intern Med 1988;109:597–598.

Richards JW Jr. J Fam Pract 1992;34:687–692.

Richter WO et al. Artif Organs 1996;20:311–317.

Rimm EB et al. N Engl J Med 1993;328:1450–1456.

Ripsin CM et al. JAMA 1992;267:3317–3325. Correction in JAMA 1992;268:3074.

Robbins AS. Am J Prev Med 1993;9:31–33.

Roberts WC. Am J Cardiol 1996;78:377–378.

Rolls BJ, Miller DL. J Am Coll Nutr 1997;16:535–543.

Rouffy C. Curr Med Res Opin 1988;11:123–132.

Rubinstein A, Weintraub M. Am J Cardiol 1995;76:184–186.

Rubenstein L. Cancer 1991;68:2519–2524.

Sacks FM, Willett W. N Engl J Med 1991;324:121–123.

Said S et al. Therapie 1994;49:313–319.

Santanello NC et al. J Am Geriatr Soc 1997;45:8–14.

Sato Y, Agishi T. Artif Organs 1996;20:324–327.

Schaefer EJ et al. JAMA 1995;274:1450–1455.

Schectman G, Hiatt J. Ann Intern Med 1996;125:990–1000.

Schlesinger M et al. Nouv Presse Med 1979;8:833–837.

Schoonjans K et al. J Lipid Res 1996;37:907–925.

Schrott HG et al. JAMA 1997;277:1281–1286.

Schuff-Werner P. Z Kardiol 1997;86(suppl 1): 57–64.

Schwab RA, Bachhuber BH. Am J Emerg Med 1991;9:363–365.

Schwartz JL. Med Clin North Am 1992;76:451–476.

Scott R. Clin Exp Pharmacol Physiol 1997;24(suppl):A26–A28.

Sellers EM et al. J Clin Psychopharmacol 1987;7:417–420.

Shepherd J. Cardiology 1989;76(suppl 1):65–74.

Shepherd J. Postgrad Med J 1993;69(suppl 1): S34–S41.

Shepherd J. Br Heart J 1995a;74:13.

Shepherd J. Eur Heart J 1995b;16:5–13.

Shepherd J et al. N Engl J Med 1980;302:1219–1222.

Shih K-C et al. Diabetes Res Clin Pract 1997;36:113–119.

Simons LA et al. Aust N Z J Med 1975;5:210–219.

Singal PK et al. FASEB J 1997;11:931–936.

Sirtori CR et al. Pharmacol Res 1992;26:243–260.

Sirtori CR et al. Cardiology 1991;78:226–235.

Siscovick DS et al. JAMA 1995;274:1363–1367.

Skaar K et al. Curr Opin Oncol 1996;8:434–440.

Skaar KL et al. Behav Med 1997;23:5–13.

Sleight P. J Hypertens 1996;14(suppl 2):S35–S39.

Smith HT et al. Am J Hypertens 1993;6(suppl):375S–382S.

Spence JD. Clin Pharmacol Ther 1997;61:395–400.

Spence JD et al. Am J Cardiol 1995a;16:5–13.

Spence JD et al. Ann Intern Med 1995b;123:493–499.

Spencer CM, Barradell LB. Drugs 1996;51:982–1018.

Stack PE, Thomas E. Dig Dis 1995;13:356–364.

Staels B et al. J Clin Invest 1995;95:705–712.

Stampfer MJ et al. Am J Public Health 1993a;83:801–804.

Stampfer MJ et al. N Engl J Med 1993b;328:1444–1449.

Staprans I et al. Arterioscler Thromb Vasc Biol 1998;18:977–983.

Stein EA, Laskarzewski P. Am J Cardiol 1998;81(suppl 4A):66B–69B.

Stephens NG et al. Lancet 1996;347:781–786.

Stephenson J. JAMA 1996;275:1217–1218.

Stockley IH. Drug interactions: a source book of adverse interactions, their mechanisms, clinical importance and management, 3rd ed. Oxford: Blackwell Scientific, 1994.

Stolerman IP, Jarvis MJ. Psychopharmacology 1995;117:2–10.

Stone NJ. Circulation 1996a;94:2337–2340.

Stone NJ. Am J Med 1996b;101(suppl 4A): 40S–49S.

Subar AF et al. Am J Clin Nutr 1989;50:508–516.

Tal A et al. South Med J 1997;90:546–547.

Tamai O et al. Circulation 1997;95:76–82.

Tatami R et al. Atherosclerosis 1992;95:1–13.

Tatò F et al. Am J Cardiol 1998;81:805–807.

Tenkanen L et al. Circulation 1995;92:1779–1785.

Ter Riet G et al. Br J Gen Pract 1990;40:379–382.

Thompson GR et al. Lancet 1975;1:1208–1211.

Tikkanen MJ. Curr Opin Lipidol 1996;7:385–388.

Titanji R, Paz-Guevara A. Maryland Med J 1992;41:231–233.

Trichopoulou A, Lagiou P. Nutr Rev 1997;55:383–389.

Trichopoulou A et al. J Cardiovasc Risk 1994;1:9–15.

Tsoh JY et al. Behav Med 1997;23:5–13.

U.S. Department of Health and Human Services. The health consequences of smoking: nicotine addiction. A report of the Surgeon General. DHHS publication no. CDC 88-8406. Washington, DC: U.S. Department of Health and Human Services, 1988.

U.S. Department of Health, Education, and Welfare. Smoking and health: A report of the Surgeon General. DHEW publication no. PHS 79-50066. Washington, DC: U.S. Department of Health, Education, and Welfare, 1979.

U.S. Public Health Service. Smoking and health. A Report of the Advisory Committee to the Surgeon General of the Public Health Service. PHS publication no. 1103. Washington, DC: U.S. Government Printing Office, 1964.

U.S. Surgeon General. Physical activity and health. Washington, DC: U.S. Department of Health and Human Services, 1996.

Uno H et al. Atherosclerosis 1995;116:93–102.

Valantine HA, Schroeder JS. Circulation 1997;96:1370–1373.

van den Berg H. Eur J Clin Nutr 1997;51 (suppl 1):S64–S45.

Van Horn L. Circulation 1997;95:2701–2704.

Van Horn L et al. Am J Clin Nutr 1997;65(1 suppl):289S–304S.

Verhoef P et al. Curr Opin Lipidol 1998;9:17–22.

Walldius G et al. Am J Cardiol 1994;74:875–883.

Wardle J et al. BMJ 1996;313:75–78.

Watts GF et al. Am J Physiol 1997;273:E462–E470.

Weber P et al. Int J Vitam Nutr Res 1996;66:19–30.

Weber P et al. Nutrition 1997;13:450–460.

Whelton PK et al. In: Manson JE et al., eds. Prevention of myocardial infarction. New York: Oxford University Press, 1996:154–171.

WHO Principal Investigators. Br Heart J 1978;40:1069–1118.

WHO Principal Investigators. Lancet 1980;2:379–385.

WHO Principal Investigators. Lancet 1984;2:600–604.

Whyte JL et al. J Am Diet Assoc 1992;92:446–449.

Willett W. Nutritional epidemiology. New York: Oxford University Press, 1990.

Willett WC et al. Am J Clin Nutr 1995;61(suppl):1402S–1406S.

Williamson DF et al. N Engl J Med 1991;324:739–745.

Wilson DE et al. J Lab Clin Med 1970;75:264–274.

Woller SC et al. Wis Med J 1995;94:266–272.

Working Group for the Study of Transdermal Nicotine in Patients with Coronary Artery Disease. Arch Intern Med 1994;154:989–995.

Young MA et al. Br J Clin Pharmacol 1998;45:37–40.

Zigler JE et al. Rehabilitation. In: Levine AM et al., eds. Spine trauma. Philadelphia: W. B. Saunders, 1998:567–607.

Zimetbaum P et al. J Clin Pharmacol 1990;30:3–9.

Zuliani G et al. Aging 1997;9:335–341.

Plasma Lipid Control and Coronary Heart Disease Risk Considerations in Population Subsets

If anything is sacred, the human body is sacred.

—Walt Whitman

The NIH [is committed to] the fundamental principles of inclusion of women and racial and ethnic minority groups and their subpopulations in research. This policy should result in a variety of new research opportunities to address significant gaps in knowledge about health problems that affect women and racial/ethnic minorities and their subpopulations.

—NIH Guidelines on the Inclusion of Women and Minorities as Subjects in Clinical Research (1994)

Women themselves must be made aware of the cardiovascular problems that affect them across the lifespan and how, in partnership with health professionals, they can promote their personal cardiovascular health. . . . Health professionals . . . must be better informed about the facts concerning heart diseases in women.

—Desmond Julian and Nanette Kass Wenger (1997)

Not all groups have experienced the full benefit of research advances in the reduction of risk for CHD. Lipid-lowering clinical trials in some subpopulations are just now beginning, or have yet to begin. The lack of research, however, should not be used as reason to deny these groups the benefit of CHD prevention.

A variety of risk reduction materials that target patient subpopulations such as women, children, African Americans, and Hispanic Americans are available from organizations such as

- The National Heart, Lung, and Blood Institute
  www.nhlbi.nih.gov/nhlbi/cardio
  1-800-336-4797; 1-800-575-WELL
- The American Heart Association
  www.americanheart.org
  1-214-373-6300

Examples from the NHLBI are "Eating with Your Heart in Mind" for 7- to 10-year-olds, "Heart Health: Your Choice" for 11- to 14-year-olds, "Hearty Habits" for 15- to 18-year-olds, "Improving Cardiovascular Health in African Americans" (package of seven booklets), and bilingual educational materials from the "Salud para su Corazón" program. AHA lifestyle brochures include such titles as "What Every Woman Should Know about High Blood Pressure," "Children and Smoking: A Message to Parents," and "La 'E' Simboliza Ejercicio." Health care workers are encouraged to make these low-cost publications, which may be purchased in quantity, available to their patients. The AHA also offers materials at a reduced reading level and can help locate recordings for the visually impaired regarding heart health. Current AHA medical/scientific statements are also available at www.americanheart.org.

References for Section V (Chapters 18–21) begin on page 380.

Chapter 18

Women

Although CHD is by far the leading single killer of women in the United States, taking about 240,000 of their lives in 1995 (AHA 1997), most women estimate that their own risk for CHD is very low. In a recent survey of Stanford University graduates with a median age of 50 years, 73% placed their risk at less than 1% by age 70 years (Pilote and Hlatky 1995). In fact, 50-year-old women have a 46% risk for development of CHD and a 31% risk for death from CHD (Schenck-Gustafsson 1996). Female sex is an independent predictor of late arrival in the emergency room for symptoms compatible with MI (Meischke et al. 1993; Schmidt and Borsch 1990). Women perceive their risk for cancer as much greater than their risk for CHD or stroke, although, for example, age-adjusted death rates are about three times higher for CHD than breast cancer (Eaker et al. 1993; AHA 1997). A focus on cancer screening (pelvic and breast examinations and Pap tests) is more common than CHD prevention in office visits to physicians (Horton 1992; Meilahn et al. 1995).

The rate of decline in CHD rates in the United States has been less in women than in men since 1979 (Mosca et al. 1997; Rich-Edwards et al. 1995). Whereas the age-adjusted all-cause mortality rate is declining for men, largely because of reduced rates of death from CVD and cancer, it is essentially unchanged for women (Haas 1998).

Physicians need to educate women about CHD risk in general and about individual risk to ensure compliance with lifestyle strategies and understanding of needed medical interventions (Douglas and Ginsburg 1996). Although much less research has been carried out on the topic of CHD risk management in women than in men, the research gap between the sexes must not be allowed to affect the quality of care offered to women.

AGE

CHD in women is largely a disease of the elderly. Symptomatic CHD occurs about 10 years later and MI occurs about 20 years later in women compared with men according to Framingham data (Murabito 1995; Kannel and Wilson 1995). The incidence of CHD increases dramatically in middle age in women, although the increase is not sudden with the natural cessation of menopause as it is with surgical menopause without ERT (Rich-Edwards et al. 1995). In the Atherosclerosis Risk in Communities (ARIC) study, B-mode ultrasound showed carotid atherosclerosis in 18% of women aged 45–49 years and in 41% of women aged 60–64 years (Li et al. 1994). Carotid disease can serve as a useful surrogate in predicting coronary events (Hodis et al. 1998) and also is a marker for stroke risk (Craven et al. 1990; O'Leary et al. 1992). There is also a shift during the menopausal years toward more serious manifestations of CHD (Murabito 1995). Premature menopause without ERT or age of 55 or higher in women is a major risk factor for CHD in NCEP guidelines (Expert Panel 1993).

MODIFIABLE RISK FACTORS

Meticulous attention needs to be paid to CHD risk reduction in women. The relations of major modifiable and unmodifiable risk factors to CHD are as strong or stronger in women as in men (Murabito 1995), and risk factor analysis may have greater predictive value in women, particularly in young women (Douglas and Ginsburg 1996). Risk factors are highly prevalent in U.S. women, and prevalence is greatest among women in disadvantaged socioeconomic circumstances and with the least education, indicating a target group for intensive risk factor modification (Wenger 1997).

In an autopsy series, Burke et al. (1998) found that traditional risk factors may have distinct effects on sudden cardiac death in women. Most of the acute coronary thrombi caused by plaque erosion rather than rupture (see Chapters 6 and 7) occurred in young female smokers without significantly elevated cholesterol, blood pressure, BMI, or glycohemoglobin, suggesting smoking cessation as a key risk modification in this age group. In postmenopausal women, on the other hand, coronary thrombosis arose from plaque rupture, which was associated with elevated cholesterol (mean, 270 vs. 194 mg/dL), emphasizing the need for cholesterol lowering in this group. Independent of other risk factors, vulnerable plaques in women were associated with hypercholesterolemia and age older than 50 years. In men, Burke et al. (1997) found coronary plaque rupture to be associated with an elevated TC:HDL-C ratio independent of age.

Plasma Lipids

The overwhelming majority of data supports plasma cholesterol as a risk factor for CHD in women (Lewis 1998). The TC concentration that correlates with increased risk may be somewhat higher in women because of a greater contribution of HDL-C (Lewis 1998).

Increased plasma TG and reduced HDL-C concentrations may be particularly important risk factors in women (LaRosa 1997b). The rise in CHD risk with increasing TG is much steeper in women than in men (Assmann and Schulte 1992), and a 1-mg/dL increase in HDL-C decreases

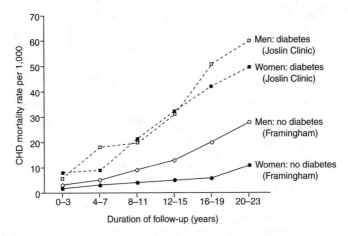

Figure 18.1. CHD mortality rate and diabetes mellitus. The presence of diabetes almost eliminates the difference between men and women. (From LaRosa 1997a; used with permission. The LaRosa figure was adapted from Krolewski et al. 1991.)

CHD risk 3% in women compared with 2% in men in observational epidemiologic data (Gordon et al. 1989).

It has been estimated on the basis of Framingham data that the 10-year CHD risk among women without CHD, diabetes, or LVH would be reduced 38% if they all obtained TC lower than 200 mg/dL and none smoked (Posner et al. 1993).

Other Risk Factors

Diabetes is a particularly strong risk factor in women, elevating CHD risk 3–7 times, in comparison with 2–3 times among men, and nearly eliminating any female premenopausal relative cardioprotection (Manson and Spelsberg 1996) (Figure 18.1). Other risk factors that appear to attenuate the premenopausal coronary disease advantage are a high TC:HDL-C ratio and LV hypertrophy (Kannel and Wilson 1995). In the Framingham study, risk for recurrent infarction was doubled by diabetes in women but there was no significant effect of diabetes in men (Abbott et al. 1988).

Half of all coronary events in women have been associated with smoking (Douglas and Ginsburg 1996); in one observational study, all the women 45 years old or younger who had sudden cardiac death were heavy smokers (Talbott et al. 1981). Hypertension in premenopausal women increases the risk for CHD death as much as 10 times, and among the elderly it is a stronger CHD predictor in women than men (Douglas and Gins-

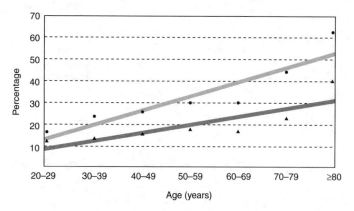

Figure 18.2.   Percentages of women (*circles*) and men (*triangles*) who reported no leisure-time physical activity in NHANES III (1988–1991). (From Limacher 1998; used with permission. Data from Crespo et al. 1996.)

burg 1996). Regarding overweight and obesity, women who gain weight chiefly around the waist are at particular risk for CHD (LaRosa 1997a); waist:hip ratio predicted risk for CHD death in women better than did BMI (Folsom et al. 1993). Although data support a 50–60% reduction in CHD risk for physically active compared with sedentary women (Rich-Edwards et al. 1995) and increased physical activity improves women's risk factor profile (Owens et al. 1990), women are more likely than men to report no physical activity (27% vs. 17%) and the difference increases with age (Crespo et al. 1996) (Figure 18.2). It is clear that quitting smoking, controlling blood pressure, avoiding obesity, and increasing physical activity will substantially reduce risk in women (Rich-Edwards et al. 1995; Hennekens 1998).

As in men, moderate alcohol consumption in women is associated with reduced risk for CHD (Stampfer et al. 1988). Women appear to be more sensitive to the toxic effects of alcohol on striated muscle, and in them the threshold dose for the development of cardiomyopathy is significantly lower (Urbano-Márquez et al. 1995). Women are more susceptible to alcoholic liver disease (Borum 1998) and perhaps alcoholic brain damage (Jacobson 1986; Mann et al. 1992). Most studies have reported an association between heavy alcohol use and risk for breast cancer (Thomas 1995). Cohort studies have reported that alcohol use and ERT act synergistically to increase risk for breast cancer (Zumoff 1998). Women who drink should do so only moderately.

Oral Contraceptives

There is general agreement that with regard to MI and stroke, modern, low-dose oral contraceptives can be used safely by women who lack risk factors for CHD (Rosenberg et al. 1997; Sidney et al. 1996, 1998). Studies of high-dose formulations showed an alarming increase in the risk for MI in smokers (Hennekens 1998). While current formulations possibly ameliorate this risk (Lewis et al. 1997), the issue must be considered undecided (Rich-Edwards et al. 1995). Any women 35 years of age or older who smokes should be advised to use a nonestrogen or nonhormonal contraceptive (Carr and Ory 1997). Meta-analysis indicated that past use of high-dose oral contraceptives does not increase CHD risk (Stampfer et al. 1990). The rapid return of risk to baseline values suggests a short-term mechanism such as increased thrombosis (Rich-Edwards et al. 1995; Stampfer et al. 1990).

Earlier, higher-dose oral contraceptives increased LDL-C and blood pressure, decreased HDL-C and glucose tolerance, and promoted clotting mechanisms (Hennekens 1998). The third-generation-progestogen, low-dose oral contraceptives have very little effect on lipid or glucose metabolism (Bagshaw 1995). According to data from a large, prospective study, current formulations continue to increase the risk for high blood pressure; risk decreases quickly with discontinuation, and past users have only a slightly increased risk (Chasan-Taber et al. 1996). Blood pressure increases are usually within the normal range (NIH 1997). In some studies, the increase in venous thromboembolism for third-generation formulations containing desogestrel or gestodene was 1.5–2.0 times higher than for second-generation formulations, but there may have been differences between users in underlying risk and in likelihood of diagnosis (Rosenberg et al. 1997; Spitzer 1997). Evidence has shown no difference between users and nonusers of oral contraceptives with regard to risk for breast cancer, although breast cancer may be discovered at an earlier age in users (Denke 1996).

TREATMENT OF DYSLIPIDEMIA

Lipid-lowering pharmacotherapy may often be delayed in premenopausal women when LDL-C does not exceed 220 mg/dL, if there is no other risk (Expert Panel 1993). In many—though not all—studies of lifestyle interventions, lipid responses have been less strong in women than in men (LaRosa 1997b). There is no evidence that lipid-lowering drugs have different efficacy or adverse effect profiles in women (LaRosa 1997a). In the Expanded Clinical Evaluation of Lovastatin (EXCEL) study, which included more than 7,000 women, efficacy and safety were equivalent in women and men (Shear et al. 1991); LDL-C lowering was somewhat greater in elderly compared with middle-aged women, and HDL-C increases from low HDL-C concentrations were somewhat greater in women than in men. The clinician may consider oral ERT (see below) for control of dyslipidemia in postmenopausal women (Expert Panel 1993).

The multicenter Heart and Estrogen-Progestin Replacement Study (HERS) recently found substantial undertreatment of hypercholesterolemia in postmenopausal women with CHD (Schrott et al. 1997). According to a 1993 national telephone survey of U.S. women, those whose family or general practitioner was a woman were more likely to receive blood cholesterol or Pap testing, and Pap testing was more common when internists were women. The sex of the physician did not affect receipt of breast examination or blood pressure screening (Cassard et al. 1997).

Results of Lipid-Lowering Clinical Trials

Women have often been excluded from lipid-lowering trials or studied only in small numbers, in part because disease typically occurs in an age group in which confounding nonatherosclerotic factors are common. In 1990, the NIH identified women as underrepresented in clinical trials, including CHD prevention trials (Palca 1991).

Testing simvastatin, 4S (see Chapter 12) convincingly demonstrated that lipid lowering reduces the risk for major coronary events in women with pre-existing CHD (Miettinen et al. 1997). The 34% reduction was the same as that in men, and the need for revascularization was reduced 49% in women, compared with 41% in men. Numbers of deaths among the 827 women (aged 35–70 years at enrollment) were too small to allow meaningful analysis of death rates. Pooling CHD mortality results in 4S with earlier secondary prevention trials that assessed CHD mortality in women (Scottish Society of Physicians and Newcastle upon Tyne clofibrate trials, each suggesting decreased mortality) yielded a summary relative risk of 0.36 (95% CI, 0.25–0.52) (Walsh and Grady 1995). In CARE, women with CHD and only average cholesterol values benefited from pravastatin therapy, in fact substantially more than men (46% vs. 20% reduction in major coronary events) (Sacks et al. 1996). In the secondary prevention LIPID trial, according to preliminary data (see Chapter 12), pravastatin therapy in patients with a wide range of baseline cholesterol values significantly reduced coronary mortality and total mortality rates; outcome in the large group of women included was consonant with benefit in the treated group as a whole.

Only a few regression lipid-lowering trials included enough women to enable separate analysis, although their results support aggressive reduction of LDL-C in women with CHD. In UCSF-SCOR, which tested diet and combination drug therapy in patients with heterozygous familial hypercholesterolemia, coronary lesion regression remained significant when analyzed in women alone (Kane et al. 1990). In CCAIT (see Chapter 10), lovastatin therapy slowed the angiographic progression of coronary disease and prevented the development of new lesions in women (Waters et al. 1995), with results similar to those in men. In CAIUS, progression of carotid disease in the control group was significantly faster in men, and pravastatin therapy effectively slowed carotid disease progression in both sexes (Mercuri et al. 1996). POSCH included 78 women among its 838 hypercholesterolemic MI survivors who underwent partial ilial bypass surgery to lower cholesterol. Coronary angiography consistently showed less disease progression in the women in the surgery group between the baseline examination and 3, 5, 7, and 10 years (Buchwald et al. 1992). In prospective pooled analysis of pravastatin regression trials, the coronary event rate was significantly reduced in women, although numbers were small (Byington et al. 1995).

AFCAPS/TexCAPS was the first large-scale primary prevention trial of LDL-C lowering to include a substantial number of women (997 of 6,605 randomized participants). Reduction in relative risk for a first major coronary event was greater among these postmenopausal, generally healthy women than among the men (46% vs. 37%), but the small numbers of events among the women precluded statistical significance (Downs et al. 1998). Although additional studies in women need to be a priority, there is no reason to think that the benefits of lipid lowering as primary prevention would not extend to women, not only to prolong life but also to postpone and diminish disability.

POSTMENOPAUSAL HORMONE REPLACEMENT

Many observational studies have demonstrated a strong and consistent relation between postmenopausal oral ERT and reduced risk for CHD (LaRosa 1997a). In 10-year data from the prospective, observational Nurses' Health Study, current estrogen use was associated, after adjustment for age and other risk factors, with a 44% decrease in risk for major CHD events as well as a 39% decrease in risk for cardiovascular death (Stampfer et al. 1991). These reductions were independent of duration of use, age, and whether menopause was natural or surgical (Stampfer et al. 1991). Cohort studies also demonstrate a reduction in risk for all-cause mortality (Schairer et al. 1997; Ettinger et al. 1996; Folsom et al. 1995; Henderson et al. 1991). The risk for stroke appears to be similar in users and nonusers (Rifkind and Rossouw 1998).

The first interventional results are now available from the Heart and Estrogen-Progestin Replacement Study (HERS) (Hulley et al. 1998). At 1-year follow-up of 2,763 postmenopausal women with CHD (mean age, 66.7 years), those assigned to conjugated equine estrogens plus medroxyprogesterone acetate (Prempro) had an increased relative risk for nonfatal MI or CHD death during the first year (RR, 1.52) and decreased risk during years 4 and 5 (RR, 0.67) compared with placebo. Overall, across the 4.1 years, the groups did not differ in CHD rate, although LDL-C was 11% lower and HDL-C was 10% higher in the hormone group. In addition, there was significantly greater risk for thromboembolic events and gallbladder disease with hormone use. Thus, it is not recommended that women with CHD start this combined hormone therapy de novo for the purpose of secondary prevention, although it may be appropriate for women already receiving replacement therapy to continue it given the favorable pattern of events after several years of therapy. Given observational findings, these results were unexpected. It is possible that in the first year thrombogenic effects dominated antiatherogenic effects, especially given that individuals with CHD are likely to have risk factors such as obesity and diabetes predisposing to thrombosis. Petitti (1998) notes, however, that only one observational study (Rosenberg et al. 1993) yielded findings consistent with the HERS MI pattern. Additional data from large interventional trials are needed to clarify the cardiovascular effects of hormone replacement therapy, including in women without established CHD. In particular, data are anticipated by 2005 from a primary prevention trial that is part of the Women's Health Initiative of the NIH (Women's Health Initiative Study Group 1998).

The beneficial effects of oral estrogens on the lipoprotein profile are a likely mechanism to account for part of any cardioprotection. Oral estrogens (0.625 mg/day of conjugated estrogen or 2 mg/day of micronized estradiol) usually increase HDL-C and decrease LDL-C, each by about 10–15% (NCEP 1994; Kushwaha 1992). Beneficially, they also increase plasma apo A-I and decrease plasma apo B and Lp[a] (see "Estrogen" in Chapter 8). In addition, however, oral estrogens may significantly increase TG, particularly when TG is already elevated (also see Chapter 8). Benefits of estrogen use may relate as well to such cardioprotective factors as lower fasting blood glucose and lower blood pressure, and there is some evidence from animal studies that estrogen might exert effects to protect the vascular wall from atherosclerosis that are independent of lipid metabolism (see Chapter 8). The selective estrogen receptor modulator raloxifene has also been shown to have beneficial effects on lipid concentrations and coagulation parameters (Walsh et al. 1998), but no data are available regarding this drug and CHD risk. Raloxifene, 60 or 120 mg/day, lowered LDL-C by 12% and did not increase TG but also did not increase HDL-C (Walsh et al. 1998).

The clinician may consider oral ERT for control of dyslipidemia in postmenopausal women (Expert Panel 1993). In some cases, ERT may obviate the need for lipid-lowering agents. Transcutaneously or percutaneously administered estrogens appear to have less effect on lipoprotein concentrations (NCEP 1994; Kushwaha 1992). Exogenous estrogens do not have an FDA indication for lowering lipids or reducing risk for CHD. If estrogen administration increases TG markedly, the estrogen should probably be discontinued.

Concomitant progestin administration reduces or eliminates the increased risk for endometrial cancer with estrogen use (Denke 1996; The Writing Group for the PEPI Trial 1996). There is far less information about the effects of the combined use of estrogen and progestin either on CHD risk or on lipoproteins, although it appears that the combination blocks some of the harmful lipid effects of progestin while allowing the beneficial lipid effects of estrogen to persist. Three-year results from the double-blind Postmenopausal Estrogen/Progestin Interventions (PEPI) trial conducted in 875 healthy postmenopausal women showed that conjugated equine estrogen alone or in combination with a progestin (cyclic micronized progesterone, or cyclic or consecutive medroxyprogesterone acetate) improves the lipoprotein profile and lowers fibrinogen concentrations without effect on blood pressure or postchallenge insulin concentrations (The Writing Group for the PEPI Trial 1995). Mean LDL-C was reduced about 20% versus placebo regardless of the hormone replacement formulation used; HDL-C was increased in all treatment groups, although the effect was blunted by the addition of progestin—substantially by medroxyprogesterone acetate, less so by micronized progesterone. As noted, it does not appear to be advisable on the basis of HERS results (Hulley et al. 1998) to start combination therapy de novo in women with established CHD.

Davidson et al. (1997) in a randomized, placebo-controlled trial in 76 hypercholesterolemic postmenopausal women found that conjugated estrogens, 0.625 mg/day, increased HDL-C 23% and TG 4% and decreased LDL-C 14%, whereas pravastatin, 20 mg/day, increased HDL-C 4% and decreased LDL-C and TG 25% and 12%. Combining the two agents retained the HDL-C raising of estrogens and the LDL-C lowering of pravastatin while keeping TG at baseline.

The decision to treat with hormone replacement therapy must be made on the basis of individualized judgment by physicians and their patients and must take into account menopausal symptoms and risks for CHD, osteoporosis, cancer, and thromboembolism (Wenger 1998; Limacher 1998b; Manson et al. 1996a) (Table 18.1). Data regarding breast cancer risk have been conflicting (Wenger 1998). By meta-analysis, long-term use of hormone replacement has been associated with a relative risk of 1.3 (Steinberg et al. 1991, ≥15 years' use; Collaborative Group 1997, ≥5 years' use), and current use with a relative risk of 1.2 (Collaborative Group 1997). Adherence to standard recommendations for breast cancer screening is prudent when ERT is used. A small increase in absolute risk but a significant increase in relative risk for venous thromboembolic disease has been described by several studies. Relative risk is as high as 3.2–3.5 for deep vein thrombosis and pulmonary embolism; absolute risk is 1/5,000 for deep vein thrombosis and 1/20,000 for pulmonary embolism, with risk higher near the initiation of therapy (Wenger 1998). A mathematical model has suggested increased survival in most women with at least one risk factor for CHD (Col et al. 1997). A postmenopausal woman is 6–10 times more likely to die of CVD than breast cancer or osteoporosis (Manson et al. 1996a).

Surveys have shown, however, that only a small percentage of postmenopausal women use ERT (Rozenberg et al. 1995; Rees 1997). In a U.S. survey, only 17% of women 65 years of age or older were current users; 27% of former users discontinued treatment because of lack of perceived benefit, and 55% who never started therapy said that they feared the medication was harmful (Salamone et al. 1996). Improved educational efforts are needed to ensure long-term compliance (Rees 1997). A U.S. survey showed higher rates of use among women physicians—60% for ages 40–49, 49% for ages 50–59, and 36% for ages 60–70—perhaps presaging greater use by U.S. women in the future (McNagny et al. 1997).

Table 18.1. POSSIBLE BENEFITS AND RISKS OF HORMONE REPLACEMENT THERAPY

	Hormone therapy regimen	
	Estrogen alone	Estrogen plus progestin
Possible benefits		
CHD	May decrease risk by 35%	May decrease risk by 20–35%, but less information than for estrogen alone
		May increase risk during first year in women with CHD
Fractures due to osteoporosis	May decrease risk for hip fracture by 25%	Same, but less information than for estrogen alone
Menopausal symptoms	Fewer hot flashes and other symptoms of menopause	Same
Bladder function	Fewer bladder problems	Same
Possible risks		
Breast cancer	May increase risk for breast cancer by 25%	Same, but less information than for estrogen alone
Uterine cancer	May increase risk	No known increase in risk
Blood clot	May increase risk in legs or lungs	Same
Side effects and vaginal bleeding	More period-like symptoms	Same

Source: Modified from Manson et al. 1996a; used with permission. The Manson et al. table was modified from Grady et al. 1992.

HYPERLIPIDEMIA IN PREGNANCY

Plasma lipids change both quantitatively and qualitatively during pregnancy (Salameh and Mastrogiannis 1994; Miller 1990). Plasma TG rises gradually throughout pregnancy, its values doubled or tripled at term and returning to prepregnancy concentrations at about 6 weeks postpartum. The rise in plasma TG parallels increases in estrogen concentration. LDL-C initially drops until about 8 weeks, after which it steadily rises to about a 50–60% increase at term; it remains elevated for up to 8 weeks after delivery. HDL_2 increases to about a twofold peak at midgestation, then falls, remaining at term about 15% above baseline; HDL_3 concentration remains fairly constant. The lipid changes are believed to be adaptive, the rise in plasma TG providing maternal fuel so that glucose is saved for the fetus. Effects of pregnancy-related diabetes on lipids are controversial (Salameh and Mastrogiannis 1994).

    VLDL particles proportionally increase their TG and cholesterol content during normal pregnancy, whereas HDL and LDL become TG enriched (Salameh and Mastrogiannis 1994; Miller 1990). The LDL profile has been reported to be altered in some individuals toward smaller, denser LDL particles, the perturbation occurring in a threshold manner at different gestational ages and TG concentrations for different women (Sattar et al. 1997).

Whether repeated exposure to the lipid changes of pregnancy increases risk for atherosclerotic disease is unclear. Data associating parity with CHD are contradictory (Salameh and Mastrogiannis 1994; Miller 1990).

Management Considerations

Common practice is to discontinue lipid-lowering drugs before conception when possible because the safety of their use in pregnancy is not proved. To condense years off medication, women with significant hypercholesterolemia should be advised to bear children over a limited number of years (Miller 1990). Bile acid resins are particularly appropriate for women considering pregnancy (NCEP 1994). In 134 women with inadvertent exposure to therapeutic dosages of lovastatin or simvastatin, no relation was found between exposure and the occurrence of adverse pregnancy outcomes (Manson et al. 1996b).

Pancreatitis during pregnancy is uncommon (1 in 1,060 to 1 in 3,000 live births), and while usually mild is potentially serious. Only 4–6% of cases are linked to hyperlipidemia, the vast majority of these accounted for by type I or type V hyperlipidemia. Most cases of pancreatitis during pregnancy are caused by cholelithiasis (Salameh and Mastrogiannis 1994). Appropriate treatment of pancreatitis in pregnancy can minimize maternal and fetal mortality (Chen 1995).

Hyperlipidemia in pregnancy could identify a patient with latent hyperlipidemia, especially if elevations are beyond the 95th percentile or fail to normalize by 6–8 weeks postpartum (Salameh and Mastrogiannis 1994). Postpartum lipid determinations should be postponed 6 months in women who were not dyslipidemic before pregnancy.

SEX DIFFERENCES IN MYOCARDIAL INFARCTION

In the Framingham Heart Study, a first MI was more likely to be fatal in women (39% vs. 31%), although the sudden death rate was only one-third of that in men (Murabito 1995). Also in Framingham, women had a higher proportion of unrecognized MI than men (35% vs. 28%) (Murabito 1995).

Excess early mortality after MI in women even after adjustment for age distribution and other variables has been reported from a number of studies (Vaccarino et al. 1995), although recent analysis of the Third International Study of Infarct Survival (ISIS 3) indicated only a small independent association (Malacrida et al. 1998). Women may have a lower case fatality rate before hospital admission (Sonke et al. 1996); however, even a small excess risk would translate into a large number of deaths in the United States (Nettleman and Klein 1998). Less aggressive care, fewer procedures, and less medication have also been reported in women with CHD (Lewis

1998). Even after adjustment for a variety of variables, women have been shown to be less likely than men to receive thrombolytic therapy, PTCA, or CABG (Weitzman et al. 1997; Giles et al. 1995). Delays in the decision to use a thrombolytic drug would complicate the delays in hospital arrival time in women (Lambrew et al. 1997).

DIAGNOSIS OF CORONARY HEART DISEASE

Because of sex differences in presentation and diminished accuracy of some diagnostic tools, the diagnosis of CHD presents a greater challenge in women (Mosca et al. 1997). However, clinicians can now more accurately assess risk for CHD in women with chest pain because of the emergence of new data (see Douglas and Ginsburg 1996, Mosca et al. 1997, and Roger and Gersh 1997 for reviews). Unrecognized ischemia is of particular concern because of the high MI fatality rate among women. When chest pain represents coronary atherosclerosis, women have a less favorable outcome than men (Wenger 1997). In the Cardiovascular Health Study, women aged 65 or older who had subclinical atherosclerotic disease (major ECG or echocardiographic changes, increased carotid wall thickness, decreased ankle/arm blood pressure index, or positive Rose questionnaire) were 2–3 times more likely than women without such findings to have an MI or stroke within 18 months (Kuller 1993).

All forms of chest pain are associated with a lower prevalence of angiographic CHD in women (Douglas and Ginsburg 1996). In the Coronary Artery Surgery Study (CASS) registry, 50% of women, compared with 17% of men, had minimal or no obstruction in their epicardial coronary arteries when referred for angiographic evaluation because of chest pain (CASS Principal Investigators 1981). Clinical history is inadequate to differentiate anginal and nonanginal chest pain in women; objective confirmatory testing is required (Wenger 1997).

During an acute MI, women are more likely than men to experience, in addition to chest pain, neck and shoulder pain, nausea and vomiting, fatigue, or dyspnea. Women with chronic stable angina are more likely than men to have chest pain while sleeping, resting, or under mental stress. Thus, the pattern of pain from ischemia is slightly different in women; the presence of other symptoms beyond typical angina during exertion or chest pain while at rest does not decrease the likelihood of CHD in women as it does in men (Douglas and Ginsburg 1996). Differences in manifestations of MI may largely reflect women's older age at presentation (Roger and Gersh 1997). However, among 36 witnessed sudden cardiac deaths (many of them in premenopausal women) in an autopsy series, only eight were preceded by chest pain (Burke et al. 1998). Twelve were preceded by nonspecific symptoms, including back pain, nausea and vomiting, dizziness, fatigue, malaise, shortness of breath, fever and chills, stomach distension, and tingling of the left shoulder. In the remaining 16 cases, witnesses reported an absence of symptoms.

Symptoms of CHD are more likely in women than in men to be attributed to psychiatric causes (Tobin et al. 1987). Women whose presentation style is exaggeratedly emotional may be perceived to be at lower risk for CHD than women with businesslike affect (Birdwell et al. 1993).

ECG stress testing has lower sensitivity and specificity in women, and ERT may induce a false-positive ST segment depression. The prognostic value of radionuclide ventriculography is limited in women; in contrast, exercise echocardiography may be valuable and is considered cost-effective in women (see Mosca et al. 1997 for a more complete discussion).

STROKE AND PERIPHERAL VASCULAR DISEASE

In the United States, stroke incidence is 19% higher in men (AHA 1997), although women are more likely to die of stroke, probably because of greater age at occurrence and greater life expectancy (Mosca et al. 1997). The incidence of ischemic stroke after a history of TIAs is higher in women than men (Whisnant et al. 1996). Recommendations for acute intervention in stroke appear to be the same for men and women (Mosca et al. 1997). PVD may be more prevalent in women than is generally appreciated (Mosca et al. 1997).

CARDIAC REHABILITATION

Differences from men in women's medical and psychosocial needs must be recognized in the design and implementation of cardiac rehabilitation programs to maximize compliance and outcome (Cargart and Ades 1998). Traditional programs were designed in the 1960s to focus on low-risk middle-aged men and do not address the needs of a variety of patients. In general, women begin cardiac rehabilitation at a lower level of cardiopulmonary fitness, related in part to their older age at MI. Women are more likely to have comorbid conditions and fewer psychosocial supports, and studies have indicated benefit in women from more social support and interactions with staff (Cargart and Ades 1998). Absence of emotional support significantly predicted the occurrence of fatal and nonfatal CVD events for 1 year after hospitalization with heart failure in elderly women but not in men (Krumholz et al. 1998). Physicians have been shown to be less likely to recommend cardiac rehabilitation to women than men despite similar severity of disease (Ades et al. 1992), and enrollment rates are lower and dropout rates higher in women (Mosca et al. 1997). Nevertheless, women achieve as much if not more benefit from cardiac rehabilitation (Mosca et al. 1997; Limacher 1998a; Balady et al. 1994). The issue of cardiac rehabilitation (see Table 18.2 for indications) is crucial for women because they have a worse prognosis after cardiac events (Mosca et al. 1997).

Table 18.2. INDICATIONS FOR PARTICIPATION IN CARDIAC REHABILITATION PROGRAMS

- CHD
  - —Multiple risk factors and poor exercise tolerance
  - —Stable angina pectoris
  - —Silent MI
  - —After MI
  - —After CABG
  - —After PTCA
- After heart transplantation
- Heart failure due to dilated cardiomyopathy or LV dysfunction
- After valve surgery
- After surgery for congenital heart disease
- Elderly patient with heart disease
- Hypertensive CVD

Source: Limacher 1998a; used with permission.

Suggested Reading

Carhart RL Jr, Ades PA. Gender differences in cardiac rehabilitation (review). Cardiol Clin 1998;16:37–43.

Douglas PS. Coronary artery disease in women. In: Braunwald E, ed. Heart disease: a textbook of cardiovascular medicine, 5th ed., vol. 1. Philadelphia: W. B. Saunders, 1997:1704–1714.

Douglas PS, Ginsburg GS. The evaluation of chest pain in women (review). N Engl J Med 1996;334:1311–1315.

Limacher MC. The role of hormone replacement therapy in preventing coronary artery disease in women (review). Curr Opin Cardiol 1998;13:139–144.

Manson JE, Ridker PM, Gaziano JM, Hennekens CH, eds. Appendix D: Postmenopausal hormone replacement therapy. In: Prevention of myocardial infarction. New York: Oxford University Press, 1996:549–553.

Mosca L, Manson JE, Sutherland SE, et al. Cardiovascular disease in women: a statement for healthcare professionals from the American Heart Association. AHA medical/scientific statement. Circulation 1997;96:2468–2482.

Rich-Edwards JW, Manson JE, Hennekens CH, Buring JE. The primary prevention of coronary heart disease in women. N Engl J Med 1995;332:1758–1766.

Roger VL, Gersh BJ. Myocardial infarction. In: Julian DG, Wenger NK, eds. Women and heart disease. St. Louis: Mosby, 1997:135–150.

Salameh WA, Mastrogiannis DS. Maternal hyperlipidemia in pregnancy (review). Clin Obstet Gynecol 1994;37:66–77.

Wenger NK. Postmenopausal hormone therapy: is it useful for coronary prevention? (review) Cardiol Clin 1998;16:17–25.

Chapter 19

The Elderly and Youths

THE ELDERLY

"You are as old as your arteries" is proverbial, and indeed CHD is the most common cause of death among the elderly in the United States. Absolute risk for CHD morbidity and mortality increases steeply with age (Castelli et al. 1992). People who are 65 years old or older, two-thirds of whom are women (LaRosa 1996), account for nearly 60% of hospital admissions for acute MI, and they have higher in-hospital and postdischarge death rates than younger patients (Forman and Aronow 1996) and are more likely to suffer sudden death (Tresch and Aronow 1996). Indeed, 85% of CHD deaths are in this age group (AHA 1997). About 35 million Americans will be older than 65 years by 2000, with the subset of those older than 85 years growing the fastest (Carroll and Pollock 1992).

CHANGES IN LIPID VALUES WITH AGE

TC rises in both men and women through middle age; in women, the rise is more gradual (Miller and Nanjee 1992). At about age 65 years in men and age 75 years in women, TC and LDL-C begin to fall (Ferrara et al. 1997). The progressive decline in cholesterol in the elderly may enrich CHD rates in mid-range cholesterol values (Denke and Winker 1995).

HDL-C values are generally higher in women than in men; they are relatively constant across age groups (Matthews et al. 1989; Johnson et al. 1993), with perhaps some decline in women after menopause (Matthews et al. 1989). Fasting TG rises gradually in both men and women, although at a slower rate in women; in middle age, it may decrease in men and continue to rise in women (The Lipid Research Clinics Program Epidemiology Committee 1979).

RISK FACTORS

The general conclusion is that major risk factors continue to be important CHD predictors when measured after age 65 years (Benfante et al. 1992;

LaRosa 1997a). Many (Aronow and Ahn 1996; Frost et al. 1996; Castelli et al. 1992; Benfante et al. 1992) although not all (Krumholz et al. 1994) studies have shown elevated plasma cholesterol to be a risk factor for CHD in older men and women, including the very old (those >80 years). There may be some diminution in relative risk as the elderly age (Shipley et al. 1991; Manolio et al. 1992), although not all analyses support a weakening of the relation (Howard et al. 1997). Nevertheless, because the absolute risk for a CHD event over a short interval is much higher in older people, the absolute risk attributable to elevated cholesterol increases with age (Malenka and Baron 1988; Expert Panel 1993). Thus, the public health impact of risk factor management may be more important in the elderly (Benfante et al. 1992).

HDL-C and plasma TG are also predictive of CHD risk in the elderly (Campbell et al. 1993; LaRosa 1997b). HDL-C may be a particularly powerful risk factor. In a large prospective cohort study of elderly men and women, low HDL-C (<35 mg/dL) compared with high HDL-C (≥60 mg/dL) quadrupled the relative risk for CHD death among people aged 71–80 years and doubled that risk among people older than 80 years (Corti et al. 1995).

LV hypertrophy is an important CHD risk factor that is often overlooked in the elderly (Lavie et al. 1996). Measures associated with its prevention and reduction include weight reduction, sodium restriction, increased dynamic exercise, and use of various drugs (e.g., ACE inhibitors, calcium antagonists, alpha-blockers, beta-blockers, indapamide) (Lavie et al. 1996).

CLINICAL TRIAL FINDINGS

Data from clinical trials limited to subjects older than 65 years are not available. Older trials that separately analyzed data in older subjects include the secondary prevention Stockholm study using clofibrate and nicotinic acid in men and women (Carlson and Rosenhamer 1988) and the Los Angeles Veterans Hospital Administration Study using diet in men with and without CHD (Dayton et al. 1969). Both found similar benefit in CHD events in younger and older patients.

Subgroup analyses of the recent statin clinical endpoint trials (see Chapter 12) support lipid lowering as both secondary and primary prevention in the elderly. Statin therapy was well tolerated by older patients in all these trials, with remarkably low rates of adverse effects.

4S: In men and women with hypercholesterolemia and a history of MI or angina, statin therapy significantly reduced all-cause mortality (34%), CHD mortality (43%), major coronary events (34%), and the need for revascularization (41%) in 518 patients who were 65 years of age or older at enrollment (70–76 years of age at the end of the study) (Miettinen et al. 1997). Lipid effects and relative risk reductions were similar in younger and older patients (the all-cause mortality reduction was somewhat better in the latter). Fewer older patients required dosage titration from 20 to 40 mg/day, which is consistent with other findings (Shear et al. 1991) suggesting enhanced response to statin therapy with increasing age. In the placebo group, all-cause and CHD mortality rates in older patients were more than double those for patients younger than 65 years; thus, the absolute risk reduction in these rates with therapy was more than doubled in older patients.

CARE: A similar approximate doubling in absolute risk reduction in older patients (65–80 years at trial's end), including in stroke or TIAs, occurred at lower cholesterol concentrations in the CARE trial of pravastatin in male and female MI survivors (Sacks et al. 1996).

LIPID: According to unpublished findings (see Chapter 12), clinical benefit at 6-year follow-up of the secondary prevention LIPID trial of pravastatin extended to patients 65–69 years of age and those 70–75 years of age at enrollment.

AFCAPS/TexCAPS: Extension of benefit to generally healthy older men and women with only average cholesterol was reported from the primary prevention AFCAPS/TexCAPS test of lovastatin (Downs et al. 1998). Analysis encompassed age above or below the baseline median (57 years in men and 62 years in women; upper limit 73 years). Lovastatin appeared to attenuate the risk conferred by age, sex, family history, hypertension, LDL-C, and below-average HDL-C.

WOSCOPS: In the hypercholesterolemic men with no history of MI who formed the study population of WOSCOPS, pravastatin therapy reduced the rate of nonfatal MI and CHD death by a significant 27% in those who were 55 years old or older at enrollment (upper limit 64 years) (Shepherd et al. 1995).

Pravastatin Atherosclerosis Intervention Program: In a prospectively planned pooled analysis of the results of four regression trials using pravastatin (KAPS, PLAC-I, PLAC-II, and REGRESS; see Chapter 10), lipid-lowering therapy significantly reduced the rate of fatal or nonfatal MI in patients 65 years of age or older as well as in those younger than 65 years (Byington et al. 1995). By 2000, the Cholesterol Treatment Trialists' Collaboration should have individual patient data on more than 60,000 subjects, including 20,000 elderly subjects (Cholesterol Treatment Trialists' Collaboration 1995).

DIAGNOSIS AND EVALUATION

It has been estimated that among the U.S. elderly, approximately 60–70% would require fasting lipoprotein analysis and 50–60% would be candidates for lipid-lowering dietary intervention (Sempos et al. 1993; Godschalk 1991). Because HDL-C tends to remain fairly stable as people age, moderately elevated TC in the elderly may represent a large proportion of HDL-C, in which case intervention is not needed.

CHD is often undiagnosed or misdiagnosed in the elderly. Failure to diagnose symptomatic CHD in the elderly may be due to differences in clinical manifestations (Tresch and Aronow 1996). Many elderly people may not experience exertional angina because of limited physical activity. Angina may be misdiagnosed as degenerative joint disease or peptic ulcer disease. Myocardial ischemia in the elderly is commonly manifested as dyspnea, or it may be manifested as acute pulmonary edema. As many as 60% of MIs in the very elderly may be unrecognized or clinically silent; a variety of explanations have been proposed, including improved collateral circulation or an inability of the elderly to verbalize the pain. Symptoms of acute MI may be very vague or atypical; dyspnea, syncope, vertigo, or abdominal pain rather than typical chest pain may occur. Acute MI should be suspected when there are unexplained behavior changes, acute signs of cerebral insufficiency, or dyspnea (Tresch and Aronow 1996).

TREATMENT

Current NCEP guidelines (Expert Panel 1993; NCEP 1994) specify that it is inappropriate to exclude the elderly from lipid-lowering therapy simply on the basis of age. High-risk but otherwise healthy elderly patients are candidates for treatment. Intervention is justified for individuals with reasonable life expectancy, and good quality of life is a relative indication. Attempts to manage multiple risk factors should be prioritized according to risk potential. Practical considerations in lipid management include motivation and understanding, food preferences and nutritional soundness, cost of drugs, potential for drug interactions, choice of antihypertensive therapy, and monitoring of renal function. Target lipid concentrations in the elderly are those used for the general adult population.

Secondary prevention is of benefit in the "young" elderly, and its use in those older than 75 years is supported by a growing consensus. Primary prevention is generally agreed to be justified in those aged 65–75 years. Its application in the older elderly should be addressed more cautiously but cannot be ruled out. Smoking cessation is prudent, and even in very old patients treatment of systolic hypertension reduces risk for stroke and CHD. Beginning lipid-lowering therapy as primary prevention in those older than 75 years is an issue of debate, but therapy begun in earlier years should be continued (Grundy et al. 1998).

Diet

Surveys have shown that the elderly are concerned about and willing to make lifestyle changes to maintain health; Soons et al. (1995) found that 60% of individuals aged 60–80 years were concerned about blood cholesterol, and 81% reported making dietary changes to reduce risk for CHD. Changes in diet appear to be as effective in the elderly as in the middle-aged (Schaefer et al. 1995). Dietary therapy needs to be carefully individualized (e.g., to accommodate rigid food preferences), particularly because elderly patients may be at risk for malnutrition because of isolation, depression, poverty, or coexisting diseases. Dietary restrictions may be viewed by the elderly as an additional deprivation at a time in life when losses can be common. An intensified (Step II) diet may not be advisable for all elderly patients, and some elderly patients may overcomply with diet, leading to caloric deficiency, calcium deficiency, or constipation or even bowel obstruction from excessive intake of fiber (NCEP 1994).

Exercise

Older patients should be encouraged to undertake regular physical exercise, but there is no evidence that slight overweight in the elderly requires correction (NCEP 1994). Current exercise recommendations emphasizing the importance of total amount of exercise, citing the benefits of intermittent exercise, and advocating lower-intensity independent exercise are particularly relevant to the elderly (Wenger 1996). It is never too late to begin exercising. Relative risks for CHD and all-cause death were reduced 26% and 20% in men and women 84 years of age or older who exercised at least three times a week (Fraser and Shavlik 1997). An important noncoronary benefit is an increase in bone density (Reid 1996). Greater emphasis must be placed on and more time allotted for warm-up and cool-down activities (Wenger 1996). Brisk walking is an excellent prototype, and it constitutes a substantial percentage of the lower maximal oxygen uptake in the elderly (Bruce et al. 1989). Because of reduced efficiency of temperature regulation, the elderly should be cautioned to reduce the intensity of their exercise in hot or humid conditions (Wenger 1996).

The target heart rate for the elderly is slightly lower than for younger people: 40–80% of maximal heart rate reserve versus 50–85% (Pollock et al. 1994). Strength and resistance training is also recommended (Limacher 1998). Clinical features are available to identify patients who should have ECG monitoring during exercise (see Fletcher et al. 1995; Parmley 1986).

Concern has been expressed that increased longevity may simply mean increased disability. Vita et al. (1998) in a longitudinal study found that exercise pattern, BMI, and smoking (preselected stratification variables) in the middle aged and elderly predicted subsequent disability. Better health habits postponed disability more than 5 years and compressed it into fewer years at the end of life.

Pharmacotherapy

Particular caution should be used in proceeding to lipid-lowering pharmacotherapy in the elderly. These patients may be especially vulnerable to the adverse effects of drugs (NCEP 1994). Concern for adverse drug reactions in the elderly arises in large measure from polypharmacy (in both prescription and over-the-counter drugs). Also, patient error is common (noncompliance or dosing error), and drug metabolism is altered in the elderly (reduced removal of drug by the liver or kidneys and hence a prolonged half-life of active drug) (Denke 1993). Gibson et al. (1996) found the equivalent maximum concentration of atorvastatin to be 43% higher and the drug half-life to be 36% longer in elderly men and women (66–92 years) than in young subjects (19–35 years). Therapeutic effects of gemfibrozil were more pronounced in elderly patients (Brosche and Kipf-muller 1996).

Secondary prevention is of great importance, since most patients with established atherosclerotic disease are 65 years old or older, and clinical judgment is crucial in deciding whether to use aggressive therapy. Well-tolerated lipid-lowering drugs for older patients are fibric acid derivatives and statins (NCEP 1994). Beyond the clinical endpoint statin trial results reviewed above, a number of small trials have shown long- and short-term efficacy and safety of statin use in the elderly (Lansberg et al. 1995; Chan et al. 1995; Baggio et al. 1994). However, most cases of severe myopathy with statin use have occurred in older patients, in particular in those with coexisting disease (e.g., renal insufficiency) (NCEP 1994). The occurrence of gallstones may be increased with fibrate use, and cholecystectomy carries more risk in older patients. Other possible side effects with fibrate use are gastrointestinal distress, impotence, and, in patients with renal insufficiency, myopathy (NCEP 1994).

With resins use, associated constipation may be a particular problem, and absorption of other drugs may be decreased. The common side effects of nicotinic acid (e.g., flushing, dry skin) may be more pronounced, and nicotinic acid may aggravate impaired glucose tolerance and raise uric acid levels (NCEP 1994). In a large series of military veterans, most of them elderly men, nicotinic acid had to be discontinued in 49% (Gray et al. 1994). Most discontinuations represented adverse effects (notably, poor glycemic control).

The cost-effectiveness of pharmacotherapy may be more difficult to prove in the elderly, because savings from averted employment losses are not available in retired people, representing, from a health policy perspective, discrimination against the elderly (Denke 1993; Jecker 1991).

Several patient strategies may remove barriers to successful lipid-lowering drug therapy in the elderly: (1) moral support, (2) simplification of therapy, and (3) minimization of side effects (Bonow et al. 1996).

HYPOTHYROIDISM

Thyroid dysfunction is relatively common among the elderly (Finucane and Anderson 1995). However, classic clinical features of hypothyroidism are often absent in the hypothyroid in this age group (Gomberg-Maitland and Frishman 1998). Because hypothyroidism can lead to elevated plasma concentrations of LDL-C, it should be considered in elderly hypercholesterolemic patients even when other symptoms and signs are lacking; screening in these patients will be relatively high yield (Barzel 1995; Mokshagundam and Barzel 1993). Hypothyroid patients have been shown to have an intrinsic defect of receptor-mediated LDL catabolism (Thompson et al. 1981). Other lipid changes reported in hypothyroidism include hypertriglyceridemia (from elevated VLDL) and increased Lp[a] and HDL-C (Becker 1985; Gomberg-Maitland and Frishman 1998). Subclinical hypothyroidism as well may be associated with lipid abnormalities

(Gomberg-Maitland and Frishman 1998). The prevalence of hypertension is also increased in hypothyroidism, and both overt hypothyroidism and subclinical dysfunction may be risk factors for CHD. However, MI and angina are low in incidence, perhaps in part because of decreased metabolic demands on the heart (Gomberg-Maitland and Frishman 1998).

Thyroxine replacement can reduce TC and LDL-C in patients with overt or subclinical hypothyroidism (Gomberg-Maitland and Frishman 1998; Arem et al. 1995; Miura et al. 1994). Tanis et al. (1996) assessed the results of intervention studies in adult patients published from 1976 to 1995 and found that in overt hypothyroidism the average reduction in TC depended on baseline cholesterol: –46 mg/dL with baseline no more than 309 mg/dL and –131 mg/dL with baseline greater than 309 mg/dL; HDL-C was also decreased (6 mg/dL). In subclinical hypothyroidism, cholesterol decreased only 15 mg/dL, independent of baseline cholesterol, when thyrotropin was restored to normal; effects on HDL-C were inconsistent. Most of the trials assessed used levothyroxine (LT4), which is the preferred agent (Mokshagundam and Barzel 1993). Thyroxine replacement appears to have little effect on fasting TG (Gomberg-Maitland and Frishman 1998), and no effect was found on Lp[a] (Arem et al. 1995).

Thyroid hormone replacement should be used cautiously in patients with CHD to avoid precipitating acute MI or precipitating or aggravating angina, ventricular arrhythmias, or congestive heart failure (Aronow 1995). In the Coronary Drug Project, conducted in male survivors of acute MI, dextrothyroxine (DT4) was discontinued because of a higher incidence of adverse cardiovascular effects, including death (Coronary Drug Project 1972). The availability of potent antianginal medications and of bypass surgery may enable prescription of effective therapy for coexisting hypothyroidism and angina (Barzel 1995).

CHILDREN AND ADOLESCENTS

PREVENTIVE CARDIOLOGY

The keystone of pediatric preventive cardiology is the understanding that lifestyle behaviors begin in childhood and that most CHD risk factors, at least in the extreme percentiles, track into adulthood (Strong and Kelder 1996). In addition to recognition and management of lipid risk (see later), smoking should be discouraged, obesity should be avoided and reduced, regular exercise should be encouraged, hypertension should be identified and treated, and diabetes mellitus should be identified and treated (American Academy of Pediatrics 1998; Strong et al. 1992). An integrated approach for the physician's office to cardiovascular health promotion in youths is shown in Table 19.1. Most youths are at only moderate risk, but these eventually will account for most adult CHD cases (Strong and Kelder 1996). Because parents of school-age children or younger children often do not receive any routine medical care except for gynecologic care, identification of risk factors in chil-

Table 19.1. PEDIATRIC CARDIOVASCULAR HEALTH SCHEDULE: RECOMMENDATIONS OF THE AHA COUNCIL ON CARDIOVASCULAR DISEASE IN THE YOUNG

Age	Actions
Birth	• Family history for early CHD, hyperlipidemia; if positive, introduce risk factors, parental referral • Start growth chart • Parental smoking history → smoking cessation referral
0–2 years	• Update family history, growth chart • With introduction of solid foods, begin teaching about healthy diet (nutritionally adequate, low in saturated fat, low in sodium) • Recommend healthy snacks as finger foods • Change to whole milk from formula or breast-feeding at ~1 year of age
2–6 years	• Update family history, growth chart → review growth chart[a] with family (concept of weight for height) • Introduce prudent diet, including ≤30% of calories from total fat (but not <20% for the pediatric population[b]), 8–10% of calories as saturated fat • Change to low-fat milk • Start blood pressure chart at ~3 years of age[c]; review concept of lower sodium intake • Encourage parent-child play that develops coordination • Lipid determination in child if parent has hypercholesterolemia, familial dyslipidemia, or family history of premature CVD → initiate lifestyle changes if abnormal
6–10 years	• Update family history, blood pressure and growth charts • Complete cardiovascular health profile of child: family history, smoking history, blood pressure percentile, weight for height, lipid determination in indicated patients, level of fitness/activity • Reinforce prudent diet and begin active antismoking counseling • Introduce fitness for health → life sport activities for child and family • Discuss role of television viewing in sedentary lifestyle and obesity
>10 years	• Update family history, blood pressure, and growth charts annually • Review prudent diet, risks of smoking, fitness benefits whenever possible • Lipid profile in indicated patients • Fitness review of personal cardiovascular health status

[a]Obesity is defined as ≥130% ideal body weight for height, 30 kg/m² (adolescents), or the 95th percentile or greater for subscapular skinfolds (Gidding et al. 1996).
[b]American Academy of Pediatrics 1998.
[c]If three consecutive interval blood pressure measurements exceed the 95th percentile (see Table 19.4) and blood pressure is not explained by weight for height, diagnosis of hypertension should be made and appropriate evaluation considered.
Source: Modified from Strong and Kelder 1996; used with permission.

dren may enable risk factor management in the entire family, with parents altering their behavior for the benefit of the child (Strong and Kelder 1996).

Nearly all smokers start smoking before the age of 18 years, and large numbers of children begin smoking at age 10 or 11 years (Gidding et al.

Table 19.2. SUGGESTIONS FOR HEALTH PROFESSIONALS TO PRE-VENT ONSET OF SMOKING IN CHILDREN

- **Anticipate** smoking risks associated with the child's developmental stage.
- **Ask** about smoking by the patient, peers, or members of the patient's family.
- **Advise** those who are trying, experimenting with, or smoking cigarettes to stop.
- **Assist** in the smoking cessation process.
- **Arrange** for follow-up on smoking status.

Source: Gidding et al. 1994; used with permission. Based on data from Epps and Manley 1991.

1994). Adverse lipid and other effects occur not only from active smoking but also from passive exposure (Gidding et al. 1994). Suggestions for health professionals to prevent onset of smoking in children are shown in Table 19.2.

Obesity is now the most common nutritional and behavioral disorder in American children and adolescents (Feinstein and Quivers 1997). In the Bogalusa Heart Study, prevalence of overweight among schoolchildren and young adults doubled between 1974 and 1994 (Freedman et al. 1997). NHANES data confirm the trend toward increasing weight and indicate that the obesity prevalence is highest in Hispanic boys and in black and Hispanic girls (Rosner et al. 1998). Emphasis on weight control in children should be on primary prevention, since 80–90% return to their original weight percentile after weight reduction efforts. In individual therapy of most obese children, the emphasis of treatment should be the prevention of weight gain above that appropriate for expected increases in height (Gidding et al. 1996). Television viewing is a sedentary activity and promotes unnecessary caloric intake; the American Academy of Pediatrics (1986) recommends that young people view no more than 2 hours of television each day. A definite role for body fat patterning (e.g., increased abdominal fat) in children is controversial (Porkka and Raitakari 1996). AHA recommendations for medical evaluation of the obese pediatric patient are shown in Table 19.3.

Only half of young people aged 12–21 years regularly participate in vigorous physical activity, and participation in all types of physical activity declines as age increases (U.S. Surgeon General 1996). Learning motor skills at the appropriate age and stage of development is an important step in how adult physical activity is determined (Strong and Kelder 1996).

Detailed recommendations regarding recognition and management of pediatric hypertension can be found in the 1996 report by the NHBPEP Working Group on Hypertension Control in Children and Adolescents. Blood pressure at the 95th percentile (or higher) on three separate occasions is considered elevated; definitions take into account age and height according to sex (Table 19.4). The fifth Korotkoff sound is now used in all ages to define DBP (NIH 1997). Attention should be paid to proper cuff size. Clinicians should be alert to identifiable causes of hypertension. Use of anabolic steroids for bodybuilding should be strongly discouraged. Lifestyle interventions should be recommended for hypertension, with pharmacotherapy (with carefully adjusted dosages) used for higher blood

Table 19.3. AHA RECOMMENDATIONS FOR MEDICAL EVALUATION OF AN OBESE CHILD OR ADOLESCENT

- History for hypoventilation (snoring, apnea, morning headaches, somnolence during the day)
- History of dysmenorrhea in adolescent females
- Careful blood pressure measurement with attention to proper cuff size
- Physical assessment for orthopedic abnormalities
- Fasting lipoprotein profile
- Fasting glucose
- Consider if evaluation suggests an abnormality:
  —Insulin and/or glucose tolerance test
  —Sleep study
  —Echocardiographic evaluation of cor pulmonale and left ventricular mass

Note: Obesity is defined as ≥130% ideal body weight for height, 30 kg/m² (adolescents), or the 95th percentile or greater for subscapular skinfolds.
Source: Gidding et al. 1994; used with permission.

pressure levels and when there is lack of response to lifestyle changes (NIH 1997). About 1% of children are hypertensive, and the younger the child, the more likely the condition is secondary (Strong and Kelder 1996).

LIPID RISK

The U.S. NCEP Expert Panel on Blood Cholesterol Levels in Children and Adolescents in 1991 issued detailed guidelines for the recognition and treatment of hypercholesterolemia in young people (aged 2–19 years) (NCEP 1991; Expert Panel 1992).

Dyslipidemia before adulthood is of concern because atherosclerosis begins in childhood. The Pathobiological Determinants of Atherosclerosis in Youth (PDAY) autopsy study has correlated specific risk factors with lesion extent in particular arteries in subjects aged 15–34 years (McGill et

Table 19.4. 95TH PERCENTILE OF BLOOD PRESSURE ACCORDING TO SELECTED AGES IN GIRLS AND BOYS

Age (years)	Girls' SBP/DBP (mm Hg)		Boys' SBP/DBP (mm Hg)	
	50th percentile for height	75th percentile for height	50th percentile for height	75th percentile for height
1	104/58	105/59	102/57	104/58
6	111/73	112/73	114/74	115/75
12	123/80	124/81	123/81	125/82
17	129/84	130/85	136/87	138/88

Source: NIH 1997; used with permission. Adapted from National High Blood Pressure Education Program 1996.

al. 1997). Smoking was associated with lesions in the abdominal aorta, and increased LDL-C and VLDL and decreased HDL-C were associated with lesions in the aorta and right coronary artery. Children and adolescents with cholesterol elevation are more likely than their peers in the general population to have cholesterol elevation as adults (Lauer et al. 1988; Lauer and Clarke 1990; Webber et al. 1991). It has been estimated that 25% of American children have high or borderline-high cholesterol (Williams and Bollella 1995). Detection of genetic dyslipidemias associated with premature CHD is already crucial during childhood to retard or prevent the atherosclerotic process (Porkka and Raitakari 1996).

Although this manual focuses on the individualized approach for clinicians, the population approach is the major emphasis in cholesterol control for children and adolescents and should include a low-fat, low-cholesterol diet and physical activity for all individuals in this age group. The AHA (Fisher et al. 1997) and the American Academy of Pediatrics (1998) have both endorsed the Step I Diet (prudent diet) in children 2 years of age or older. Safety of its use has been amply demonstrated in both survey and prospective studies (Fisher et al. 1997). Total fat intake should not be less than 20% in the pediatric population (American Academy of Pediatrics 1998). After the second birthday, when the diet becomes more varied, a heart-healthy diet can be achieved by replacing foods high in fat with grains, fruits, lean meat, and other foods low in fat and high in complex carbohydrates and protein (Fisher et al. 1997). Schools, health professionals, the food industry, the mass media, and others play important roles in providing information and influencing behavior.

Detection

In the pediatric population, screening is selective rather than universal (Table 19.5). Screening should be performed in the context of continuing health care; mass screening should be discouraged. Blood sampling may be performed any time after the second birthday: Before then, more calories as fat are needed for growth; after that age, TC and LDL-C concentrations are reasonably consistent. These screening recommendations are especially directed toward physicians who care for adults, since it is they who know the parents' risk status.

Evaluating lipids may be considered as well in a child or adolescent when a family history cannot be obtained, the patient has other risk for CHD, or the patient is receiving a medication that can alter lipid concentrations. As in adults, lipid determinations may be misleading if the patient is actively ill or has an infectious disease; testing should be avoided in these circumstances.

Evaluation

TC and LDL-C cutpoints for pediatric patients (Table 19.6) are lower than in adults. As in adults, cutpoints are to be interpreted flexibly, in the context of total risk. The NCEP values expressly apply to children and adoles-

Table 19.5. LIPID SCREENING IN CHILDREN AND ADOLESCENTS AGED 2–19 YEARS

- Screening should be performed selectively.
- Measure nonfasting TC (and HDL-C if accuracy can be ensured*) if parent has TC >240 mg/dL. Physician may choose full fasting lipoprotein analysis as the initial assessment.
- Perform full fasting lipoprotein analysis if
  —TC >200 mg/dL, or averages >170 mg/dL by two measurements,
  —Family history of early CVD, or
  —Parent has familial dyslipidemia.*

*Authors' addition.
Source: Data from NCEP 1991; Expert Panel 1992.

cents from families with inherited cholesterol problems or premature CVD. The clinical focus is LDL-C, and any intervention requires establishment of an elevation of LDL-C concentration by at least two fasting determinations. In some families with early CHD, the inherited risk factor seems to be low HDL-C (<35 mg/dL). The significance of TG elevation in children for eventual CHD risk remains uncertain.

As in adults, a full clinical evaluation should be performed if LDL-C proves to be high. Possible causes of secondary dyslipidemia considered in adults are also considered in children and adolescents. Some conditions to consider in particular are overweight and use of oral contraceptives,

Table 19.6. MAJOR LIPID CUTPOINTS IN CHILDREN AND ADOLESCENTS, AGED 2–19 YEARS[a]

Lipid	Values (mg/dL)
TC	
High	>200
Borderline-high	170–200
Acceptable	<170
LDL-C	
High	>130
Borderline-high	110–130
Acceptable	<110
HDL-C	
Low	<35
TG	
Quite elevated	>150
Moderately elevated[b]	Males: ~120; females: ~130

[a]Lipid values are for children and adolescents from families with inherited cholesterol problems or premature CVD.
[b]Authors' note: In pediatric patients, TG >200 mg/dL is often related to obesity and TG >500 mg/dL is usually due to a genetic disorder (International Task Force 1992).
Source: Data from NCEP 1991; Expert Panel 1992.

isotretinoin, or anabolic steroids. The two most common familial dyslip-idemias expressed as LDL-C elevations that are currently recognized in children are FH and FCH. It has been estimated that 1 in 25 children with LDL-C higher than 130 mg/dL has heterozygous FH. In heterozygous FH, hypercholesterolemia is typically detectable at birth. In homozygous FH, which occurs in only about 1 in 1 million people, cutaneous xanthomas develop within the first few months or years of life; treatment (e.g., LDL apheresis) is by lipid specialists. Humphries et al. (1997) reviewed issues of genetic testing for FH; their recommendations include testing in immediate family members of patients with FH. Hyperlipidemia in FCH may or may not be expressed in childhood; it has been estimated that FCH is about three times more common in children and adolescents than het-erozygous FH. Other genetic dyslipidemias, such as hypoalphalipopro-teinemia (which entails very low HDL-C concentrations), are discussed in detail in the report of the NCEP Expert Panel on Blood Cholesterol Lev-els in Children and Adolescents. Early diagnosis of familial disorders such as FH and FCH is hampered by the absence of specific phenotypic mark-ers and the cumbersome nature of pedigree examination (Porkka and Raitakari 1996). Although clinical manifestations of FH are not common before the age of 20 years, ultrasound examination of Achilles tendons may be useful in children (Porkka and Raitakari 1996). Koivunen-Niemala et al. (1994) found hypoechoic infiltration of the normal tendon structure in 38% of pediatric patients (aged 3–18 years) with heterozygous FH. Sonographic abnormalities were not found in control patients, and the mean thickness of the tendon was greater in the children with FH (7.1 mm vs. 5.8 mm). Although specific molecular diagnosis is at present available only for FH, it is hoped that early diagnosis of other common lipid disor-ders will be possible within a few years (Porkka and Raitakari 1996).

Treatment

After causes of secondary dyslipidemia have been ruled out or treated, dietary therapy is the primary intervention (Table 19.7). The diets pre-scribed are those used in adults; calorie levels are selected to support growth and development and to reach or maintain desirable body weight. Consultation with a dietitian may be needed to achieve dietary compli-ance. When children are placed on an intensified lipid-lowering diet (Step II Diet), it is important to ensure adequacy of nutrients.

Pharmacotherapy may be considered in pediatric patients 10 years of age or older when LDL-C remains very high despite vigorous dietary ther-apy, especially when multiple risk factors are present. The age cutpoint reflects the fact that early lesions of atherosclerosis begin to occur at about age 10 years; however, drug therapy may be warranted in younger patients when hyperlipidemia is severe. The only lipid-lowering drugs generally rec-ommended at present for use in children are the bile acid sequestrants (resins). Bile acid resins are effective and appear to be well tolerated in chil-dren, although compliance is low because of unpalatability. Low dosages

Table 19.7. TREATMENT OF HYPERCHOLESTEROLEMIA IN CHILDREN AND ADOLESCENTS, AGED 2–19 YEARS

LDL-C (mg/dL)[a]	Action[b]
<110	**Counsel** on healthy diet and on risk factor reduction; repeat lipoprotein analysis within 5 years.
110–130	**Provide Step I Diet** and other risk factor intervention; re-evaluate status in 1 year.
>130	**Perform full clinical evaluation** (family history, physical examination, laboratory tests); assess for causes of secondary dyslipidemia and for familial disorders. Some patients with familial disorders will require referral to a lipid specialist. Screen family members.
	Initiate dietary therapy (see next) and other risk reduction.
Refractory >190 or >160 + either positive family history of early CVD or ≥2 other persistent risk factors[c]	**Consider bile acid resin to supplement diet in patients ≥10 years of age.** It is usual to provide folic acid supplementation with resins in these patients. Nicotinic acid may be used in a very limited number of pediatric patients, but only by a lipid specialist. Monitor at 6 weeks and then every 3 months by lipoprotein analysis; every 6 months to 1 year after LDL-C goal achieved.
<130 (ideally, <110)	**LDL-C goal** of diet or diet + drug therapy

[a]For intervention: established by the average of at least two consecutive fasting determinations.
[b]Calorie levels in children and adolescents are to promote normal growth and development and to reach or maintain desirable body weight.
[c]The NCEP notes that cutpoints that minimize misclassification between pediatric patients with and without FH are about 164 mg/dL for LDL-C and 235 mg/dL for TC.
Source: Data from NCEP 1991; Expert Panel 1992.

are preferred and vitamin supplementation is prudent (Tonstad 1997). Nicotinic acid may be used in a limited number of pediatric patients, but should be administered in these patients only by a lipid specialist. Data on HMG-CoA reductase inhibitors and fibrates remain insufficient to enable their recommendation in pediatric patients (Tonstad 1997).

For elevated plasma TG in pediatric patients, dietary and other lifestyle measures should be recommended unless the elevation is extreme. Chylomicronemia (LPL deficiency or apo C-II deficiency) may be a cause for concern because of the danger for pancreatitis. Low HDL-C is generally managed by lifestyle measures.

Diabetic Patients

In children 2 years of age or older with diabetes, a lipid profile should be obtained after the diagnosis of diabetes and establishment of glucose control (ADA 1998a). When values fall within acceptable risk levels according to NCEP guidelines for pediatric patients, redetermination should be done every 5 years. Abnormal or borderline values should be confirmed by repeat testing, with therapy according to NCEP pediatric guidelines. In children with diabetes, blood pressure should be reduced to the corresponding age-adjusted 90th percentile values (ADA 1998a).

Suggested Reading

The Elderly

Barzel US. Hypothyroidism: diagnosis and management (review). Clin Geriatr Med 1995;11:239–249.

Gomberg-Maitland M, Frishman WH. Thyroid hormone and cardiovascular disease (review). Am Heart J 1998;135:187–196.

LaRosa JC. Cholesterol management in women and the elderly (review). J Intern Med 1997;241:307–316.

Children and Adolescents

American Academy of Pediatrics. Cholesterol in childhood. Policy statement. Pediatrics 1998;101:141–147.

Expert Panel on Blood Cholesterol Levels in Children and Adolescents. National Cholesterol Education Program: report of the Expert Panel on Blood Cholesterol Levels in Children and Adolescents. Pediatrics 1992;89:525–584.

Fisher EA, Van Horn L, McGill HC. Nutrition and children: a statement for healthcare professionals from the Nutrition Committee, American Heart Association. AHA medical/scientific statement. Circulation 1997;95:2332–2333.

Gidding SS, Leibel RL, Daniels S, et al. Understanding obesity in youth. A statement for healthcare professionals from the Committee on Atherosclerosis and Hypertension in the Young of the Council on Cardiovascular Disease in the Young and the Nutrition Committee, American Heart Association. AHA medical/scientific statement. Circulation 1996;94:3383–3387.

Gidding SS, Morgan W, Perry C, et al. Active and passive tobacco exposure: a serious pediatric health problem. A statement from the Committee on Atherosclerosis and Hypertension in Children, Council on Cardiovascular Disease in the Young, American Heart Association. AHA medical/scientific statement. Circulation 1994;90:2581–2590.

Strong WB, Deckelbaum RJ, Gidding SS, et al. Integrated cardiovascular health promotion in childhood: a statement for health professionals from the Subcommittee on Atherosclerosis and Hypertension in Childhood of the Council on Cardiovascular Disease in the Young, American Heart Association. Circulation 1992;85:1638–1650.

Strong WB, Kelder SH. Pediatric preventive cardiology. In: Manson JE, Ridker PM, Gaziano JM, Hennekens CH, eds. Prevention of myocardial infarction. New York: Oxford University Press, 1996:433–459.

Chapter 20

U.S. Ethnic Minorities

The U.S. Department of Health and Human Services' Task Force on Black and Minority Health called for increased amounts of focused research into CVD to identify differences in etiology and the relations of risk factors and disease in minority populations, including racial/ethnic minorities (Task Force 1986). According to U.S. Bureau of the Census estimates for May 1, 1998, the U.S. population is 72.4% non-Hispanic white, 12.1% non-Hispanic black, 11.2% Hispanic, 3.6% non-Hispanic Asian and Pacific Islander, and 0.7% non-Hispanic American Indian, Eskimo, and Aleut (http://www.census.gov; accessed June 1998).

Issues in CHD prevention and treatment in racial/ethnic minorities include culturally sensitive and focused education and intervention as well as changing risk for CHD as immigrant populations acculturate. The influence of race on pharmacokinetics or pharmacodynamics has only recently become a focus of interest, and data remain very limited (Wood and Zhou 1991; Matthews 1995; Johnson 1997). Most studies have evaluated differences between Asian and white subjects (Johnson 1997). Johnson (1997) suggested that differences in drug kinetics between racial groups are more likely to occur with drugs that undergo significant gut or hepatic first-pass metabolism and that are highly bound to AGP than with drugs that are eliminated entirely by the kidneys through filtration and reabsorption and that are not highly bound to plasma proteins (or that are bound to albumin).

AFRICAN AMERICANS

CHD strikes early and may be particularly severe in African Americans. CHD death rates are 7% higher among black males and 35% higher among black females compared with their white counterparts (AHA 1997), and the CHD mortality rate is not declining as rapidly in blacks as in whites (Kochanek et al. 1994; Gillum 1994). In the National Hospital Discharge Survey, median age at death from MI was 5 years lower in African Americans than white Americans (Roig et al. 1987). A variety of reasons could potentially account for these differences, such as different risk factor profiles and access to health care, which are among the priority research areas identified by the Working Group on Research in Coronary Heart Disease in Blacks convened by the NHLBI (Francis 1997).

African Americans are less likely than whites to receive interventional therapy for CHD, even after adjustment for factors such as ability to pay (Ford and Cooper 1995; Giles et al. 1995; Curry 1994). Whether factors such as physician bias or patient willingness to accept procedures are important has not yet been determined (Ford and Cooper 1995). Blacks have generally been slower to seek professional care for symptoms of MI (Lee 1997). In an office-based family medicine residency training program in Rochester, New York, blacks were less likely than whites to be screened for hypercholesterolemia and less likely to be diagnosed as hypercholesterolemic when TC exceeded 240 mg/dL (Naumburg et al. 1993).

RISK FACTORS

Blacks and whites share much of the same group of risk factors for CHD but there are clinically important racial differences in emphasis (Hutchinson et al. 1997). The prevalence of hypertension among African Americans is among the highest in the world (NIH 1997), and the prevalence of LV hypertrophy is higher than in whites (Clark and Emerole 1995). Blacks are more likely than whites to be diabetic or physically inactive, and black women are more likely to be overweight or obese and black men somewhat more likely to smoke than their white counterparts (AHA 1997). Blacks may be more likely to have poor glycemic control in diabetes (Auslander et al. 1997; Weatherspoon et al. 1994; Eberhardt et al. 1994) and to have higher rates of complications of diabetes (Tull et al. 1994). Rural blacks are even more likely to be hypertensive, diabetic, or obese (Willems et al. 1997). Lower socioeconomic status is an important contributor to premature morbidity and mortality (Williams 1998), and in 1996, according to the U.S. Bureau of the Census, 28.4% of blacks lived below the poverty line, compared with 11.2% of whites (http://www.census.gov; accessed June 1998). Socioeconomic differences in mortality appear to be due to an array of factors, including hostility, depression, and social isolation, and may persist even with improved health behaviors among the disadvantaged (Lantz et al. 1998; Williams 1998). The burden of traditional major risk factors and the risk from socioeconomic and psychosocial factors are considered to place African Americans in a precarious position with regard to CHD risk (Curry 1994).

In the Atherosclerosis Risk in Communities (ARIC) study, clustering of major risk factors was more common in blacks, and a prevalence of no risk factors was greatest in whites (Hutchinson et al. 1997); analysis of NHANES I follow-up data showed a higher burden of comorbidities considered (stroke, CHD, hypertension, and diabetes) in blacks compared with whites (McGee et al. 1996). Compared with white physicians, African-American physicians 23–35 years after medical school had higher CVD risk, higher CHD incidence, and a much higher case fatality rate (51.5% vs. 9.4%); the best predictor of risk for the black physicians was blood pressure, whereas the best predictors in whites were smoking, cholesterol concentration, and paternal history (Thomas et al. 1997).

Blood Pressure

Hypertension not only is more prevalent in American blacks than whites (35% vs. 24% among men and 34% vs. 19% among women) but also develops earlier in life and is more severe at any decade of life (AHA 1997). African Americans have higher rates of stage 3 hypertension (NIH 1997). Black men and women are 2.5 times more likely to die of stroke compared with white Americans, and as many as 30% of all deaths in black men with hypertension and 20% of all deaths in black women with hypertension can be attributed to the hypertension (AHA 1997). It is not established whether genetic mechanisms are responsible in part for the high prevalence of hypertension; environmental factors such as obesity and health care access account for some of the difference (Douglas et al. 1996). In the ARIC study, the percentages of black patients on treatment whose blood pressure was under control were lower than in whites (56% vs. 73% for men, 63% vs. 74% for women) (Hutchinson et al. 1997).

Plasma Lipids

The prevalence of hypercholesterolemia is roughly similar between U.S. adult blacks and whites (AHA 1997). About 27% of black adults compared with 30% of white adults would be candidates for lipid-lowering dietary intervention by current NCEP guidelines (Sempos et al. 1993). In recent ARIC data (Hutchinson et al. 1997), LDL-C values were essentially the same in black and white adults, although some studies have reported slightly lower LDL-C in black men and women (e.g., Evans County Study—Tyroler et al. 1975) or black men alone (NHANES III—Johnson et al. 1993). In ARIC, as in NHANES III, HDL-C was virtually the same between black and white women but was substantially higher in black men than in white men (50 vs. 43 mg/dL). TG was lower in black men (120 vs. 148 mg/dL) and black women (110 vs. 129 mg/dL). Among MRFIT screenees, the relation between TC and CHD mortality rate at 12 years' follow-up was virtually identical between black and white men (Stamler et al. 1986).

The atherogenic potential of Lp[a] may vary between blacks and other populations. In whites and Asians, the population distribution of Lp[a] is highly skewed, with most people having low concentrations, and an elevated concentration has been associated in many although not all studies with increased prevalence and severity of CHD. In Africans and African Americans, however, the distribution is more symmetric, and the mean

Lp[a] concentration is twice as high as in whites or Asians (Moliterno et al. 1995; Utermann 1989). Several studies have reported no association between Lp[a] concentration and atherosclerotic risk in African Americans (Moliterno et al. 1995), but other evidence suggests atherogenicity in this population (Schreiner 1994).

EVALUATION AND TREATMENT

Blacks have been described as having a lower incidence of classic chest pain but an increased incidence of dyspnea with MI (Lee 1997).

Considering their substantially increased risk for CVD mortality, aggressive risk factor management seems appropriate in African Americans. Weight loss may be particularly difficult to achieve in this population (Kumanyika et al. 1992; Bild et al. 1996; Wing and Anglin 1996). Between 1987 and 1992 in the United States, total and saturated fat intakes declined among whites and Hispanics, but only minimal changes occurred among blacks (Norris et al. 1997). Pravastatin (Jacobson et al. 1995) and lovastatin (Fong and Ward 1997; Prisant et al. 1996) have been studied in African Americans with primary hypercholesterolemia and were found to be safe and effective.

For hypertension, monotherapy with beta-blockers or ACE inhibitors is less effective in African Americans (Matthews 1995), but when specific indications are present, these agents are indicated regardless of ethnicity and the addition of diuretics markedly improves response. Diuretics are the agents of first choice in African Americans in the absence of conditions that prohibit their use; calcium antagonists and alpha-beta-blockers are also effective (NIH 1997). Sodium restriction may be emphasized since blacks have a higher prevalence of salt sensitivity (Douglas et al. 1996).

HISPANIC AMERICANS

Hispanics are the second largest minority group in the United States and, with a population increasing at about eight times the rate of non-Hispanic Americans, are expected to become the largest minority group early in the 21st century (Liao et al. 1997; U.S. Bureau of the Census 1993). The group is culturally and demographically diverse. Among 22.4 million Hispanic Americans, Mexican Americans are the largest group (13 million), followed by Puerto Ricans (3 million) and Cuban Americans (1 million) (U.S. Bureau of the Census 1993). According to 1992 data, higher percentages of all deaths are from CVD among Cuban Americans (37.1% in males and 44.6% in females) than among Mexican Americans (26.7% and 35.1%), Puerto Ricans (24.6% and 35.1%), or Hispanic Americans with origins in Central or South America (19.8% and 26.3%) (AHA 1998b).

Compared with adult non-Hispanic whites, adult Hispanics have an adverse CHD risk profile: substantially higher prevalences of overweight and obesity (in particular among women) and diabetes mellitus as well as an increased prevalence of physical inactivity (AHA 1997). In addition, more central obesity, lower HDL-C, and higher plasma TG are described (Liao et al. 1997). Despite these factors, prevalence is fairly equivalent between Hispanics and whites for high blood pressure and hypercholesterolemia (≥240 mg/dL); smoking prevalence is lower (in particular among women) (AHA 1997). Differences between Hispanics and non-Hispanic whites in insulin, glucose, BMI, and other risk factors occur as early as age 8–10 years (Tortolero et al. 1997). The estimated prevalence of CHD among Hispanic adults, however, is lower than in other groups: 5.6% for Mexican Americans compared with 7.5% for non-Hispanic whites and 6.9% for non-Hispanic blacks (AHA 1997). The San Luis Valley Diabetes Study described similar CHD incidences in nondiabetic Hispanics and non-Hispanic whites and a lower incidence in diabetic Hispanics (Rewers et al. 1993). Sudden cardiac death has been estimated to be about 50% lower in both Hispanic men and women compared with their white counterparts (whereas black men and women had rates about 30% higher than whites) (Gillum 1997).

The lower-than-expected CHD rates have led to the proposal of a "Hispanic paradox" (Markides and Coreil 1986). However, while Liao et al. (1997) in a large national sample found CHD and CVD mortality rates to be approximately 20% lower among adult Hispanics than among whites, the proportion of deaths due to CHD was similar between the groups, since the all-cause mortality rate was also 20% lower among Hispanics. The San Antonio Heart Study found no evidence for a diminished effect of major risk factors in Mexican Americans. Current smoking, diabetes, high cholesterol, and hypertension together accounted for 45% of their all-cause mortality and 55% of their CVD mortality (Wei et al. 1996). In the Northern Manhattan Stroke Study, Hispanics had significantly less carotid plaque than blacks or whites, but increasing LDL-C produced a greater impact (Sacco et al. 1997).

In adjusted analyses, Hispanics have been described as receiving fewer drugs after MI (Herholz et al. 1996) and undergoing fewer invasive cardiovascular procedures (Carlisle 1995). Hispanics as a group use fewer preventive services than whites and have reduced levels of health insurance coverage and socioeconomic status (Liao et al. 1997). According to the 1990 U.S. census, 78% of Hispanics older than 5 years speak a language other than English in the home and 37% of Hispanics report that they speak English poorly or not at all (U.S. Bureau of the Census 1993). It is critical that culturally sensitive risk reduction initiatives in Spanish be instituted; as noted at the beginning of the chapter, a variety of materials in Spanish are available from the AHA and the NHLBI.

In Puerto Rico, CHD and stroke mortality rates have been reported to be increasing rather than decreasing (Ramirez 1994). Recent lifestyle changes may be contributing to this problem (Ramirez 1994).

ASIAN/PACIFIC-ISLANDER AMERICANS

CHANGING RISK WITH ACCULTURATION: THE JAPANESE-AMERICAN EXPERIENCE

At the start of the Seven Countries Study, which assessed disease risk in middle-aged men beginning between 1958 and 1964, only 7% of the men studied in Japan had TC greater than 250 mg/dL, compared with 39% of the U.S. cohort (Keys 1970). The low prevalence of hypercholesterolemia in Japan reflected a diet in which only 3% of total calories were provided by saturated fat. Prevalence of CHD in the cohorts of the study was directly related to TC concentration, and the 5-year age-standardized annual CHD death rate was five times higher in the American than in the Japanese population studied (Keys 1970). The migration Ni-Hon-San Study begun in the mid-1960s provided a "natural experiment," also in middle-aged men, and found that the serum cholesterol concentration and CHD death rate in Honolulu were both intermediate between Japan (Nippon) and San Francisco (Benfante 1992). Saturated fat intake was about four times higher among the Japanese Americans than among the men living in Japan. Thus, it appeared that the gradient in cardiovascular death rate reflected the gradient of westernization of the men of Japanese ancestry (Benfante 1992). Long-term follow-up in the Honolulu Heart Study of Japanese-American men living in Hawaii has confirmed the long-term CHD predictive utility of major risk factors in this population (Goldberg et al. 1995; Yano et al. 1984).

Rapid westernization of the lifestyle in Japan has led to drastic increases in plasma cholesterol, particularly in urban areas and among younger Japanese (Yamada et al. 1997). Between 1963–1966 and 1980–1983 in Japan, the age-adjusted mean cholesterol concentration rose 22 mg/dL (to 179 mg/dL) in middle-aged men and 29 mg/dL (to 192 mg/dL) in middle-aged women (Shimamoto et al. 1989), and a rapid increase continued between 1980 and 1990 (Sakata and Labarthe 1996). A large, multicenter study in Japan showed that TC and TG concentrations had become higher in Japanese 30 years of age or older than in their American counterparts (Sekimoto et al. 1983; Goto 1980; Lipid Research Clinics Program Epidemiology Committee 1979). Although in most Asian countries there has been a rapid increase in the incidence of CHD in association with economic development (Singh et al. 1996; Hughes 1986), in Japan CHD mortality rates have remained low despite higher blood pressure than in most other developed countries and a high prevalence of smoking among men (Yamada et al. 1997). Whether the apparent inconsistency in Japan represents a greater stability of lifestyle in older people (so that the lifestyle changes have not yet contributed to mortality rates) or perhaps the protective effect of other dietary factors remains unclear. However, data from a large, community-based screening registry in Okinawa showed TC (determined in 1983) to be an independent predictor of acute MI 5–8 years later (Wakugami et al. 1997); risk for MI increased proportionally with cholesterol concentration. In a series of 330 Japanese patients with established CHD, predictors of cardiac events during 4 years were serum cholesterol, obesity, and the number of diseased vessels (Takahashi et al. 1997).

RISK PROFILES

CVD and cancer were the leading killers of Asian/Pacific-Islander Americans in a 1992 survey in seven states conducted by the National Center for Health Statistics (Hoyert and Kung 1997) and in 1995 U.S. data (AHA 1998a). Data compiled by the AHA (1997) show Asian or Pacific-Islander adults in the United States to be substantially less likely than non-Hispanic whites to have high blood pressure (although 73% of Japanese-American men aged 71–93 years have high blood pressure) or to be overweight or obese (prevalence of 10.8% in men, 10.1% in women, vs. 59.5% and 45.5%). Compared with their white counterparts, Asian/Pacific-Islander men are about as likely to smoke (20.4% vs. 28.0%) and more likely to have cholesterol greater than 240 mg/dL (27.4% vs. 17.3%) and diabetes (3.4% vs. 2.5%), whereas Asian/Pacific-Islander women are less likely to smoke (7.5% vs. 24.7%), somewhat more likely to have high cholesterol (25.8% vs. 20.2%), and equally as likely to have diabetes (2.4%).

This population, however, is extremely heterogeneous and socioeconomically bipolar (Kwon and Bae 1995). Asian/Pacific Americans come from more than 43 countries and speak more than 100 languages and dialects (Kwon and Bae 1995). Asian Americans, about two-thirds of whom are foreign born, represent at least 16 distinct ethnic groups (e.g., Chinese, Indian, Japanese, Korean, Vietnamese, Filipino) (http://www.census.gov; accessed June 1998). Ethnic differences in CVD risk factors among different groups of Asian Americans have been described. Klatsky et al. (1996) in adjusted analysis of data on 13,000 Asian Americans in northern California found the highest TC among Japanese-American men and women, the greatest prevalence of hypertension among Filipino-American men and women, and the lowest BMI and smoking prevalence among Chinese-American men and women.

At one end of the CHD risk spectrum are immigrants who have maintained traditional lifestyles associated with low rates of CHD. Choi et al. (1990) in a survey in the early 1980s of elderly Chinese immigrants living in Boston found a risk factor profile resembling that in mainland China, including a low-fat diet, a high level of physical activity, a low prevalence of obesity, lower blood cholesterol than among white counterparts, and, among men, a high rate of cigarette smoking (39%). In a population in Shanghai with an average TC concentration of only 162 mg/dL, only 7% of deaths over 8–13 years of follow-up were the result of CHD (Chen et al. 1991). There was a strong, positive relation between cholesterol concentration and CHD mortality rate, and cholesterol did not contribute to other causes of death.

Native Hawaiians represent the other end of the risk spectrum. Today accounting for only 13% of the population of the islands of Hawaii, they have one of the poorest health profiles in the United States (Mokuau et al. 1995). Life expectancy is about 5 years less than for the state of Hawaii as a whole, and prevalences of diabetes, hypertension, obesity, and smoking are high (Mokuau et al. 1995; Mau et al. 1997); 65.5% of men and 62.6% of women are overweight or obese (AHA 1997). The CHD mortality and diabetes mortality rates are 44% and 200% higher than in the total U.S. population (Mokuau et al. 1995). Many native Hawaiians live in isolated rural communities, and access to preventive health care programs is often limited (Mokuau et al. 1995). Samoans are also among the most overweight people in the world and suffer from high rates of weight-related illnesses such as heart disease, hypertension, and diabetes (Shovic 1994). The prevalence of overweight in Samoan women in Hawaii is 80%, compared with 46% in Western Samoa (McGarvey 1991). The frequency of obesity among Samoans in American Samoa, Hawaii, and Western Samoa increased in the 1980s as they held more modern jobs (Bindon and Baker 1985). In Western Samoa between 1978 and 1991, the "epidemiologic transition" included prevalence increases in obesity, type 2 diabetes, and hyperlipidemia; in the capital, Apia, cholesterol higher than 212 mg/dL increased in prevalence from 18% to 36% and TG greater than 175 mg/dL increased from 9% to 15% (Hodge et al. 1997).

CHD is an important cause of death in Asian Indian Americans (Wild et al. 1995). A study by Enas et al. (1996) of Asian Indian physicians who were first-generation immigrants to the United States and their family members found the age-adjusted prevalence of MI and angina to be about three times higher in the men than in white men in the Framingham Offspring Study; the prevalence was similar between Indian and white women. This and several other studies have suggested that insulin resistance, type 2 diabetes, reduced HDL-C, and increased plasma TG may be particularly important risk factors in this racial group (Dhawan 1996). In the Enas et al. study, Asian Indians, despite a very low prevalence of obesity (4.2%), were seven times more likely than whites to have type 2 diabetes; the prevalence of cigarette smoking was also low (1.3%). In India, diabetes and CVD have rapidly increased in prevalence, particularly in urban areas, in association with rapid lifestyle changes (Singh et al. 1997).

ANTIHYPERTENSIVE DRUG THERAPY IN ASIAN AMERICANS

South Asians appear to be more sensitive than whites to various antihypertensive agents (NIH 1997; Matthews 1995). Key points as reviewed by Hui and Pasic (1997) include that many of the differences between Asians and whites have been described regarding beta-blockers. Isradipine was shown to be more effective in Chinese than in white patients. Usual dosages of carvedilol in Japan are about half those in the United States.

In Korean patients, the response was similar to that of white patients when enalapril maleate was given as monotherapy but exceeded that of white patients when hydrochlorothiazide was added. In their series of 396 patients in Los Angeles, Hui and Pasic found that medication changes, dosage reduction, and side effects were significantly more frequent in Asian than in white patients. The authors noted that consideration in prescribing must be given to body weight and dietary habits; for example, the Chinese tend to eat more vegetables, and they often use herbs that may be pharmacologically active.

AMERICAN INDIANS AND ALASKA NATIVES

AMERICAN INDIANS

CVD is now the leading cause of death among American Indians, although it appears that heart disease was uncommon before lifestyle modernization. Overall CVD mortality rate remains lower than in the U.S. population as a whole, although rates vary distinctly among tribes—for example, CVD mortality rates in Northern Plains Indians are as high as or higher than U.S. rates, whereas rates are low (but appear to be increasing) in some southwestern tribes such as the Pima and Navajo (Howard et al. 1996). Ongoing changes in lifestyle are expected to affect CVD risk adversely (Robbins et al. 1996). Overall, the health status of American Indians both on or near reservations and in urban settings is far below that of other Americans (Grossman et al. 1994; Rhoades et al. 1987).

A number of studies are focusing on CVD risk factors in American Indians, including the large Strong Heart Study of American Indians aged 45–74 years living in Oklahoma, North and South Dakota, and Arizona. This study has confirmed a high prevalence of diabetes (46–72%) (Lee et al. 1995). Diabetes appeared to have, as it does in whites, a greater effect on women, although the prevalence of MI or definite CHD was greater in men (Howard et al. 1995). BMI in the Strong Heart Study participants was 19–36% higher than in the general U.S. population (Welty et al. 1995), and rates of obesity are increasing in tribes throughout North America (Robbins et al. 1996). Participants in the study reported higher intakes of fat and cholesterol than participants in NHANES III (general U.S. population) (Zephier et al. 1997). In contrast, the traditional diet of the Pima Indians of the Gila River Community in Arizona was very low in fat: approximately 8–12% fat, 70–80% carbohydrate, and 12–18% protein (Boyce and Swinburn 1993).

All three regional populations in the Strong Heart Study had greater percentages of people with cholesterol values less than 200 mg/dL and fewer with values of 240 mg/dL or higher compared with the U.S. population; mean cholesterol values were similar in diabetic and nondiabetic subjects, with the expected higher TG and lower HDL-C among diabetic subjects (Robbins et al. 1996). Mean TC was 20 mg/dL lower among the men and 27 mg/dL lower among the women than national mean concentrations for the same age group; the mean concentration was 20 mg/dL lower in Arizona than in the North and South Dakota. Mean HDL-C was lower than for the United States, and HDL-C was a significant predictor of CHD. Hypertension was more prevalent in the Arizona and Oklahoma tribes than in the United States as a whole, but blood pressure was significantly lower in North and South Dakota tribes. Smoking prevalence was higher in all Indian groups except Arizona women, but smoking frequency was lower than in the United States as a whole (Welty et al. 1995; Howard et al. 1995). Smokeless tobacco has a high rate of use among American Indians (Spangler and Salisbury 1995).

In Arizona Indians in the Strong Heart Study, obesity, hypertension, and insulin values were higher than in the other Indian centers studied, yet CHD rates were lower (Howard et al. 1995). Previous studies have shown the incidence of fatal CHD in the Pima to be less than half that in the Framingham population after control for age, sex, and diabetes (Nelson et al. 1990). Pima Indians have the world's highest rates of type 2 diabetes, with an incidence of end-stage renal disease more than 20 times that of the general U.S. population (Nelson et al. 1996). Possible explanations for the apparent paradox include a lower and more favorable lipoprotein profile (including low TC and LDL-C), lower frequency of smoking, and higher degree of Indian heritage; the subject remains one of intense scrutiny (Howard et al. 1995). The emergence of the diabetes epidemic in the Pima has been associated with profound lifestyle changes. It is considered likely that a genetic susceptibility accounts for the epidemic (Charles et al. 1997). Segregation analysis suggests a major gene effect, with expression of the gene perhaps dependent on environmental factors that have increased in prevalence in younger cohorts (Hanson et al. 1995). Obesity is considered a major factor interacting with the presumed genetic susceptibility (Knowler et al. 1993).

Intensive risk factor education and intervention are needed in American Indian communities. Careful attention needs to be given to the readability and cultural relevance of educational materials (e.g., a human figure, because drawn as bald, was viewed as non-Indian) (Hosey et al. 1990). The many barriers to compliance with nutrition guidelines include high cost or even unavailability of fresh fruits and vegetables at stores and trading posts that serve many American Indian communities (Zephier et al. 1997).

ALASKA NATIVES

Traditionally, CHD mortality rates have been low among the indigenous peoples of Greenland, Alaska, and Canada, perhaps related to protective environmental factors, such as consumption of marine omega-3 fatty acids with beneficial effects on the plasma lipid profile. The profile of low CHD risk also included a diet low in saturated fat, rare obesity, uncommon hypertension, and a high level of physical activity, although smoking was common (Sassen et al. 1994). Westernization of lifestyle has contributed to an increase in hypertension, diabetes, and CVD in Alaska Natives (Schraer et al. 1996, 1997; Davidson et al. 1993). CVD is now the leading cause of death among Alaska Natives (Ellis and Campos-Outcalt 1994), although deaths from all cardiac diseases and CHD recently remained 80% and 61% of levels in Alaskan whites (Davidson et al. 1993). Although it has also been suggested that death from other causes before middle age in Alaska Natives may dictate CHD rates, autopsy investigation has shown a significantly lower prevalence and extent of raised atherosclerotic lesions in the abdominal aorta and coronary arteries of Alaska Natives compared with non-natives (Newman et al. 1993, 1997). Tobacco use is the leading preventable cause of death among Alaska Natives; prevalence of use is high for both cigarettes and smokeless tobacco (Kaplan et al. 1997).

Suggested Reading

African Americans

Hutchinson RG, Watson RL, Davis CE, et al., for the ARIC Study Group. Racial differences in risk factors for atherosclerosis: the ARIC study. Angiology 1997;48:279–290.

Livingston IL, ed. Handbook of black American health: the mosaic of conditions, issues, policies, and prospects. Westport, CT: Greenwood Press, 1994.

Hispanic Americans

Liao Y, Cooper RS, Cao G, et al. Mortality from coronary heart disease and cardiovascular disease among adult U.S. Hispanics: findings from the National Health Interview Survey (1986 to 1994). J Am Coll Cardiol 1997;30:1200–1205.

Asian/Pacific-Islander Americans

Benfante R. Studies of cardiovascular disease and cause-specific mortality trends in Japanese-American men living in Hawaii and risk factor comparisons with other Japanese populations in the Pacific region: a review. Hum Biol 1992;64:791–805.

Hui KK, Pasic J. Outcome of hypertension management in Asian Americans. Arch Intern Med 1997;157:1345–1348.

Klatsky AL, Tekawa IS, Armstrong MA. Cardiovascular risk factors among Asian Americans. Public Health Rep 1996;111(suppl 2):62–64.

Mokuau N, Hughes CK, Tsark JU. Heart disease and associated risk factors among Hawaiians: culturally responsive strategies. Health Soc Work 1995;20:46–51.

American Indians and Alaska Natives

Howard BV, Lee ET, Cowan LD, et al. Coronary heart disease prevalence and its relation to risk factors in American Indians. The Strong Heart Study. Am J Epidemiol 1995;142:254–268.

Welty TK, Lee ET, Yeh J, et al. Cardiovascular disease risk factors among American Indians. The Strong Heart Study. Am J Epidemiol 1995;142:269–287.

Chapter 21

Adults with Diabetes Mellitus and Patients with Concomitant Dyslipidemia and Hypertension

ADULTS WITH DIABETES MELLITUS

This section includes a summary of recommendations for the treatment of dyslipidemia in diabetes that was recently added to the ADA's clinical practice recommendations (ADA 1998c). The rationale for the dyslipidemia recommendations is discussed in detail in an ADA technical report (Haffner 1998), which forms an additional basis for the present review and provides full referencing. Because of their high risk for CHD (see Chapter 8), the ADA considers optimal in adult patients with diabetes an LDL-C value of 100 mg/dL or lower, that is, the target recommended in the NCEP guidelines for patients with CHD (Expert Panel 1993). This is in keeping with the NCEP's position that clinicians may wish to use aggressive management in primary prevention when a patient is at very high risk because of concomitant risk factors such as diabetes. The ADA also emphasizes management of low HDL-C and elevated plasma TG in patients with diabetes.

Treatment of type 2 diabetes mellitus should emphasize multiple risk management including medical nutrition therapy; exercise; weight reduction as needed; and use of oral glucose-lowering agents, insulin, or both, with careful attention to all cardiovascular risk factors, including not only dyslipidemia but also hypertension, smoking, and family history (ADA 1998a). Blood pressure in adults with diabetes should be reduced to less than 130/85 mm Hg (ADA 1998a; NIH 1997). The ADA recommends initial lifestyle modifications unless hypertension is at an urgent level, with stepwise addition of drugs as needed (ADA 1998a). Blood pressure should be measured in the supine, sitting, and standing positions in all patients with diabetes to detect evidence of autonomic dysfunction and orthostatic hypotension; automated ambulatory monitoring may be particularly helpful (NIH 1997). The JNC (NIH 1997) has recommended antihypertensive drug choices in diabetes. ACE inhibitors, alpha-blockers, calcium antagonists, and diuretics at low dosages are preferred because of fewer adverse effects on glucose homeostasis, the lipid profile, and renal function. Beta-blockers may prolong hypoglycemia, adversely affect peripheral blood flow, and mask symptoms of hypoglycemia; however, treatment with diuretics and beta-blockers has yielded as much or more reduction of CVD risk in diabetic as in nondiabetic patients. ACE inhibitors are preferred in patients with diabetic nephropathy; angiotensin II receptor blockers may be considered if ACE inhibitors are contraindicated or not well tolerated, and renoprotection has also been reported with use of a calcium antagonist.

DYSLIPIDEMIA IN DIABETES

In type 2 diabetes, the most common pattern of dyslipidemia is elevated TG and decreased HDL-C. Median TG, however, is less than 200 mg/dL, and TG is less than 400 mg/dL in 85–95% of patients. Familial disorders such as FCH and FH, which occur frequently in diabetic subjects, may contribute to the severe TG elevations seen in some patients with diabetes, as may renal disease, hypothyroidism, use of alcohol, and use of estrogens. Typically, LDL-C concentration is not different from that in subjects without diabetes, although LDL particles are more likely to be small and dense in diabetes, perhaps increasing risk for atherosclerosis. In many studies, the dyslipidemia in diabetes is more severe in women than in men, which is consistent with relatively greater risk for CHD in diabetic women compared with diabetic men (Haffner 1998).

CLINICAL TRIAL RESULTS

No reported lipid-lowering trial has been restricted to patients with diabetes, but post hoc analyses of results in diabetic patients are available from 4S and CARE in secondary prevention and from the Helsinki Heart Study in primary prevention. The 4S trial provided the first evidence that lipid lowering significantly reduces risk for new CHD events in diabetic patients with hypercholesterolemia and CHD; treatment with simvastatin reduced CHD risk 55% (compared with 32% in patients without diabetes) and reduced all-cause mortality 43% (compared with 28% in nondiabetic subjects), the latter result not quite statistically significant (Pyörälä et al. 1997). In the placebo group in 4S, CHD risk was 2.5 times higher in diabetic subjects than in nondiabetic subjects; simvastatin treatment reduced the risk in diabetic subjects to slightly below the risk in the nondiabetic placebo group. Also, treatment was effective in all lipid subgroups, including those with elevated TG and low HDL-C, although 4S excluded subjects with baseline TG above 220 mg/dL. CARE, in which pravastatin was used, also showed significant CHD risk reduction in diabetic patients with CHD, but extended benefit to patients with lower LDL-C concentrations (Sacks et al. 1996). CHD risk reduction was similar between diabetic and nondiabetic subjects (25% and 23%). In the primary prevention Helsinki Heart Study, significant reduction of CHD risk with the gemfibrozil therapy was enhanced in patients with a high LDL-C:HDL-C ratio and elevated TG (Manninen et al. 1992) and in overweight subjects with additional risk factors known to contribute to insulin resistance syndrome (Tenkanen et al. 1995). Gemfibrozil reduced CHD risk 60% in Helsinki subjects with diabetes, although the reduction was not significant because of the small patient numbers (Koskinen et al. 1992).

Because of these data from trials of LDL-C lowering, the ADA places primary emphasis on intervention against LDL-C, although it notes that interventions to lower TG and raise HDL-C may also be useful. In observational studies (although relatively few prospective data are available), HDL-C may be the best predictor of CHD in type 2 diabetes, followed by TG and TC.

As an addition to the ADA report, we note that the LIPID trial, which by a factor of 2 is the largest randomized trial of cholesterol lowering in patients with CHD, included 777 patients with diabetes (9% of the study population) (The LIPID Study Group 1995). Unpublished data indicate that reduction of CHD risk in the diabetic subjects was similar to that in nondiabetic subjects with treatment; subjects had relatively normal cholesterol concentrations (presented by Andrew Tonkin, MD, at the 47th Annual Scientific Session of the American College of Cardiology, March 29–April 1, 1998, Atlanta, Georgia). Five percent of the subjects in the separately published substudy that examined carotid progression in the LIPID trial were diabetic, and there were no significant differences in the size of the B-mode ultrasound effects between diabetic and nondiabetic subjects (MacMahon et al. 1998). Treatment with pravastatin prevented any detectable increase in carotid wall thickening over 4 years of follow-up.

TREATMENT

The ADA recommends that a full fasting lipoprotein profile be obtained every year in adult patients with diabetes. Optimal LDL-C for adults with diabetes is no more than 100 mg/dL. Action limits for LDL-C reduction in adult patients are shown in Table 21.1; priorities for treatment of diabetic dyslipidemia are listed in Table 21.2. Borderline or abnormal values should be confirmed by repeat testing. Aggressive LDL-C lowering in primary prevention derives in part from the high death rate from a first MI among diabetic subjects. Risk in adults according to HDL-C concentration is considered higher at less than 35 mg/dL, borderline at 35–45 mg/dL, and lower at greater than 45 mg/dL (even higher HDL-C may be advisable in women). Risk in adults according to fasting TG concentration is considered higher at 400 mg/dL or more, borderline at 200–399 mg/dL, and lower at less than 200 mg/dL.

Table 21.1. TREATMENT DECISIONS BASED ON LDL-C CONCENTRATION (mg/dL) IN ADULTS WITH DIABETES MELLITUS—ADA RECOMMENDATIONS

	Medical nutrition therapy		Drug therapy	
	Initiation	LDL-C goal	Initiation	LDL-C goal
With known athero-sclerotic disease	>100	≤100	>100	≤100
Without known athero-sclerotic disease	>100	≤100	≥130	130*

Note: Caveats are that (1) medical nutrition therapy should be attempted before starting pharmacologic therapy; (2) because diabetic men and women are considered to have equal risk for CVD, age and sex are not considered risk factors.

*Optimal LDL-C for adults with diabetes is ≤100 mg/dL. For diabetic patients with one or more CHD risk factors (HDL-C <35 mg/dL, hypertension, smoking, family history of premature CVD, or microalbuminuria or proteinuria), some authorities recommend an LDL-C goal ≤100 mg/dL in primary prevention.

Source: ADA 1998c; used with permission.

Table 21.2. ORDER OF PRIORITIES FOR TREATMENT OF DIABETIC DYSLIPIDEMIA IN ADULTS—ADA RECOMMENDATIONS

I. LDL-C lowering
—First choice: HMG-CoA reductase inhibitors (statins)
—Second choice: bile acid resins
II. HDL-C raising
—Behavioral interventions such as weight loss, increased physical activity, and smoking cessation may be helpful
—Difficult except with nicotinic acid, which has relative contraindication
III. TG lowering
—Glycemic control first priority
—Fibric acid derivative (gemfibrozil)
—Statins are moderately effective at high dosage in hypertriglyceridemic subjects who also have high LDL-C
IV. Combined hyperlipidemia
—First choice: improved glycemic control plus statin at high dosage
—Second choice: improved glycemic control plus statin plus gemfibrozil*
—Third choice: improved glycemic control plus resin plus gemfibrozil OR improved glycemic control plus statin plus nicotinic acid* (nicotinic acid may significantly worsen hyperglycemia; glycemic control must be carefully monitored)

Note: The decision to treat elevated LDL-C before elevated TG is based on clinical trial data indicating safety and efficacy of available agents.

*The combination of a statin with nicotinic acid and especially with gemfibrozil may confer increased risk for myopathy.

Source: ADA 1998c; used with permission.

Nutritional Therapy and Physical Activity

The ADA has made detailed recommendations for both medical nutrition therapy (ADA 1998b) and physical activity (ADA 1998d) (available at www.diabetes.org). Nutritional recommendations are similar to those of the NCEP in specifying a reduction in saturated fat and, in the overweight, weight loss, but differ from the NCEP in permitting either a higher-carbohydrate diet or a higher-fat diet enriched in polyunsaturated or (if TG and VLDL are the primary concerns) monounsaturated fat. Polyunsaturated fats of the omega-3 series provided naturally in fish and other seafood need not be curtailed in people with diabetes. Fish oil supplementation, the major effect of which is to reduce plasma TG, has been reported to lead to deterioration of glucose homeostasis in diabetic patients, although worsening glycemic control has not materialized in recent studies (Harris 1996). The area remains controversial. There is evidence from some (although not all) studies that metabolic effects may be better in diabetic subjects eating a diet high in monounsaturated fat rather than one high in carbohydrates, although any high-fat diet may make weight loss difficult. It appears that long-term programs of regular exercise are feasible for patients with uncomplicated type 2 diabetes or impaired glucose tolerance, with special precautions as stipulated in the ADA recommendations (e.g., thorough screening, precautions regarding the feet, careful warm-up and cool-down, proper hydration, avoidance of high-resistance exercise in older individuals and those with long-standing diabetes, exercises appropriate when there is loss of protective sensation).

Weight loss and increased physical activity should lower TG and raise HDL-C and may modestly decrease LDL-C. When averaged LDL-C at the beginning of therapy exceeds the LDL-C goal by more than 25 mg/dL, the physician may decide to begin lipid-lowering pharmacotherapy at the same time as behavioral therapy in patients at high risk (i.e., patients with a history of MI or with other risk factors). Otherwise, effectiveness of behavioral interventions may be evaluated every 6 weeks, with consideration of pharmacotherapy at 3–6 months.

Glucose-Lowering Agents

Previous debates about the lipid effects of particular diabetic agents may be of reduced relevance because combined therapy with several agents is now common (Haffner 1998). Glycemic control improves the lipid profile, especially TG concentrations, in diabetes, whether achieved with sulfonylurea, insulin, acarbose, or troglitazone therapy (Haffner 1998). Effects on TG usually reflect the degree of glycemic control; effects on HDL-C are more variable (Haffner 1998), although HDL composition may be altered in a direction believed to be antiatherogenic (ADA 1998c). With glycemic control, LDL-C may also decrease modestly ($\leq$10–15%), although LDL composition may change favorably with decreased plasma TG (ADA 1998c).

Troglitazone may modestly increase TC, LDL-C, and HDL-C without changing the TC:HDL-C or LDL-C:HDL-C ratio (*Physicians' Desk Reference* 1998). Unlike the sulfonylurea agents, metformin has consistently been shown to yield beneficial lipid changes, including not only TG lowering but also apparently LDL-C lowering and possibly HDL-C raising, all of the changes modest; its effects on the fibrinolytic system would be expected to enhance fibrinolysis (Howes et al. 1996).

Pharmacotherapy

Low-Density Lipoprotein Cholesterol

The ADA's recommendations for treatment of elevated LDL-C (see Table 21.1) generally follow the NCEP (Expert Panel 1993) and the ADA consensus panel on dyslipidemia (ADA 1993). In the NCEP adult guidelines, drug therapy is considered in patients with atherosclerotic disease when LDL-C remains at least 130 mg/dL despite lifestyle intervention; whether to intervene if LDL-C remains greater than 100 mg/dL is left to clinical judgment about overall risk. The ADA in effect advises physicians that diabetes confers enough risk in patients with atherosclerotic disease that drug therapy is appropriate at the lower action limit. The ADA also considers LDL-C of 100 mg/dL or lower optimal in primary prevention, with pharmacotherapy to be considered after lifestyle measures and glucose control if LDL-C remains 130 mg/dL or higher, that is, the NCEP drug action limit for secondary prevention. The goal of drug therapy in primary prevention is less than 130 mg/dL, or, according to clinical judgment, no more than 100 mg/dL. Lipid-lowering pharmacotherapy should be begun at the same time as behavioral therapy in diabetic patients when clinical atherosclerotic disease is present or LDL-C is 200 mg/dL or higher. As noted, glucose control will only modestly decrease LDL-C. The ADA gives LDL-C management first priority in lipid-altering pharmacotherapy (see Table 21.2) in part because data from clinical trials are more convincing for the statins than for gemfibrozil.

High-Density Lipoprotein Cholesterol

Pharmacologically raising HDL-C in patients with diabetes is difficult because nicotinic acid, the most effective agent for increasing HDL-C, has a relative contraindication in this disease. Weight loss, smoking cessation, and increased physical activity may increase HDL-C.

Triglyceride

As in the report of the ADA consensus panel (ADA 1993), increased fasting TG is recognized as a target for intervention. Initial therapy consists of lifestyle measures: weight loss as needed, increased physical activity, and moderation of alcohol consumption. Improved glycemic control is very effective for reducing TG and should be employed aggressively before a fibrate is introduced. TG greater than 1,000 mg/dL requires prompt, aggressive action, including pharmacotherapy and severe dietary fat restriction, to reduce risk for pancreatitis.

When glycemic control has been improved as much as is likely, addition of a fibrate may be considered. As an addition to the ADA recommendations, it should be noted that fibrates should be used with caution if at all in the presence of diabetic nephropathy with renal insufficiency because of risk for myopathy (Gotto et al. 1995). The ADA advises that strong consideration should be given to pharmacotherapy when TG remains greater than 400 mg/dL; physicians are referred to clinical judgment for values of 200–400 mg/dL. A statin at a higher dosage may be moderately effective in TG reduction when TG exceeds 300 mg/dL. High-dosage statin therapy may reduce LDL-C to 80 mg/dL or less, for which there are no safety data. Gemfibrozil should not be initiated alone in diabetic patients who have increased concentrations of both LDL-C and TG. Combination drug therapy may be initiated in some cases; several options are shown in Table 21.2. Changes in pharmacotherapy should be made at intervals of about 4–6 weeks on the basis of laboratory findings.

CONSIDERATIONS IN TYPE 1 DIABETES IN ADULTS

Plasma lipid concentrations tend to be normal and sometimes are even better than normal in patients with type 1 diabetes mellitus who have good glycemic control. Lipoproteins may be abnormal in composition but the clinical significance of the changes is unknown. Although no clinical trial data and few observational epidemiologic data are available regarding lipid concentrations and CHD risk in type 1 diabetes, the ADA considers aggressive treatment reasonable if LDL-C concentrations are above the goals recommended in type 2 diabetes. For CHD risk reduction, improved glycemic control may be even more important in type 1 diabetes mellitus, as suggested by data from the Wisconsin Epidemiologic Study of Diabetic Retinopathy (Klein 1995).

PATIENTS WITH CONCOMITANT DYSLIPIDEMIA AND HYPERTENSION

Hyperlipidemic individuals have a higher than expected prevalence of hypertension, and hypertensive individuals have a higher than expected prevalence of hyperlipidemia (NCEP 1994). The two conditions increase CHD risk synergistically and should be treated aggressively when they coexist (NCEP 1994; NIH 1997). The principles for lifestyle modification are similar for both conditions: Weight reduction in the overweight and increased physical activity are very important, in addition to reducing dietary fat, sodium, and alcohol.

Several antihypertensive agents affect plasma lipid concentrations. As reviewed by the JNC (NIH 1997), thiazide and loop diuretics in high dosages can induce at least short-term increases in TC, LDL-C, and plasma TG. The effects can be reduced or eliminated by dietary modifications. Beta-blockers may increase plasma TG transiently and decrease HDL-C; nonetheless, beta-blockers have been demonstrated in clinical trials to reduce total mortality, sudden death, and recurrent MI rates in MI survivors (Yusuf et al. 1985). Alpha-blockers may modestly decrease TC and increase HDL-C. ACE inhibitors, angiotensin II receptor blockers, calcium antagonists, and central adrenergic agonists are neutral with regard to effects on plasma lipid concentrations. The NCEP (1994) notes that beta-blockers with intrinsic sympathomimetic activity and labetalol produce no appreciable changes in lipid concentrations.

Post hoc analyses of data through 1995 from clinical studies revealed no clinically important interactions between any of the statins and diuretics, ACE inhibitors, or calcium channel blockers (Garnett 1995). However, the selective calcium channel inhibitor mibefradil (Posicor), approved by the FDA in June 1997 and chemically unlike other approved agents in its class, was voluntarily withdrawn from the U.S. market in June 1998 because of the potential for interaction with other drugs, including lovastatin and simvastatin, that depend on the same liver enzyme as mibefradil (FDA 1998). Small decreases in bioavailability of lovastatin and pravastatin when coadministered with propranolol are unlikely to have a meaningful impact on the clinical effects of these statins (Garnett 1995). Maximum serum concentration but not the serum concentration-time curve of simvastatin was decreased with propranolol, although the clinical relevance is not known (*Physicians' Desk Reference* 1998). Neither bioavailability nor clearance of fluvastatin was affected by propranolol (Garnett 1995). In clinical studies, cerivastatin was used concomitantly with diuretics, ACE inhibitors, calcium channel blockers, and beta-blockers, and atorvastatin with various antihypertensives, without evidence of clinically important adverse interactions (*Physicians' Desk Reference* 1998). Resins may delay or decrease absorption of concomitant oral medications such as thiazide diuretics and propranolol (*Physicians' Desk Reference* 1998). Both diuretics and nicotinic acid can induce hyperuricemia and sometimes gout (Scott 1991). Nicotinic acid may potentiate the effects of antihypertensive agents (International Task Force 1993). For full information about potential drug interactions, refer to manufacturers' production information.

Although the trial was designed to assess the effects of pravastatin therapy, post hoc analysis of REGRESS data (see Chapter 10) showed a synergistic effect of cotreatment with calcium channel blockers in enhancing benefits in the progression of coronary lesions and the development of new lesions (Jukema et al. 1996). The mechanisms for such an effect, if confirmed, are unknown; speculations include amelioration of endothelial dysfunction or antioxidant properties of calcium channel blockers (Jukema et al. 1996). There was not a difference in effect between dihydropyridine and nondihydropyridine agents.

Suggested Reading

American Diabetes Association. Management of dyslipidemia in adults with diabetes (position statement). Diabetes Care 1998;21(suppl 1):S36–S39.

American Diabetes Association. Standards of medical care for patients with diabetes mellitus (position statement). Diabetes Care 1998;21(suppl 1): S23–S31.

American Diabetes Association. Nutrition recommendation and principles for people with diabetes mellitus (position statement). Diabetes Care 1998; 21(suppl 1):S32–S35.

American Diabetes Association. Diabetes and exercise (position statement). Diabetes Care 1998;21(suppl 1):S40–S44.

American Diabetes Association. Detection and management of lipid disorders in diabetes (consensus statement). Diabetes Care 1993;16(suppl 2):106–112.

Haffner SM. Management of dyslipidemia in adults with diabetes (technical review). Diabetes Care 1998;21:160–178.

Pyörälä K, Pedersen TR, Kjeksus J, et al. Cholesterol lowering with simvastatin improves prognosis of diabetic patients with coronary heart disease: a subgroup analysis of the Scandinavian Simvastatin Survival Study (4S). Diabetes Care 1997;20:614–620.

REFERENCES

Abbott RD et al. JAMA 1988;260:3456–3460.

Ades PA et al. Arch Intern Med 1992;152:1033–1035.

American Academy of Pediatrics. Television and the family. Elk Grove Village, IL: American Academy of Pediatrics, 1986.

American Academy of Pediatrics. Pediatrics 1998;101:141–147.

American Diabetes Association. Diabetes Care 1993;16(suppl 2):106–112.

American Diabetes Association. Diabetes Care 1998a;21(suppl 1):S23–S31.

American Diabetes Association. Diabetes Care 1998b;21(suppl 1):S32–S35.

American Diabetes Association. Diabetes Care 1998c;21(suppl 1):S36–S39.

American Diabetes Association. Diabetes Care 1998d;21(suppl 1):S40–S44.

American Heart Association. 1998 heart and stroke statistical update. Dallas: American Heart Association, 1997.

American Heart Association. Biostatistical fact sheet: Asian/Pacific Islanders and cardiovascular diseases. Dallas: American Heart Association, 1998a.

American Heart Association. Biostatistical fact sheet: Hispanics and cardiovascular diseases. Dallas: American Heart Association, 1998b.

Arem R et al. Metab Clin Exp 1995;44:1559–1563.

Aronow WS. Clin Geriatr Med 1995;11:219–229.

Aronow WS, Ahn C. Am J Cardiol 1996;77:864–866.

Assmann G, Schulte H. Am J Cardiol 1992;8:99–103.

Auslander WF et al. Diabetes Care 1997;20:1569–1575.

Baggio G et al. Drugs 1994;47(suppl 2):59–63.

Bagshaw S. Drug Safety 1995;12:91–96.

Balady GJ et al. Circulation 1994;90:1602–1610.

Barzel US. Clin Geriatr Med 1995;11:239–249.

Becker C. Endocrinol Rev 1985;6:432–440.

Benfante R. Hum Biol 1992;64:791–805.

Benfante R et al. Ann Epidemiol 1992;2:273–282.

Bild DE et al. Int J Obes Relat Metab Disord 1996;20:47–55.

Bindon JR, Baker PT. Ann Hum Biol 1985;12:67–76.

Birdwell BG et al. Arch Intern Med 1993;153:1991–1995.

Bonow RO et al. Am J Med 1996;101(suppl 4A): 17S–24S.

Borum ML. Med Clin North Am 1998;82:51–75.

Boyce VL, Swinburn BA. Diabetes Care 1993;16:369–371.

Brosche T, Kipfmuller G. Fortschr Med 1996;114:157–160.

Bruce RA et al. J Cardiopulmonary Rehabil 1989;9:24–29.

Buchwald H et al. Ann Surg 1992;216:389–398.

Burke AP et al. N Engl J Med 1997;336:1276–1282.

Burke AP et al. Circulation 1998;97:2110–2116.

Byington RP et al. Circulation 1995;92:2419–2425.

Campbell AJ et al. J Am Geriatr Soc 1993;41:1333–1338.

Carhart RL Jr, Ades PA. Cardiol Clin 1998;16:37–43.

Carlisle DM et al. Am J Public Health 1995;85:352–356.

Carlson LA, Rosenhamer G. Acta Med Scand 1988;223:405–418.

Carr BR, Ory H. Contraception 1997;55:267–272.

Carroll JF, Pollock ML. In: Lowenthal DT, ed. Geriatric cardiology. Cardiovascular clinics. Philadelphia: FA Davis, 1992.

CASS Principal Investigators. Circulation 1981;63(suppl I):I1–I81.

Cassard SD et al. J Womens Health 1997;6:199–207.

Castelli WP et al. Ann Epidemiol 1992;2:23–28.

Chan P et al. Am J Hypertens 1995;8:1099–1104.

Charles MA et al. Diabetes Metab 1997;23 (suppl 4):6–9.

Chasan-Taber L et al. Circulation 1996;94:483–489.

Chen CP et al. Acta Obstet Gynecol Scand 1995;74:607–610.

Chen Z et al. BMJ 1991;303:276–282.

Choi ES et al. Arch Intern Med 1990;150:413–418.

Cholesterol Treatment Trialists' Collaboration. Am J Cardiol 1995;75:1130–1134.

Clark LT, Emerole O. Cleve Clin J Med 1995;62:285–292.

Col NF et al. JAMA 1997;277:1140–1147.

Collaborative Group on Hormonal Factors in Breast Cancer. Lancet 1997;350:1047–1059.

Coronary Drug Project. JAMA 1972;220:996–1008.

Corti M-C et al. JAMA 1995;274:539–544.

Craven TE et al. Circulation 1990;82:1230–1242.

Crespo CJ et al. Arch Intern Med 1996;156:93–98.

Curry C. In: Livingston IL, ed. Handbook of black American health: the mosaic of conditions, issues, policies, and prospects. Westport, CT: Greenwood Press, 1994:24–32.

Davidson M et al. Int J Epidemiol 1993;22:62–71.

Davidson MH et al. Arch Intern Med 1997;157:1186–1192.

Dayton S et al. Circulation 1969;40(suppl 2):1–63.

Denke MA. Curr Opin Lipidol 1993;4:56–62.

Denke MA. Curr Opin Lipidol 1996;7:369–373.

Denke MA, Winker MA. JAMA 1995;274:575–577.

Dhawan J. Curr Opin Lipidol 1996;7:196–198.

Douglas JG et al. J Assoc Acad Minor Phys 1996;7:16–21.

Douglas PS, Ginsburg GS. N Engl J Med 1996;334:1311–1315.

Downs JR et al. JAMA 1998;279:1615–1622.

Eaker ED et al. Circulation 1993;88:1999–2009.

Eberhardt MS et al. J Clin Epidemiol 1994;47:1181–1189.

Ellis JL, Campos-Outcalt D. Am J Prev Med 1994;10:295–307.

Enas EA et al. Indian Heart J 1996;48:343–353.

Epps RP, Manley MW. Pediatrics 1991;88:140–144.

Ettinger B et al. Obstet Gynecol 1996;87:6–12.

Expert Panel on Blood Cholesterol Levels in Children and Adolescents. Pediatrics 1992;89:525–584.

Expert Panel on Detection, Evaluation, and Treatment of High Blood Cholesterol in Adults. JAMA 1993;269:3015–3023.

Feinstein JA, Quivers ES. Curr Opin Cardiol 1997;12:70–77.

Ferrara A et al. Circulation 1997;96:37–43.

Finucane P, Anderson C. Drugs Aging 1995;6:268–277.

Fisher EA et al. Circulation 1997;95:2332–2333.

Fletcher GF et al. Circulation 1995;91:580–615.

Folsom AR et al. JAMA 1993;269:483–487.

Folsom AR et al. Am J Public Health 1995;85:1128–1132.

Fong RL, Ward HJ. Am J Med 1997;102:387–391.

Food and Drug Administration. FDA talk paper: Roche Laboratories announces withdrawal of Posicor from the market. June 8, 1998. http://www.fed.gov.

Ford ES, Cooper RS. Health Serv Res 1995;30:237–252.

Forman R, Aronow WS. Clin Geriatr Med 1996;12:169–180.

Francis CK. J Health Care Poor Underserved 1997;8:250–269.

Fraser GE, Shavlik DJ. Arch Intern Med 1997;157:2249–2258.

Freedman DS et al. Pediatrics 1997;99:420–426.

Frost PH et al. Circulation 1996;94:26–34.

Garnett WR. Am J Health Syst Pharm 1995;52:1639–1645.

Gibson DM et al. J Clin Pharmacol 1996;36:242–246.

Gidding SS et al. Circulation 1994;90:2581–2590.

Gidding SS et al. Circulation 1996;94:3383–3387.

Giles WH et al. Arch Intern Med 1995;155:318–324.

Gillum RF. J Am Coll Cardiol 1994;23:1273–1277.

Gillum RF. Am J Public Health 1997;87:1461–1466.

Godschalk MF. Va Med Q 1991;118:99–101.

Goldberg RJ et al. Arch Intern Med 1995;155:686–694.

Gomberg-Maitland M, Frishman WH. Am Heart J 1998;135:187–196.

Gordon DJ et al. Circulation 1989;79:8–15.

Goto Y. Atherosclerosis 1980;36:341–349.

Gotto AM Jr et al. The ILIB lipid handbook for clinical practice: blood lipids and coronary heart disease. Houston: International Lipid Information Bureau, 1995.

Grady D et al. Ann Intern Med 1992;117:1016–1037.

Gray DR et al. Ann Intern Med 1994;121:252–258.

Grossman DC et al. JAMA 1994;271:845–850.

Grundy SM et al. Circulation 1998;97:1876–1887.

Haas J. N Engl J Med 1998;338:1694–1695.

Haffner SM. Diabetes Care 1998;21:160–178.

Hanson RL et al. Am J Hum Genet 1995;57:160–170.

Harris WS. Curr Opin Lipidol 1996;7:3–7.

Henderson BE et al. Arch Intern Med 1991;151:75–78.

Hennekens CH. Cardiol Clin 1998;16:1–8.

Herholz H et al. J Clin Epidemiol 1996;49:279–287.

Hodge AM et al. Int J Epidemiol 1997;26:297–306.

Hodis HN et al. Ann Intern Med 1998;128:262–269.

Horton JA, ed. The women's health data book: a profile of women's health in the United States. New York: Jacobs Institute of Women's Health/Elsevier, 1992.

Hosey GM et al. Diabetes Educator 1990;16:407–414.

Howard BV et al. Am J Epidemiol 1995;142:254–268.

Howard G et al. Stroke 1997;28:1693–1701.

Howes LG et al. Clin Exp Pharmacol Physiol 1996;23:201–206.

Hoyert DL, Kung HC. Mon Vital Stat Rep 1997;46(1 suppl):1–63.

Hughes K. Int J Epidemiol 1986;15:44–50.

Hui KK, Pasic J. Arch Intern Med 1997;157:1345–1348.

Hulley S et al. JAMA 1998;280:605–613.

Humphries SE et al. Q J Med 1990;76:169–181.

Hutchinson RG et al. Angiology 1997;48:279–290.

International Task Force. Nutr Metab Cardiovasc Dis 1992;2:113–156.

International Task Force. Guidelines of the European Atherosclerosis Society: a desktop guide to the management of risk factors for coronary heart disease. London: Current Medical Literature, 1993.

Jacobson R. Psychol Med 1986;16:547–549.

Jacobson TA et al. Arch Intern Med 1995;155:1900–1906.

Jecker N. JAMA 1991;266:3012–3015.

Johnson CL et al. JAMA 1993;269:3002–3008.

Johnson JA. J Pharm Sci 1997;86:1328–1333.

Jukema JW et al. Arterioscler Thromb Vasc Biol 1996;16:425–430.

Kane JP et al. JAMA 1990;264:3007–3012.

Kannel WB, Wilson PW. Arch Intern Med 1995;155:57–61.

Kaplan SD et al. Prev Med 1997;26:460–465.

Keys A. Circulation 1970;41/42(suppl I): I186–I195.

Klatsky AL et al. Public Health Rep 1996;111(suppl 2):62–64.

Klein R. Diabetes Care 1995;18:258–268.

Knowler WC et al. Diabetes Care 1993;16:216–227.

Kochanek KD et al. Am J Public Health 1994;84:938–944.

Koivunen-Niemela T et al. Acta Pediatr 1994;83:1178–1181.

Koskinen P et al. Diabetes Care 1992;15:820–825.

Krolewski AS et al. Am J Med 1991;90(suppl 2A): 56S–61S.

Krumholz HM et al. JAMA 1994;272:1335–1340.

Krumholz HM et al. Circulation 1998;97:958–964.

o

Kuller LH et al. Circulation 1993;88(suppl, part 2):I-261–I-270.

Kumanyika S et al. Ethn Dis 1992;2:166–175.

Kushwaha RS. Curr Opin Lipidol 1992;3:167–172.

Kwon IW, Bae M. Mo Med 1995;92:648–652.

Lambrew CT et al. Arch Intern Med 1997;157:2577–2582.

Lansberg PJ et al. Atherosclerosis 1995;116:153–162.

Lantz PM et al. JAMA 1998;279:1703–1708.

LaRosa JC. Clin Geriatr Med 1996;12:33–40.

LaRosa JC. J Intern Med 1997a;241:307–316.

LaRosa JC. Arch Intern Med 1997b;157:961–968.

Lauer RM, Clarke WR. JAMA 1990;264:3034–3038.

Lauer RM et al. Pediatrics 1988;82:309–318.

Lavie CJ et al. Clin Geriatr Med 1996;12:57–68.

Lee ET et al. Diabetes Care 1995;18:599–610.

Lee HO. Am J Crit Care 1997;6:7–13.

Lewis MA et al. Contraception 1997;56:129–140.

Lewis SJ. Cardiol Clin 1998;16:9–15.

Li R et al. Stroke 1994;25:2377–2383.

Liao Y et al. J Am Coll Cardiol 1997;30:1200–1205.

Limacher MC. Cardiol Clin 1998a;16:27–36.

Limacher MC. Curr Opin Cardiol 1998b;13:139–144.

The LIPID Study Group. Am J Cardiol 1995;76:474–479.

The Lipid Research Clinics Program Epidemiology Committee. Circulation 1979;60:427–439.

MacMahon S et al. Circulation 1998;97:1784–1790.

Malacrida R et al. N Engl J Med 1998;338:8–14.

Malenka DJ, Baron JA. Arch Intern Med 1988;148:2247–2252.

Mann K et al. Alcohol Clin Exp Res 1992;16:1052–1056.

Manninen V et al. Circulation 1992;85:37–45.

Manolio TA et al. Ann Epidemiol 1992;2:161–176.

Manson JE, Spelsberg A. In: Manson JE, et al., eds. Prevention of myocardial infarction. New York: Oxford University Press, 1996a:241–273.

Manson JE et al., eds. Prevention of myocardial infarction. New York: Oxford University Press, 1996a:549–553.

Manson JM et al. Reprod Toxicol 1996b;10:439–446.

Markides KS, Coreil J. Public Health Rep 1986;101:253–265.

Matthews HW. Drug Metab Drug Interact 1995;12:77–91.

Matthews KA et al. N Engl J Med 1989;321:641–646.

Mau MK et al. Diabetes Care 1997;20:1376–1380.

McGarvey ST. Am J Clin Nutr 1991;53(6 suppl):1586S–1594S.

McGee D et al. Ann Epidemiol 1996;6:381–385.

McGill HC Jr et al. Arterioscler Thromb Vasc Biol 1997;17:95–106.

McNagny SE et al. Ann Intern Med 1997;127:1093–1096.

Meilahn EN et al. Cardiology 1995;86:286–298.

Meischke H et al. Ann Emerg Med 1993;22:1597–1601.

Mercuri M et al. Am J Med 1996;101:627–634.

Miettinen TA et al. Circulation 1997;96:4211–4218.

Miller NE, Nanjee MN. Cardiovasc Risk Factors 1992;2:158–169.

Miller VT. Endocrinol Metab Clin North Am 1990;19:381–398.

Miura S et al. Intern Med 1994;33:413–417.

Mokshagundam S, Barzel US. J Am Geriatr Soc 1993;41:1361–1369.

Mokuau N et al. Health Soc Work 1995;20:46–51.

Moliterno DJ et al. Arterioscler Thromb Vasc Biol 1995;15:850–855.

Mosca L et al. Circulation 1997;96:2468–2482.

Murabito JM. J Am Med Womens Assoc 1995;50:35–39.

National Cholesterol Education Program. Report of the Expert Panel on Blood Cholesterol Levels in Children and Adolescents. NIH publication no. 91-2732. Bethesda, MD: U.S. Department of Health and Human Services, 1991.

National Cholesterol Education Program. Circulation 1994;89:1329–1445.

National High Blood Pressure Education Program Working Group on Hypertension Control in Children and Adolescents. Pediatrics 1996;98:649–658.

National Institutes of Health. The sixth report of the Joint National Committee on Prevention, Detection, Evaluation, and Treatment of High Blood Pressure. NIH publication no. 98-4080. Bethesda, MD: National Institutes of Health, 1997.

Naumburg EH et al. J Fam Pract 1993;36:425–430.

Nelson RG et al. Circulation 1990;81:987–995.

Nelson RG et al. N Engl J Med 1996;335:1636–1642.

Nettleman MD, Klein WS. N Engl J Med 1998;338:1543–1544.

Newman WP et al. Lancet 1993;341:1056–1057.

Newman WP III et al. Arch Pathol Lab Med 1997;121:1069–1075.

Norris J et al. Am J Public Health 1997;87:740–746.

O'Leary DH et al. Stroke 1992;23:1752–1760.

Owens JF et al. Prev Med 1990;19:147–157.

Palca J. Science 1991;254:792.

Parmley WW. J Am Coll Cardiol 1986;7:451–453.

Petitti DB. JAMA 1998;280:650–652.

Physicians' desk reference, ed. 52. Montvale, NJ: Medical Economics Company, 1998.

Pilote L, Hlatky MA. Am Heart J 1995;129:1237–1238.

Pollock ML et al. South Med J 1994;87:S88–S95.

Porkka KVK, Raitakari OT. Curr Opin Lipidol 1996;7:183–187.

Posner BM et al. Arch Intern Med 1993;153:1549–1556.

Prisant LM et al. Am J Cardiol 1996;78:420–424.

Pyörälä K et al. Diabetes Care 1997;20:614–620.

Ramirez EA. Bol Asoc Med P R 1994;86:28–36.

Rees MC. Br J Obstet Gynecol 1997;104 (suppl 16):1–3.

Reid IR. Am J Med Sci 1996;312:278–286.

Rewers M et al. Ethn Dis 1993;3:44–54.

Rhoades ER et al. Public Health Rep 1987;102:361–368.

Rich-Edwards JW et al. N Engl J Med 1995;332:1758–1766.

Rifkind BM, Rossouw JE. JAMA 1998;279:1483–1484.

Robbins DC et al. Curr Opin Lipidol 1996;7:188–195.

Roger VL, Gersh BJ. In: Julian DG, Wenger NK, eds. Women and heart disease. St. Louis: Mosby, 1997:135–150.

Roig E et al. Circulation 1987;76:280–288.

Rosenberg L et al. Am J Epidemiol 1993;137:54–63.

Rosenberg L et al. Am J Obstet Gynecol 1997;177:707–715.

Rosner B et al. J Pediatr 1998;132:211–222.

Rozenberg S et al. Int J Fertil Menopausal Stud 1995;40(suppl 1):23–32.

Sacco RL et al. Stroke 1997;28:929–935.

Sacks FM et al. N Engl J Med 1996;335:1001–1009.

Sakata K, Labarthe DR. J Epidemiol 1996;6:93–107.

Salameh WA, Mastrogiannis DS. Clin Obstet Gynecol 1994;37:66–77.

Salamone LM et al. Arch Intern Med 1996;156:1293–1297.

Sassen LMA et al. Cardiovasc Drugs Ther 1994;8:179–191.

Sattar N et al. J Clin Endocrinol Metab 1997;82:2483–2491.

Schaefer EJ et al. Arterioscler Thromb Vasc Biol 1995;15:1079–1085.

Schairer C et al. Epidemiology 1997;8:59–65.

Schenck-Gustafsson K. Eur Heart J 1996;17(suppl D):2–8.

Schmidt SB, Borsch MA. Am J Cardiol 1990;65:1411–1415.

Schraer CD et al. Public Health Rep 1996;111:51–52.

Schraer CD et al. Diabetes Care 1997;20:314–321.

Schreiner PJ. Chem Phys Lipids 1994;67–68:405–410.

Schrott HG et al. JAMA 1997;277:1281–1286.

Scott JT. Baillieres Clin Rheumatol 1991;5:39–60.

Sekimoto H et al. Jpn Circ J 1983;47:1351–1358.

Sempos CT et al. JAMA 1993;269:3009–3014.

Shear CL et al. Circulation 1991;85:1293–1303.

Shepherd J et al. N Engl J Med 1995;333:1301–1307.

Shimamoto T et al. Circulation 1989;79:503–515.

Shipley MJ et al. BMJ 1991;303:89–92.

Shovic AC. J Am Diet Assoc 1994;94:541–543.

Sidney S et al. Obstet Gynecol 1996;88:939–944.

Sidney S et al. Circulation 1998;98:1058–1063.

Singh RB et al. J Cardiovasc Risk 1996;3:489–494.

Singh RB et al. J Cardiovasc Risk 1997;4:201–208.

Sonke GS et al. BMJ 1996;313:853–855.

Soons KR et al. Gerontology 1995;41:57–62.

Spangler JG, Salisbury PL III. Am Fam Physician 1995;52:1421–1430.

Spitzer WO. Hum Reprod 1997;12:2347–2357.

Stamler J et al. JAMA 1986;256:2823–2828.

Stampfer MJ et al. N Engl J Med 1988;319:267–273.

Stampfer MJ et al. Am J Obstet Gynecol 1990;163:285–291.

Stampfer MJ et al. N Engl J Med 1991;325:756–762.

Steinberg KK et al. JAMA 1991;265:1985–1990.

Strong WB, Kelder SH. In: Manson JE, et al., eds. Prevention of myocardial infarction. New York: Oxford University Press, 1996:433–459.

Strong WB et al. Circulation 1992;85:1638–1650.

Takahashi T et al. Jpn Circ N 1997;61:139–144.

Talbott E et al. Am J Epidemiol 1981;114:671–681.

Tanis BC et al. Clin Endocrinol 1996;44:643–649.

Task Force on Black and Minority Health. Report of the Secretary's Task Force on Black and Minority Health, vol. 4. Cardiovascular and cerebrovascular disease. Washington, DC: U.S. Department of Health and Human Services, 1986.

Tenkanen L et al. Circulation 1995;92:1779–1785.

Thomas DB. Environ Health Perspect 1995;103(suppl 8):153–160.

Thomas J et al. J Health Care Poor Underserved 1997;8:270–283.

Thompson GR et al. Proc Natl Acad Sci U S A 1981;78:2591–2595.

Tobin JN et al. Ann Intern Med 1987;19–25.

Tonstad S. Drug Safety 1997;16:330–341.

Tortolero SR et al. Circulation 1997;96:418–423.

Tresch DD, Aronow WS. Clin Geriatr Med 1996;12:89–100.

Tull ES et al. In: Livingston IL, ed. Handbook of black American health: the mosaic of conditions, issues, policies, and prospects. Westport, CT: Greenwood Press, 1994:94–109.

Tyroler HA et al. Prev Med 1975;4:541–549.

Urbano-Márquez A et al. JAMA 1995;274:149–154.

U.S. Bureau of the Census. We the American . . . Hispanics. Washington, DC: U.S. Government Printing Office, 1993.

U.S. Surgeon General. Physical activity and health: a report of the Surgeon General. Washington, DC: U.S. Department of Health and Human Services, 1996.

Utermann G. Science 1989;246:904–910.

Vaccarino V et al. Circulation 1995;91:1861–1871.

Vita AJ et al. N Engl J Med 1998;338:1035–1041.

Wakugami K et al. Serum cholesterol and risk of acute myocardial infarction in a cohort of mass screening in Okinawa, Japan. In: Unpublished abstracts book of the Fourth International Conference on Preventive Cardiology, Montreal, June 29–July 3, 1997.

Walsh BW et al. JAMA 1998;279:1445–1451.

Walsh JME, Grady D. JAMA 1995;274:1152–1158.

Waters D et al. Circulation 1995;92:2404–2410.

Weatherspoon LJ et al. Diabetes Care 1994;17:1148–1153.

Webber LS et al. Am J Epidemiol 1991;133:884–899.

Wei M et al. Am J Epidemiol 1996;144:1058–1065.

Weitzman S et al. Am J Cardiol 1997;79:722–726.

Welty TK et al. Am J Epidemiol 1995;142:269–287.

Wenger NK. Clin Geriatr Med 1996;12:79–88.

Wenger NK. In: Julian DG, Wenger NK, eds. Women and heart disease. St. Louis: Mosby, 1997:21–38.

Wenger NK. Cardiol Clin 1998;16:17–25.

Whisnant JP et al. Neurology 1996;47:1420–1428.

Wild SH et al. Ann Epidemiol 1995;5:432–439.

Willems JP et al. South Med J 1997;90:814–820.

Williams CL, Bollella M. J Pediatr Health Care 1995;9:153–161.

Williams RB. JAMA 1998;279:1745–1746.

Wing RR, Anglin K. Diabetes Care 1996;19:409–413.

Women's Health Initiative Study Group. Control Clin Trials 1998;19:61–109.

Wood AJ, Zhou HH. Clin Pharmacokinet 1991;20:350–373.

The Writing Group for the PEPI Trial. JAMA 1995;273:199–208.

The Writing Group for the PEPI Trial. JAMA 1996;275:370–375.

Yamada M et al. J Clin Epidemiol 1997;50:425–434.

Yano K et al. Am J Epidemiol 1984;119:653–666.

Yusuf S et al. Prog Cardiovasc Dis 1985;27:335–371.

Zephier EM et al. Prev Med 1997;26:508–515.

Zumoff B. Proc Soc Exp Biol Med 1998;217:30–37.

Index

Note: Page numbers followed by *f* indicate figures;
page numbers followed by *t* indicate tables.

Chart 1. LIPID CONVERSIONS, WITH NCEP INITIAL CLINICAL ACTION LIMITS IN ADULTS

Cholesterol (conversion factor 0.02586)			Triglyceride (conversion factor 0.01129)		
mg/dL		mmol/L	mg/dL		mmol/L
20		0.5	50		0.6
35	**Low HDL-C[a]**	**0.9**	80		0.9
40		1.0	100		1.1
50		1.3	120		1.4
60	High (protective) HDL-C	1.6	150		1.7
			180		2.0
85		2.2	**200**	**Borderline-high[a]**	**2.3**
100	**Elevated LDL-C in 2° prevention[a]**	**2.6**	250		2.8
			300		3.4
130	**Borderline-high LDL-C in 1° prevention[a]**	**3.4**	400	High	4.5
			500		5.6
160	**High LDL-C in 1° prevention[a]**	**4.1**	800		9.0
			1,000	**Very high[b]**	**11.3**
190		4.9			
200	Borderline-high TC in 1° prevention	5.2			
220	Severe LDL-C elevation	5.7			
240	High TC in 1° prevention	6.2			
300		7.8			
350		9.1			
500		12.9			

Note: Primary (1°) prevention = patients known to have atherosclerotic disease; secondary (2°) prevention = patients not known to have atherosclerotic disease.
[a]**Action limit for initiation of lipid-regulating lifestyle changes** (in the case of LDL-C 130–159 mg/dL in 1° prevention, if ≥2 other risk factors). For drug action limits, see Chart 2.
[b]**Requires immediate, vigorous intervention because of the risk for acute pancreatitis.**

Chart 2. CUTPOINTS IN ADULT CLINICAL PRACTICE GUIDELINES

Risk factor (guidelines)	Category	Cutpoint(s)
Smoking		No level acceptable
Hyperlipidemia action limits for consideration of lipid-lowering drugs[a] (NCEP 1993)	**No CHD, <2 other RF**	**LDL-C ≥190 mg/dL**
	No CHD, ≥2 other RF	**LDL-C ≥160 mg/dL**
	Atherosclerotic disease	**LDL-C ≥130 mg/dL**
	Any patient	TG ≥200 mg/dL with high risk for CHD
		TG ≥1,000 mg/dL immediate attention (pancreatitis risk)
Hypertension (JNC VI 1997)	Optimal blood pressure	<120/80 mm Hg
	Normal blood pressure	<130/85 mm Hg
	High normal blood pressure	SBP 130–139 mm Hg or DBP 85–89 mm Hg
	Hypertension	**SBP ≥140 mm Hg or DBP ≥90 mm Hg**
Diabetes according to fasting glucose (ADA 1997)	Normal fasting glucose	<110 mg/dL
	Impaired fasting glucose[b]	110–125 mg/dL
	Diabetes (fasting glucose)	**≥126 mg/dL**
Overweight and obesity (NIH—NHLBI and NIDDK 1998)	Normal weight	BMI 18.5–24.9 kg/m²
	Overweight	**BMI 25.0–29.9 kg/m²**
	Obesity	**BMI ≥30.0 kg/m²**
	Extreme obesity	**BMI ≥40.0 kg/m²**

[a]Action limits for initiation of lifestyle changes in dyslipidemia are shown in Chart 1. Use clinical judgment as to whether to use drugs in 2° prevention for LDL-C 100–129 mg/dL.
[b]Authors' note: Regardless of the HgbA$_{1c}$ value, fasting glucose >110 mg/dL (and perhaps even >90 mg/dL) confers high risk for macrovascular disease (see Chapter 16).